ACSM's
HEALTH & FITNESS
CERTIFICATION
REVIEW

ACSM Group Exercise Leader$_{SM}$
ACSM Health/Fitness Instructor$_{SM}$

$.2(26.8)(5) + (.9(26.8)(5)(.05) + 3.5$
$26.8 \quad + 6.03 \quad 36,33$

ACSM's
HEALTH & FITNESS
CERTIFICATION
REVIEW

ACSM GROUP EXERCISE LEADER_{SM}
ACSM HEALTH/FITNESS INSTRUCTOR_{SM}

AMERICAN COLLEGE OF SPORTS MEDICINE

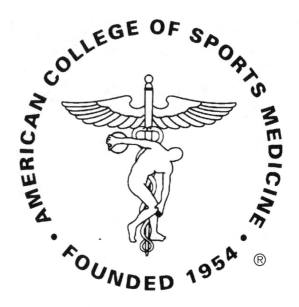

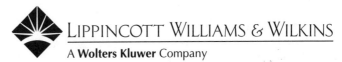
LIPPINCOTT WILLIAMS & WILKINS
A **Wolters Kluwer** Company

Philadelphia · Baltimore · New York · London
Buenos Aires · Hong Kong · Sydney · Tokyo

Editor: Peter Darcy
Editorial Director of Development: Julie P. Scardiglia
Development Editors: Rosanne Hallowell and Linda Weinerman
Managing Editor: Amy G. Dinkel
Illustrator: Holly R. Fischer
ACSM Publications Committee Chair: W. Larry Kenney, PhD, FACSM
ACSM Group Publisher: D. Mark Robertson

CONTRIBUTORS

ELAINE FILUSCH BETTS, PhD, PT, FACSM
Professor
Physical Therapy
Central Michigan University
Mt. Pleasant, Michigan
Chapter 1, Anatomy and Biomechanics

JEFFERY J. BETTS, PhD
Associate Professor
Director of Exercise and Health Sciences Division
Department of Health Promotion and Rehabilitation
Central Michigan University
Mt. Pleasant, Michigan
Chapter 1, Anatomy and Biomechanics

KHALID W. BIBI, PhD
Associate Professor, Sports Medicine, Health and
   Human Performance
Director, Health and Human Performance Center
Canisius College
Buffalo, New York
Chapter 11, Metabolic Calculations

DAVID S. CRISWELL, PhD
Assistant Professor
Department of Kinesiology
Texas Woman's University
Denton, Texas
Chapter 3, Human Development and Aging

FREDERICK S. DANIELS, MS
President
CPTE Health Group, Inc.
Nashua, New Hampshire
Chapter 7, Safety, Injury Prevention, and Emergency Care
Chapter 10, Program and Administration / Management

ANDREA L. DUNN, PhD, FACSM
Associate Director
Division of Epidemiology and Clinical Applications
The Cooper Institute
Dallas, Texas
Chapter 5, Human Behavior and Psychology

BETH H. MARCUS, PhD
Associate Professor of Psychiatry and Human Behavior
Brown University Center for Behavioral and
   Preventive Medicine
The Miriam Hospital
Providence, Rhode Island
Chapter 5, Human Behavior and Psychology

MAUREEN SMITH PLOMBON, MS, RD, FACSM,
FADA
President
Integrated Health Consultants
Oakton, Virginia
Chapter 9, Nutrition and Weight Management

SUSAN M. PUHL, PhD
Associate Professor of Kinesiology
Department of Physical Education and Kinesiology
California Polytechnic State University
San Luis Obispo, California
Chapter 4, Pathophysiology / Risk Factors
Chapter 6, Health Appraisal and Fitness Testing

JEFFREY C. RUPP, PhD
Associate Professor and Chair
Department of Kinesiology & Health
Georgia State University
Atlanta, Georgia
Chapter 2, Exercise Physiology

JANET R. WOJCIK, PhD
Research Scientist
Center for Research in Health Behavior
Virginia Polytechnic Institute and State University
Blacksburg, Virginia
Chapter 9, Nutrition and Weight Management

JOHN W. WYGAND, MA
Director of Adult Fitness Programs
Department of Health, Physical Education and Human
   Performance Science
Adelphi University
Garden City, New York
Chapter 8, Exercise Programming

CONTENTS

FOREWORD

Starting in 1975, the American College of Sports Medicine (ACSM) developed certification programs to serve and recognize those providing leadership in the delivery of health-related and rehabilitation-based programs in which exercise prescription was a major part. The ACSM certification programs are recognized as the "gold standards" by health professionals and other health-profession organizations. The fact that the content of some of ACSM's certifications have been incorporated substantially into the fitness certifications of other organizations confirms the old adage that imitation is the sincerest form of flattery. ACSM's certification programs were developed and are sustained by the efforts of ACSM volunteers. The behind-the-scenes work of volunteers includes the ongoing development of behavioral objectives or KSAs (knowledge, skills, and abilities), examinations, workshops, and educational materials that support the certification programs. They are, without question, the hardest working volunteers I have had the pleasure to be around over the past 25 years.

This text, *ACSM's Health & Fitness Certification Review,* is part of that legacy to serve those who plan to take one of the examinations in the Health & Fitness track. The text pulls together, in a review format, information that bears directly on the content of the health and fitness objectives as they are spelled out in the sixth edition of the *ACSM's Guidelines for Exercise Testing and Prescription.* This review should be very helpful to candidates who have already completed formal coursework in the major areas covered on the examinations. At the same time, this review will assist those getting started by pointing out weaknesses that can be corrected by additional coursework

Knowledgeable professionals were recruited to organize the material for this text in a coherent manner, and write about it in a style that facilitates learning. I believe that this text will provide insights into the various KSAs associated with the health and fitness certifications of ACSM. I encourage young fitness professionals to achieve ACSM certification and to become active in the regional chapters of the ACSM. This may lead to volunteer opportunities in the ACSM to pass along this legacy to the next generation of health and fitness professionals.

Best wishes for a successful career!

Edward T. Howley, PhD, FACSM
Professor and Head
Exercise Science and Sport Management
The University of Tennessee
Knoxville, Tennessee

PREFACE

The *ACSM's Health & Fitness Certification Review* is one of two review books for ACSM certification; the other book is the *ACSM's Clinical Certification Review*. Along with the *ACSM's Resource Manual for Guidelines for Exercise Testing and Prescription, 3rd edition,* these review books present materials relevant to ACSM certification in an organized and user-friendly fashion.

The information in the *ACSM's Health & Fitness Certification Review* covers almost all of the knowledge, skills, and abilities (KSAs) for both the ACSM Group Exercise Leader$_{SM}$ (GEL) and the ACSM Health/Fitness Instructor$_{SM}$ (HFI) certifications. Although it does not include those KSAs that are solely ACSM Health/Fitness Director KSAs, it does cover the ACSM Health/Fitness Director "prerequisites" with the GEL and HFI KSAs.

Features. The chapters in the *ACSM's Health & Fitness Certification Review* coincide with the major categories of the KSAs and are presented in **outline form** to allow quick, topical review of each area. This type of presentation is possible because of the new organization of the KSAs. **Tables and figures** supplement the outline text and allow for easy access to supporting information. At the conclusion of each chapter there is a **Review Test** consisting of multiple-choice study questions written in the same format and at about the same difficulty level as the examination questions in the ACSM's Health & Fitness Track certification exam. A **Comprehensive Examination** is presented at the end of the book for additional practice. It too has been formulated using the same "blueprint" as the certification examination so that candidates get a taste of the true written examination process. **Answers with explanations** are provided for each Review Test and Comprehensive Examination question. In the Review Tests and Comprehensive Examination, the candidate will find questions that are representative of the KSAs and applicable to each level of certification. A listing of **Recommended Readings** pertaining to each chapter can also be found at the end of the book, preceding the Comprehensive Examination; these references can be consulted for more-detailed information about the topics outlined in this review book.

How to Use This Book. The *ACSM's Health & Fitness Certification Review* is meant to be used by ACSM Health & Fitness Track certification candidates who are ready (or nearly ready) for the certification examination and want to review the KSAs. Those candidates who are just beginning the study process may want to use this book as a study guide to identify their "weak areas" where more intense study may be necessary. This book is *not* meant to be a primary resource; it is really a "skeletal" outline of the critical KSAs for the Health & Fitness Track (with the exception of the more advanced or administrative KSAs for the ACSM Health/Fitness Director ®). The reader is further advised that the two basic study books for all ACSM Certification candidates are the *ACSM's Guidelines for Exercise Testing and Prescription,* 6th edition (© 2000) and the *ACSM's Resource Manual for Guidelines for Exercise Testing and Prescription,* 3rd edition (© 1998). These are invaluable and primary resources for all certification candidates and professionals who need supplemental information about the ACSM's Guidelines and their derivation.

Summary. The features contained in the *ACSM's Health & Fitness Certification Review*—the outline format, the tables and illustrations, the practice questions for each chapter, and the comprehensive examination at the end of the book—should make this study guide a great aid to those preparing for certification. It is our hope that this type of presentation will assist all candidates for these certifications to increase their level of knowledge and preparation for the examination and certification process.

Acknowledgments. We would like to acknowledge the support and participation of our loved ones (Lana, Kay, Lindsay, and Shaia), and thank them for their patience with our participation in this project and the hours we spent away from them. We would also like to acknowledge the following manuscript reviewers:

Christopher Hubert
Moira Kelsey, RN, MS
Tom LaFontaine, PhD
Swapan Mookerjee, PhD
Brian Rieger, MS
Tracy York, MS
Nancy Zambraski, MS

Jeffrey L. Roitman, EdD, FACSM
Khalid W. Bibi, PhD

Knowledge, Skills, and Abilities (KSAs) for ACSM Group Exercise Leader_{SM} and ACSM Health/Fitness Instructor_{SM} Certifications

KSA Numbering System. The first number in the sequence denotes the certification level of the KSA. KSAs numbered "1.—" are specific to Group Exercise Leader; KSAs numbered "2.—" are specific to Health/Fitness Instructor.

The second number in the sequence denotes the content matter of the KSA. For example, KSAs numbered "—.1" are related to Anatomy and Biomechanics; KSAs numbered "—.2" are related to Exercise Physiology. The second numbers denote content matter as follows:

—.1 Anatomy and Biomechanics
—.2 Exercise Physiology
—.3 Human Development and Aging
—.4 Pathophysiology and Risk Factors
—.5 Human Behavior and Psychology
—.6 Health Appraisal and Fitness Testing
—.7 Safety and Injury Prevention
—.8 Exercise Programming
—.9 Nutrition and Weight Management
—.10 Program and Administration/Management

Example. A KSA numbered "1.3.—" is a KSA for an Exercise Leader that relates to Human Development and Aging. A KSA numbered "2.4.—" is for a Health/Fitness Instructor that relates to Pathophysiology and Risk Factors.

This numbering system allows exact determination of KSAs specific to the level of certification and the content matter.

Anatomy and Biomechanics

1.1.0	Knowledge of anatomy as it relates to exercise and health.
1.1.0.1	Knowledge of the basic structures of bone, skeletal muscle, and connective tissues.
1.1.0.2	Knowledge of the basic anatomy of the cardiovascular system and respiratory system.
1.1.0.3	Ability to identify the major bones and muscles. Major muscles include, but are not limited to, the following: trapezius, pectoralis major, latissimus dorsi, biceps, triceps, rectus abdominis, internal and external obliques, erector spinae, gluteus maximus, quadriceps, hamstrings, adductors, abductors, and gastrocnemius.
1.1.0.4	Knowledge of the definition of the following terms: supination, pronation, flexion, extension, adduction, abduction, hyperextension, rotation, circumduction, agonist, antagonist, and stabilizer.
1.1.0.5	Ability to identify the joints of the body.
1.1.1	Knowledge of biomechanical aspects of exercise participation.
1.1.1.1	Knowledge to identify the plane in which each muscle action occurs.
1.1.1.2	Knowledge of the interrelationships among center of gravity, base of support, balance, stability, and proper spinal alignment.
1.1.1.3	Ability to describe the following curvatures of the spine: lordosis, scoliosis, and kyphosis.
1.1.1.4	Knowledge of and skill to demonstrate exercises designed to enhance muscular strength and/or endurance of specific major muscle groups.
1.1.1.5	Knowledge of and skill to demonstrate exercises for enhancing musculoskeletal flexibility.
1.1.1.6	Knowledge to describe the myotatic stretch reflex.
1.1.1.7	Knowledge to identify the primary action and joint range of motion for each major muscle group.

2.1.0	Knowledge of functional anatomy and biomechanics.
2.1.0.1	Knowledge of the structure and ability to describe movements for the major joints of the body.

2.1.0.2 Ability to locate the anatomic landmarks for palpation of peripheral pulses.

2.1.0.3 Ability to locate the brachial artery and correctly place the cuff and stethoscope in position for blood pressure measurement.

2.1.0.4 Ability to locate common sites for measurement of skinfold thicknesses and circumferences (for determination of body composition and waist-hip ratio).

2.1.1 Knowledge of biomechanical principles that underlie performance of the following activities: walking, jogging, running, swimming, cycling, weight lifting, and carrying or moving objects.

EXERCISE PHYSIOLOGY

1.2.0 Basic knowledge of exercise physiology as it relates to exercise prescription.

1.2.1 Ability to define aerobic and anaerobic metabolism.

1.2.2 Knowledge of the role of aerobic and anaerobic energy systems in the performance of various activities.

1.2.3 Knowledge of the following terms: ischemia, angina pectoris, tachycardia, bradycardia, arrhythmia, myocardial infarction, cardiac output, stroke volume, lactic acid, oxygen consumption, hyperventilation, systolic blood pressure, diastolic blood pressure, and anaerobic threshold.

1.2.4 Knowledge of the role of carbohydrates, fats, and proteins as fuels for aerobic and anaerobic metabolism.

1.2.5 Knowledge of the components of fitness: cardiorespiratory fitness, muscular strength, muscular endurance, flexibility, and body composition.

1.2.6 Knowledge to describe normal cardiorespiratory responses to static and dynamic exercise in terms of heart rate, blood pressure, and oxygen consumption.

1.2.7 Knowledge of how heart rate, blood pressure, and oxygen consumption responses change with adaptation to chronic exercise training.

1.2.8 Knowledge of the physiological adaptations associated with strength training.

1.2.9 Ability to identify and apply to both groups and individuals methods used to monitor exercise intensity, including heart rate and rating of perceived exertion.

1.2.10 Knowledge of the physiological principles related to warm-up and cool-down.

1.2.11 Knowledge of the common theories of muscle fatigue and delayed onset muscle soreness (DOMS).

2.2.0 Knowledge of exercise physiology including the role of aerobic and anaerobic metabolism, muscle physiology, cardiovascular physiology, and respiratory physiology at rest and during exercise. In addition, demonstrate an understanding of the components of physical fitness, the effects of aerobic and strength and/or resistance training on the fitness components and the effects of chronic disease.

2.2.1 Knowledge of the physiological adaptations that occur at rest and during submaximal and maximal exercise following chronic aerobic and anaerobic exercise training.

2.2.2 Knowledge of the differences in cardiorespiratory response to acute graded exercise between conditioned and unconditioned individuals.

2.2.3 Knowledge of the structure of the skeletal muscle fiber and the basic mechanism of contraction.

2.2.4 Knowledge of the characteristics of fast and slow twitch fibers.

2.2.5 Knowledge of the sliding filament theory of muscle contraction.

2.2.6 Knowledge of twitch, summation, and tetanus with respect to muscle contraction.

2.2.7 Ability to discuss the physiological principles involved in promoting gains in muscular strength and endurance.

2.2.8 Ability to define muscular fatigue as it relates to task, intensity, duration, and the accumulative effects of exercise.

2.2.9 Knowledge of the relationship between the number of repetitions, intensity, number of sets, and rest with regard to strength training.

2.2.10 Knowledge of the basic properties of cardiac muscle and the normal pathways of conduction in the heart.

2.2.11 Knowledge of the response of the following variables to acute exercise: heart rate, stroke volume, cardiac output, pulmonary ventilation, tidal volume, respiratory rate, and arteriovenous oxygen difference.

2.2.12 Knowledge of the differences in the cardiorespiratory responses to static exercise compared with dynamic exercise, including possible hazards and contraindications.

2.2.13 Ability to describe how each of the following differs from the normal condition: premature atrial contractions and premature ventricular contractions.

2.2.14 Knowledge of blood pressure responses associated with acute exercise, including changes in body position.

2.2.15 Knowledge of and ability to describe the implications of ventilatory threshold (anaerobic threshold) as it relates to exercise training and cardiorespiratory assessment.

2.2.16 Knowledge of and ability to describe the physiological adaptations of the respiratory system that occur at rest and during submaximal and maximal exercise following chronic aerobic and anaerobic training.

2.2.17 Ability to describe how each of the following differs from the normal condition: dyspnea, hypoxia, and hypoventilation.

2.2.18 Knowledge of and ability to discuss the physiological basis of the major components of physical fitness: flexibility, cardiovascular fitness, muscular strength, muscular endurance, and body composition.

2.2.19 Ability to explain how the principle of specificity relates to the components of fitness.

2.2.20 Ability to explain the concept of detraining or reversibility of conditioning and its implications in fitness programs.

2.2.21 Ability to discuss the physical and psychological signs of overtraining and to provide recommendations for these problems.

2.2.22 Ability to describe the physiological and metabolic responses to exercise associated with chronic disease (heart disease, hypertension, diabetes mellitus, and pulmonary disease).

HUMAN DEVELOPMENT AND AGING

1.3.0 Knowledge of the benefits and risks associated with exercise training in prepubescent and postpubescent youth.

1.3.1 Knowledge of the benefits and precautions associated with resistance and endurance training in older adults.

1.3.2 Ability to describe specific leadership techniques appropriate for working with participants of all ages.

2.3.0 Knowledge of the changes that occur during growth and development from childhood to old age.

2.3.0.1 Ability to modify cardiovascular and resistance exercises based on age and physical condition.

2.3.0.2 Knowledge of and ability to describe the changes that occur in maturation from childhood to adulthood for the following: skeletal muscle, bone structure, reaction time, coordination, heat and cold tolerance, maximal oxygen consumption, strength, flexibility, body composition, resting and maximal heart rate, and resting and maximal blood pressure.

2.3.0.3 Knowledge of the effect of the aging process on the musculoskeletal and cardiovascular structure and function at rest, during exercise, and during recovery.

2.3.0.4 Ability to characterize the differences in the development of an exercise prescription for children, adolescents, and older participants.

2.3.0.5 Knowledge of and ability to describe the unique adaptations to exercise training in children, adolescents, and older participants with regard to strength, functional capacity, and motor skills.

2.3.0.6 Knowledge of common orthopedic and cardiovascular considerations for older participants and the ability to describe modifications in exercise prescription that are indicated.

PATHOPHYSIOLOGY/RISK FACTORS

1.4.0 Knowledge of cardiovascular, respiratory, metabolic, and musculoskeletal risk factors that may require further evaluation by medical or allied health professionals before participation in physical activity.

1.4.0.1 Ability to determine those risk factors that may be favorably modified by physical activity habits.

1.4.0.2   Knowledge to define the following terms: total cholesterol (TC), high-density lipoprotein cholesterol (HDL-C), TC/HDL-C ratio, low-density lipoprotein cholesterol (LDL-C), triglycerides, hypertension, and atherosclerosis.

1.4.0.3   Knowledge of plasma cholesterol levels for adults as recommended by the National Cholesterol Education Program (NCEP II).

2.4.0   Knowledge of the pathophysiology of atherosclerosis and how this process is influenced by physical activity.

2.4.1   Knowledge of the risk factor concept of CAD and the influence of heredity and lifestyle on the development of CAD.

2.4.2   Knowledge of the atherosclerotic process, the factors involved in its genesis and progression, and the potential role of exercise training in treatment.

2.4.3   Ability to discuss in detail how lifestyle factors, including nutrition, physical activity, and heredity, influence lipid and lipoprotein profiles.

2.4.4   Knowledge of cardiovascular risk factors or conditions that may require consultation with medical personnel before testing or training, including inappropriate changes in resting or exercise heart rate and blood pressure, new onset discomfort in chest, neck, shoulder, or arm, changes in the pattern of discomfort during rest or exercise, fainting or dizzy spells, and claudication.

2.4.5   Knowledge of respiratory risk factors or conditions that may require consultation with medical personnel before testing or training, including asthma, exercise-induced bronchospasm, extreme breathlessness at rest or during exercise, bronchitis, and emphysema.

2.4.6   Knowledge of metabolic risk factors or conditions that may require consultation with medical personnel before testing or training, including body weight more than 20% above optimal, BMI 1 30, thyroid disease, diabetes or glucose intolerance, and hypoglycemia.

2.4.7   Knowledge of musculoskeletal risk factors or conditions that may require consultation with medical personnel before testing or training, including acute or chronic back pain, osteoarthritis, rheumatoid arthritis, osteoporosis, tendonitis, and low back pain.

Human Behavior and Psychology

1.5.0   Ability to identify and define at least five behavioral strategies to enhance exercise and health behavior change (i.e., reinforcement, goal setting, social support).

1.5.1   Ability to list and define the five important elements that should be included in each counseling session.

1.5.2   Knowledge of specific techniques to enhance motivation (e.g., posters, recognition, bulletin boards, games, competitions). Define extrinsic and intrinsic reinforcement and give examples of each.

1.5.3   Knowledge of the stages of motivational readiness.

1.5.4   Ability to list and describe three counseling approaches that may assist less motivated clients to increase their physical activity.

2.5.0   Ability to list and describe the specific strategies aimed at encouraging the initiation, adherence, and return to participation in an exercise program.

2.5.1   Knowledge of symptoms of anxiety and depression that may necessitate referral.

2.5.2   Knowledge of the potential symptoms and causal factors of test anxiety (i.e., performance, appraisal threat during exercise testing) and how it may affect physiological responses to testing.

Health Appraisal and Fitness Testing

1.6.1   Knowledge of the importance of a health/medical history.

1.6.2   Knowledge of the value of a medical clearance prior to exercise participation.

1.6.3   Skill to measure pulse rate accurately both at rest and during exercise.

2.6.0   Knowledge, skills, and abilities to assess the health status of individuals and the ability to conduct fitness testing.

2.6.0.1   Ability to obtain a health history and risk appraisal that includes past and current medical history, family history of cardiac disease, orthopedic limitations, prescribed medications, activity patterns, nutritional habits, stress and anxiety levels, and smoking and alcohol use.

2.6.0.2   Ability to describe the categories of participants who should receive medical clearance prior to administration of an exercise test or participation in an exercise program.

2.6.0.3   Ability to identify relative and absolute contraindications to exercise testing or participation.

2.6.0.4   Ability to discuss the limitations of informed consent and medical clearance prior to exercise testing.

2.6.0.5   Ability to obtain informed consent.

2.6.0.6   Ability to explain the purpose and procedures for monitoring clients prior to, during, and after cardiorespiratory fitness testing.

2.6.0.7   Skill in instructing participants in the use of equipment and test procedures.

2.6.0.8   Ability to describe the purpose of testing, select an appropriate submaximal or maximal protocol, and conduct an assessment of cardiovascular fitness on the cycle ergometer or the treadmill.

2.6.0.9   Skill in accurately measuring heart rate, blood pressure, and obtaining rating of perceived exertion (RPE) at rest and during exercise according to established guidelines.

2.6.0.10   Ability to locate and measure skinfold sites, skeletal diameters, and girth measurements used for estimating body composition.

2.6.0.11   Ability to describe the purpose of testing, select appropriate protocols, and conduct assessments of muscular strength, muscular endurance, and flexibility.

2.6.0.12   Skill in various techniques of assessing body composition.

2.6.0.13   Knowledge of the advantages/disadvantages and limitations of the various body composition techniques.

2.6.0.14   Ability to interpret information obtained from the cardiorespiratory fitness test and the muscular strength and endurance, flexibility, and body composition assessments for apparently healthy individuals and those with stable disease.

2.6.0.15   Ability to identify appropriate criteria for terminating a fitness evaluation and demonstrate proper procedures to be followed after discontinuing such a test.

2.6.0.16   Ability to modify protocols and procedures for cardiorespiratory fitness tests in children, adolescents, and older adults.

2.6.0.17   Knowledge of common drugs from each of the following classes of medications and describe the principal action and the effects on exercise testing and prescription:

2.6.0.17.1   Antianginals
2.6.0.17.2   Antihypertensives
2.6.0.17.3   Antiarrhythmics
2.6.0.17.4   Bronchodilators
2.6.0.17.5   Hypoglycemics
2.6.0.17.6   Psychotropics
2.6.0.17.7   Vasodilators

2.6.0.18   Ability to identify the effects of the following substances on exercise response: antihistamines, tranquilizers, alcohol, diet pills, cold tablets, caffeine, and nicotine.

2.6.0.19   Skill in techniques for calibration of a cycle ergometer and a motor-driven treadmill.

SAFETY, INJURY PREVENTION, AND EMERGENCY CARE

1.7.0   Knowledge of and skill in obtaining basic life support and cardiopulmonary resuscitation certification.

1.7.1   Knowledge of appropriate emergency procedures (i.e., telephone procedures, written emergency procedures, personnel responsibilities) in the group exercise setting.

1.7.2 Knowledge of basic first aid procedures for exercise-related injuries, such as bleeding, strains/sprains, fractures, and exercise intolerance (dizziness, syncope, heat injury).

1.7.3 Knowledge of basic precautions taken in a group exercise setting to ensure participant safety.

1.7.4 Ability to identify the physical and physiological signs and symptoms of overtraining.

1.7.5 Ability to list the effects of temperature, humidity, altitude, and pollution on the physiological response to exercise.

1.7.6 Knowledge of the following terms: shin splints, sprain, strain, tennis elbow, bursitis, stress fracture, tendonitis, patellar femoral pain syndrome, low back pain, plantar fasciitis, and rotator cuff tendonitis.

1.7.7 Skill to demonstrate exercises used for people with low back pain.

1.7.8 Knowledge of hypothetical concerns and potential risks that may be associated with the use of exercises such as straight leg sit-ups, double leg raises, full squats, hurdlers stretch, yoga plough, forceful back hyperextension, and standing bent-over toe touch.

2.7.0 Skill in demonstrating appropriate emergency procedures during exercise testing and/or training.

2.7.1 Knowledge of safety plans, emergency procedures, and first aid techniques needed during fitness evaluations, exercise testing, and exercise training.

2.7.2 Ability to identify the components that contribute to the maintenance of a safe environment.

2.7.3 Knowledge of the health/fitness instructor's responsibilities, limitations, and the legal implications of carrying out emergency procedures.

2.7.4 Ability to describe potential musculoskeletal injuries (e.g., contusions, sprains, strains, fractures), cardiovascular/pulmonary complications (e.g., tachycardia, bradycardia, hypotension/hypertension, tachypnea) and metabolic abnormalities (e.g., fainting/syncope, hypoglycemia/hyperglycemia, hypothermia/hyperthermia).

2.7.5 Knowledge of the initial management and first aid techniques associated with open wounds, musculoskeletal injuries, cardiovascular/pulmonary complications, and metabolic disorders.

2.7.6 Knowledge of the components of an equipment maintenance/repair program and how it may be used to evaluate the condition of exercise equipment to reduce the potential risk of injury.

EXERCISE PROGRAMMING

1.8.0 Knowledge of the recommended intensity, duration, frequency, and type of physical activity necessary for development of cardiorespiratory fitness in an apparently healthy population.

1.8.1 Ability to differentiate between the amount of physical activity required for health benefits and the amount of exercise required for fitness development.

1.8.2 Ability to describe exercises designed to enhance muscular strength and/or endurance of specific major muscle groups.

1.8.3 Knowledge of the principles of overload, specificity, and progression and how they relate to exercise programming.

1.8.4 Skill to teach and demonstrate appropriate exercises used in the warm-up and cool-down of a variety of group exercise classes.

1.8.5 Ability to teach the components of an exercise session (i.e., warm-up, aerobic stimulus phase, cool-down, muscular strength/endurance, flexibility).

1.8.6 Knowledge of the following terms: progressive resistance, isotonic/isometric, concentric, eccentric, atrophy, hypertrophy, sets, repetitions, plyometrics, Valsalva maneuver.

1.8.7 Skill to teach class participants how to monitor intensity of exercise using heart rate and rating of perceived exertion.

1.8.8 Skill to teach participants how to use RPE and heart rate to adjust the intensity of the exercise session.

1.8.9 Ability to calculate training heart rates using two methods: percent of age-predicted maximum heart rate and heart rate reserve (Karvonen).

1.8.10 Skill to teach and demonstrate appropriate modifications in specific exercises for the following groups: older adults, pregnant and postnatal women, obese persons, and persons with low back pain.

1.8.11 Ability to recognize proper and improper technique in the use of resistive equipment such as stability balls, weights, bands, resistance bars, and water exercise equipment.

1.8.12 Ability to recognize proper and improper technique in the use of cardiovascular conditioning equipment (e.g., steps, cycles, slides).

1.8.13 Skill to teach and demonstrate appropriate exercises for improving range of motion of all major joints.

1.8.14 Ability to modify exercises in the group setting for apparently healthy persons of various fitness levels.

1.8.15 Ability to teach a progression of exercises for all major muscle groups to improve muscular strength and endurance.

1.8.16 Knowledge to describe the various types of interval, continuous, and circuit training programs.

1.8.17 Knowledge to describe various ways a leader can take a position relative to the group to enhance visibility, participant interactions, and communication.

1.8.18 Ability to communicate effectively with exercise participants in the group exercise session.

1.8.19 Knowledge to describe partner resistance exercises that can be used in a group class setting.

1.8.20 Ability to demonstrate techniques for accommodating various fitness levels within the same class.

1.8.21 Knowledge of the properties of water that affect the design of a water exercise session.

1.8.22 Knowledge of basic music fundamentals, including downbeat, 8 count, and 32 count.

1.8.23 Skill to effectively use verbal and nonverbal cues in the group exercise setting, including anticipatory, motivational, safety, and educational.

1.8.24 Skill to demonstrate the proper form, alignment, and technique in typical exercises used in the warm-up, stimulus, muscle conditioning and cool-down phases of the group session.

1.8.25 Ability to evaluate specific exercises in terms of safety and effectiveness for various participants.

1.8.26 Ability to demonstrate a familiarity with a variety of group exercise formats (e.g., traditional, step, slide, muscle conditioning, flexibility, indoor cycling, water fitness, walking).

2.8.0 Knowledge, skills, and abilities to prescribe and administer exercise programs for apparently healthy individuals, individuals at higher risk, and individuals with known disease.

2.8.0.1 Ability to design, implement, and evaluate individualized and group exercise programs based on health history and physical fitness assessments.

2.8.0.2 Ability to modify exercises based on age and physical condition.

2.8.0.3 Knowledge, skills, and abilities to calculate energy cost, $\dot{V}O_2$, METs, and target heart rates and apply the information to an exercise prescription.

2.8.0.4 Ability to convert weights from pounds (lb) to kilograms (kg) and speed from miles per hour (mph) to meters per minute (m · min^{-1}).

2.8.0.5 Ability to convert METs to $\dot{V}O_2$ expressed as mL · kg^{-1} · min^{-1}, L · min^{-1}, and/or mL · kg FFW^{-1} · min^{-1}.

2.8.0.6 Ability to calculate the energy cost in METs and kilocalories for given exercise intensities in stepping exercise, cycle ergometry, and during horizontal and graded walking and running.

2.8.0.7 Knowledge of approximate METs for various sport, recreational, and work tasks.

2.8.0.8 Ability to prescribe exercise intensity based on $\dot{V}O_2$ data for different modes of exercise, including graded and horizontal running and walking, cycling, and stepping exercise.

2.8.0.9 Ability to explain and implement exercise prescription guidelines for apparently healthy clients, increased risk clients, and clients with controlled disease.

2.8.0.10 Ability to adapt frequency, intensity, duration, mode, progression, level of supervision, and monitoring techniques in exercise programs for patients with controlled chronic disease (heart disease, diabetes mellitus, obesity, hypertension), musculoskeletal problems, pregnancy and/or postpartum, and exercise-induced asthma.

2.8.0.11 Ability to understand the components incorporated into an exercise session and the proper sequence (i.e., pre-exercise evaluation, warm-up, aerobic stimulus phase, cool-down, muscular strength and/or endurance, and flexibility).

2.8.0.12 Skill in the use of various methods for establishing and monitoring levels of exercise intensity, including heart rate, RPE, and METs.

2.8.0.13 Knowledge of special precautions and modifications of exercise programming for participation at altitude, different ambient temperatures, humidity, and environmental pollution.

2.8.0.14 Ability to design resistive exercise programs to increase or maintain muscular strength and/or endurance.

2.8.0.15 Ability to evaluate flexibility and prescribe appropriate flexibility exercises for all major muscle groups.

2.8.0.16 Knowledge of the importance of recording exercise sessions and performing periodic evaluations to assess changes in fitness status.

2.8.0.17 Knowledge of the advantages and disadvantages of implementation of interval, continuous, and circuit training programs.

2.8.0.18   Ability to design training programs using interval, continuous, and circuit training programs.
2.8.0.19   Ability to discuss the advantages and disadvantages of various commercial exercise equipment in developing cardiorespiratory fitness, muscular strength, and muscular endurance.
2.8.0.20   Knowledge of the types of exercise programs available in the community and how these programs are appropriate for various populations.

NUTRITION AND WEIGHT MANAGEMENT

1.9.0   Knowledge to define the following terms: obesity, overweight, percent fat, lean body mass, anorexia nervosa, bulimia, and body fat distribution.
1.9.1   Knowledge of the relationship between body composition and health.
1.9.2   Knowledge of the effects of diet plus exercise, diet alone, and exercise alone as methods for modifying body composition.
1.9.3   Knowledge of the importance of an adequate daily energy intake for healthy weight management.
1.9.4   Ability to differentiate between fat-soluble and water-soluble vitamins.
1.9.5   Ability to describe the importance of maintaining normal hydration before, during, and after exercise.
1.9.6   Knowledge of the USDA Food Pyramid.
1.9.7   Knowledge of the importance of calcium and iron in women's health.
1.9.8   Ability to describe the myths and consequences associated with inappropriate weight loss methods (e.g., saunas, vibrating belts, body wraps, electric simulators, sweat suits, fad diets).
1.9.9   Knowledge of the number of kilocalories in one gram of carbohydrate, fat, protein, and alcohol.
1.9.10   Knowledge of the number of kilocalories equivalent to losing 1 pound of body fat.

2.9.0   Knowledge, skills, and abilities to provide information concerning nutrition and the role of diet and exercise on body composition and weight control.
2.9.0.1   Ability to describe the health implications of variation in body fat distribution patterns and the significance of the waist to hip ratio.
2.9.0.2   Knowledge of the guidelines for caloric intake for an individual desiring to lose or gain weight.
2.9.0.3   Knowledge of common nutritional ergogenic aids, the purported mechanism of action, and any risk and/or benefits (e.g., carbohydrates, protein/amino acids, vitamins, minerals, sodium bicarbonate, creatine, bee pollen).
2.9.0.4   Knowledge of nutritional factors related to the female athlete triad syndrome (i.e., eating disorders, menstrual cycle abnormalities, and osteoporosis).
2.9.0.5   Knowledge of the NIH Consensus statement regarding health risks of obesity, Nutrition for Physical Fitness Position Paper of the American Dietetic Association, and the ACSM Position Stand on proper and improper weight loss programs.
2.9.0.6   Knowledge of NCEP II guidelines for lipid management.

PROGRAM AND ADMINISTRATION/MANAGEMENT

2.10.0   Knowledge, skills, and ability to administer and deliver health/fitness programs.
2.10.0.1   Knowledge of the health/fitness instructor's supportive role in administration and program management within a health/fitness facility.
2.10.0.2   Ability to administer fitness-related programs within established budgetary guidelines.
2.10.0.3   Ability to develop marketing materials for the purpose of promoting fitness-related programs.
2.10.0.4   Ability to use various sales techniques for prospective program clients/participants.
2.10.0.5   Ability to describe and use the documentation required when a client shows signs or symptoms during an exercise session and should be referred to a physician.

2.10.0.6   Ability to create and maintain records pertaining to participant exercise adherence, retention, and goal setting.

2.10.0.7   Ability to develop and administer educational programs (e.g., lectures, workshops) and educational materials.

2.10.0.8   Knowledge of management of a fitness department (e.g., working within a budget, training exercise leaders, scheduling, running staff meetings).

2.10.0.9   Knowledge of the importance of tracking and evaluating member retention.

CHAPTER 1

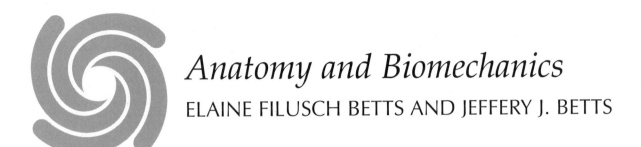

Anatomy and Biomechanics
ELAINE FILUSCH BETTS AND JEFFERY J. BETTS

I. INTRODUCTION

A. GROSS ANATOMY

–can be learned as **regional or topographic anatomy,** in which study is organized according to regions, parts, or divisions of the body (e.g., the hand, the mouth).

–can be learned as **systemic anatomy,** in which study is organized according to organ systems (e.g., respiratory system, nervous system).

–**This chapter uses the systemic anatomy approach,** and discusses anatomy of the following systems only: skeletal, muscular (skeletal muscles), cardiovascular, and respiratory.

B. BIOMECHANICS

–is the field of study concerned with the principles of physics related to energy and force as they apply to the human body.

–is discussed in this chapter as it applies to specific movements or activities.

C. TERMS OF ORIENTATION

–Superior, inferior, proximal, distal, anterior, posterior, lateral, medial (**Figure 1-1**)

D. BODY PLANES

1. There are **three cardinal planes** of the body (**Figure 1-2**). Each plane is perpendicular to each of the others.

   –The **sagittal plane** makes a division into right and left portions.

   –The **frontal plane** makes a division into front (anterior) and back (posterior) portions.

   –The **transverse plane** makes a division into upper (superior) and lower (inferior) portions.

2. These planes can be applied to the whole body or to parts of the body.

3. Movement is described in relation to these planes.

II. THE SKELETAL SYSTEM

A. DIVISIONS (Figure 1-3)

1. **Axial skeleton**

   –includes the bones of the head, vertebral column, ribs, and sternum.

   –forms the longitudinal axis of the body.

   –supports and protects organ systems.

   –provides surface area for the attachment of muscles.

   –**The spine,** also called the **vertebral column** (**Figure 1-4**), serves as the main axial support for the body.

   a. **The vertebrae**

      –There are commonly 33 vertebrae in the human spine: 7 cervical, 12 thoracic, 5 lumbar, 5 sacral (fused into one bone, the sacrum), and 4 coccygeal (fused into one bone, the coccyx).

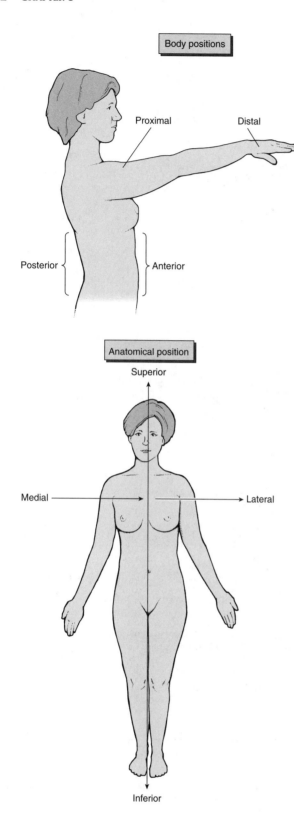

Body positions

Anatomical position

FIGURE 1-1 Terms of orientation. (Adapted from *ACSM's Resource Manual for Guidelines for Exercise Testing and Prescription,* 3rd ed. Baltimore, Williams & Wilkins, 1998, p. 90.)

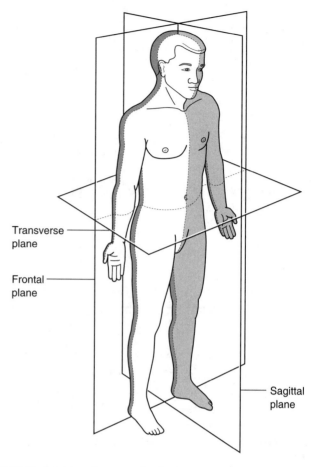

FIGURE 1-2 The three cardinal planes of the body: sagittal, frontal, and transverse.

   b. The intervertebral discs

–are flat, round, plate-like structures composed of fibrocartilaginous tissue.

(1) The outer, fibrocartilaginous portion of the disc is the annulus fibrosus.

(2) The inner gelatinous portion is the nucleus pulposus.

–unite the vertebral bodies.

–serve as **shock absorbers.**

   c. The adult vertebral column has **four major curvatures** (see Figure 1-4).

–Two primary curves: thoracic and sacral

–Two secondary curves: cervical and lumbar

   d. Commonly found abnormal curves (Figure 1-5) include **scoliosis** (lateral deviation), **kyphosis** (posterior thoracic curvature), and **lordosis** (anterior lumbar curvature).

2. Appendicular skeleton

–includes the bones of the arms and legs and the pectoral and pelvic girdles.

–functions to attach the limbs to the trunk.

B. BONE

–is an **osseous tissue:** a supporting connective tissue composed of calcium salts and resistant to tensile and compressive forces.

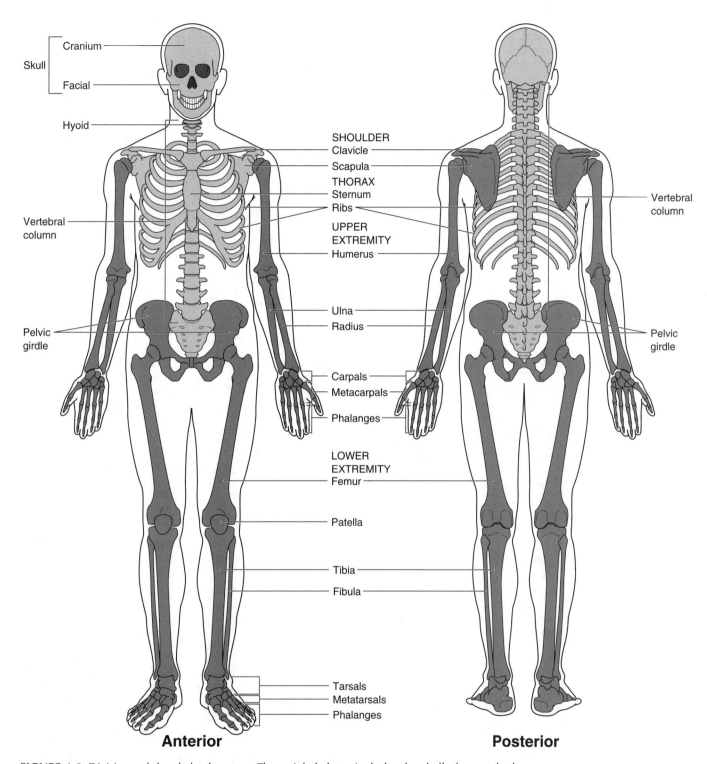

FIGURE 1-3 Divisions of the skeletal system. The *axial skeleton* includes the skull, the vertebral column, the hyoid, and the thorax. The *appendicular skeleton* includes the shoulder, the pelvic girdle, and the upper and lower extremities. (Adapted from Tortora G, Anagnostakos N: *Principles of Anatomy and Physiology,* 6th ed. New York, Harper & Row, 1992, p.163. Reprinted by permission of John Wiley & Sons, Inc.)

–is covered by a **periosteum** that isolates it from the surrounding tissues and provides for circulatory and nervous supply.

–includes **compact** (cortical, dense) and **cancellous** (trabecular, spongy) types.

   1. Functions of bones

a. Provide structural support for the entire body

b. Protect organs and tissues of the body

c. Serve as levers that can change the magnitude and direction of forces generated by skeletal muscles

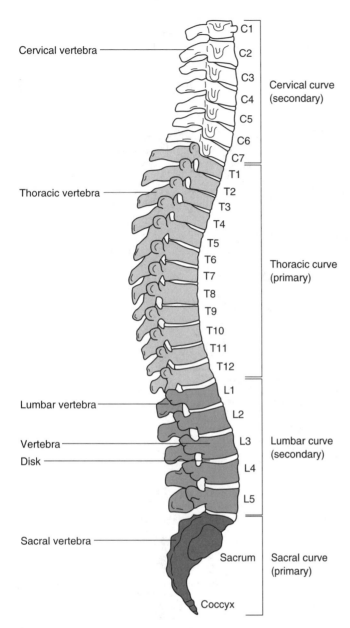

Cervical vertebra
C1
C2
C3
C4
C5
C6
C7

Cervical curve (secondary)

Thoracic vertebra
T1
T2
T3
T4
T5
T6
T7
T8
T9
T10
T11
T12

Thoracic curve (primary)

Lumbar vertebra
L1
L2
L3
L4
L5

Vertebra
Disk

Lumbar curve (secondary)

Sacral vertebra

Sacrum

Sacral curve (primary)

Coccyx

FIGURE 1-4 Lateral view of the spine, showing the vertebrae and discs.

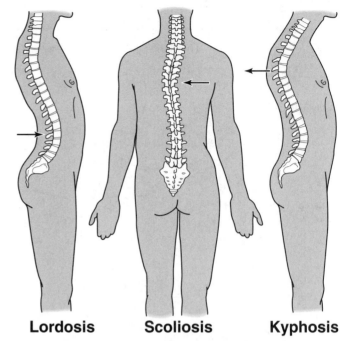

Lordosis   **Scoliosis**   **Kyphosis**

FIGURE 1-5 Abnormal curvatures of the spine. (Adapted from Ignatavicius DD, Workman ML, Mishler MA: *Medical–Surgical Nursing: A Nursing Process Approach,* 2nd ed. Philadelphia, WB Saunders, 1995, p 1399.)

(2) Epiphysis

–consists of cancellous bone surrounded by a layer of compact bone.

–contains **red bone marrow** in the porous chambers of spongy bone. **Hematopoiesis** (production of red blood cells, white blood cells, and platelets) occurs within red bone marrow.

–articulates with adjoining bones and is covered with **articular (hyaline) cartilage,** which facilitates joint movement.

3. Epiphyseal plate

–in immature long bones, the junction between the epiphysis and the diaphysis where **growth** of long bone **occurs**

b. Short bones

–are almost cuboidal in shape (e.g., bones of the wrist and ankle).

–are often covered with articular surfaces that interface with joints.

c. Flat bones

–are thin and relatively broad (e.g., bones of the skull, ribs, and scapulae).

d. Irregular bones

–have mixed shapes that do not fit easily into other categories (e.g., vertebrae).

d. Provide storage for calcium salts to maintain concentrations of calcium and phosphate ions in body fluids

e. Produce blood cells

2. General bone shapes

a. Long bones

–found in the appendicular skeleton

–consist of a central cylindrical shaft, or diaphysis, with an epiphysis at each end (e.g., femur)

(1) Diaphysis

–consists of compact bone surrounding a thin layer of cancellous bone, within which lies the **medullary cavity,** which is filled with **yellow bone marrow.**

C. CONNECTIVE TISSUES

–are tissues not generally exposed outside the body.

Table 1-1. Types of Synovial Joints

Type	Example	Movements
Ball and socket	Hip, shoulder	Circumduction, rotation, and angular in all planes
Condyloid	Wrist (radiocarpal)	Circumduction, abduction, adduction, flexion, and extension
Gliding	Ankle (subtalar)	Inversion and eversion
Hinge	Knee, elbow, ankle (talocrural)	Flexion and extension in one plane
Pivot	Atlas/axis	Rotation around central axis
Saddle	Thumb	Flexion, extension, abduction, adduction, circumduction, and opposition

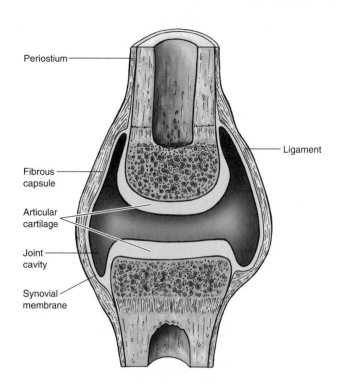

FIGURE 1-6 Synovial joint characteristics. (Adapted from Moore KL: *Clinically Oriented Anatomy,* 3rd ed. Baltimore, Williams & Wilkins, 1992.)

1. **Basic components**

    –Specialized cells (i.e., in blood, bone, cartilage)

    –Extracellular protein fibers (i.e., elastin, collagen, fibrin)

    –Ground substance

2. **Functions**

    –Provide support and protection

    –Transport materials

    –Store energy reserves

    –Perform regulatory functions

D. JOINTS (ARTICULATIONS)

–A joint exists wherever two bones meet.

–The particular function and integrity of a joint depends on its anatomy and on the requirement for strength or mobility.

1. **Classification**

    a. **Structural classes**

       (1) Fibrous joints (e.g., sutures of the skull)

       (2) Cartilaginous joints (e.g., disc between vertebrae)

       (3) Synovial joints (e.g., hip, elbow)

    b. **Functional classes**

       (1) Immovable joints: synarthroses

       (2) Slightly movable joints: amphiarthroses

       (3) Freely movable joints: diarthroses, or synovial joints

2. **Types of synovial joints:** Table 1-1

3. **Characteristics of synovial joints** (Figure 1-6)

    –Bony surfaces are covered with **articular cartilage.**

    –Surrounding the joint is a **fibrous joint capsule.**

    –**Ligaments** join bone to bone.

    –Inner surfaces of the **joint cavity** are lined with **synovial membranes.**

    –Synovial fluid from the membrane provides lubrication to the joint.

    –Some synovial joints, such as the knee, contain **fibrocartilaginous discs** (e.g., menisci).

    –**Bursae** reduce friction and act as shock absorbers.

4. **Movements at synovial joints** (see Table 1-1)

    –are determined by the structure of the joint and the arrangements of the associated muscles and bone.

    a. **Angular movements** (decrease or increase of the joint angle) include flexion, extension, hyperextension, abduction, and adduction.

    b. **Circular movements** include rotation (medial or lateral and supination or pronation) and circumduction.

       –occur at joints having bone with a rounded surface articulating with the depression of another bone.

    c. **Special movements**

       –include inversion, eversion, protraction, retraction, elevation, and depression.

III. THE MUSCULAR SYSTEM

–The muscular system includes skeletal, cardiac, and smooth muscle.

–Skeletal muscles can be controlled voluntarily.

A. GROSS ANATOMY OF SKELETAL MUSCLES

–There are three layers of connective tissue in skeletal muscle.

1. The **epimysium** is the outer layer that separates the muscle from surrounding tissues and organs.

   –The epimysium converges at the end of the muscle to form the tendon that attaches muscle to bone.

2. The **perimysium** is the central layer that divides the muscle into compartments called fascicles that contain skeletal muscle cells (muscle fibers).

3. The **endomysium** is the inner layer that surrounds each muscle fiber.

B. MUSCLE CONTROL

–A **motor neuron** controls each skeletal muscle fiber.

–The cell bodies of the motor neurons lie within the central nervous system.

–A motor neuron and all the muscle fibers it innervates comprise a **motor unit.**

–Motor units are recruited separately for muscle contraction.

–**Communication** between a motor neuron and a skeletal muscle fiber occurs at the **neuromuscular junction.**

–Each axon of the motor neuron ends at a **synaptic knob** containing the neurotransmitter **acetylcholine (ACh).**

–The **synaptic cleft** separates the synaptic knob from the sarcolemma of the skeletal muscle fiber.

–The **sarcolemma** of the motor end-plate contains chemically gated sodium channels and membrane receptors that bind ACh.

C. MICROANATOMY OF THE MUSCLE CELL

–The cytoplasm of the muscle cell is called **sarcoplasm.**

–Extensions of the **sarcolemma** form a network of tubules called transverse or **T-tubules.**

–The T-tubules extend into the sarcoplasm and communicate with the **sarcoplasmic reticulum,** which stores calcium in special sacs called **terminal cisternae.**

–**Myofibrils** contain **myofilaments,** which consist of the contractile proteins **actin** and **myosin.**

–Myofilaments are organized in repeating functional units called **sarcomeres.**

–Actin and myosin form **cross-bridges** and slide past one another during muscle contraction, thus shortening the sarcomeres.

–**Tropomyosin** covers the actin bridging site during resting condition. Tropomyosin is attached to **troponin.**

–Tropomyosin and troponin regulate bridging of actin and myosin for **muscle contraction and relaxation.**

D. MUSCLE CLASSIFICATION

–Each muscle begins at a proximal attachment **(origin),** ends at a distal attachment **(insertion),** and contracts to produce a specific **action.**

1. A **prime mover,** or **agonist,** is responsible for producing a particular movement. Prime movers, and their associated joints and movements, are outlined in **Table 1-2.**

2. An **antagonist** is a prime mover that opposes the agonist.

3. A **synergist** assists the prime mover, but is not the primary muscle responsible for the action.

IV. THE CARDIOVASCULAR SYSTEM

A. THE HEART

–receives blood from the veins and propels it into the arteries.

–is located near the center of the thoracic cavity.

–is divided into four chambers: right and left atria and right and left ventricles.

–is enclosed by connective tissues of the pericardium in the mediastinum.

1. **Surface anatomy**

   –The **atria** lie superior to the **ventricles.**

   –The **coronary sulcus** marks the border between the atria and the ventricles.

Table 1-2. Muscles That Are Prime Movers

Joint	Movement	Muscle(s) [Portion]
SHOULDER	Abduction	Deltoid [middle], supraspinatus
	Adduction	Latissimus dorsi, pectoralis major, teres major, posterior deltoid
	Extension	Latissimus dorsi, pectoralis major [sternal], teres major, posterior deltoid
	Horizontal extension	Deltoid [posterior], infraspinatus, latissimus dorsi, teres major, teres minor
	Hyperextension	Latissimus dorsi, teres major
	Flexion	Deltoid [anterior], pectoralis major [clavicular]
	Horizontal flexion	Deltoid [anterior], pectoralis major
	Lateral rotation	Infraspinatus, teres minor
	Medial rotation	Latissimus dorsi, pectoralis major, teres major, subscapularis
Shoulder girdle	Abduction (protraction)	Pectoralis minor, serratus anterior
	Adduction (retraction)	Rhomboids, trapezius [middle fibers]
	Depression	Pectoralis minor, subclavius, trapezius [lower fibers]
	Elevation	Levator scapulae, rhomboids, trapezius [upper fibers]
Scapula	Upward rotation	Serratus anterior, trapezius [upper and lower fibers]
	Downward rotation	Pectoralis minor, rhomboids
ELBOW	Flexion	Biceps brachii, brachialis, brachioradialis
	Extension	Triceps brachii
Radioulnar joint	Supination	Supinator, biceps brachii
	Pronation	Pronator quadratus, pronator teres
WRIST	Abduction (radial flexion)	Flexor carpi radialis, extensor carpi radialis longus, extensor carpi radialis brevis
	Adduction (ulnar flexion)	Flexor carpi ulnaris, extensor carpi ulnaris
	Extension/hyperextension	Extensor carpi radialis longus, extensor carpi radialis brevis, extensor carpi ulnaris
	Flexion	Flexor carpi radialis, flexor carpi ulnaris, palmaris longus
TRUNK	Flexion	Rectus abdominus, internal oblique, external oblique
	Extension/Hyperextension	Erector spinae group, semispinalis
	Lateral flexion	Internal oblique, external oblique, erector spinae group, multifidus, quadratus lumborum, rotatores
	Rotation	Internal oblique, external oblique, erector spinae group, multifidus, rotatores, semispinalis
HIP	Abductors	Gluteus medius, piriformis
	Adductors	Adductor brevis, adductor longus, adductor magnus, gracilis, pectineus
	Extensors	Biceps femoris, gluteus maximus, semimembranosus, semitendinosus
	Flexors	Iliacus, pectineus, psoas major, rectus femoris
	Lateral rotation	Gemelli, gluteus maximus, obturator externus, obturator internus
	Medial rotation	Gluteus medius, gluteus minimus
KNEE	Extension	Rectus femoris, vastus intermedius, vastus lateralis, vastus medialis
	Flexion	Biceps femoris, semimembranosus, semitendinosus
ANKLE	Extension (plantar flexion)	Gastrocnemius, soleus
	Flexion (dorsiflexion)	Extensor digitorum longus, peroneus tertius, tibialis anterior
FOOT (Intertarsal)	Eversion	Peroneus brevis, peroneus longus, peroneus tertius
	Inversion	Flexor digitorum longus, tibialis anterior, tibialis posterior

–The atria have thin muscular walls and are called **auricles** when not filled with blood.

–The ventricles have thicker muscular walls.

–The **interventricular sulcus** marks the boundary between the left and right ventricles.

–The great veins and arteries of the circulatory system are connected to the **base** of the heart.

–The **apex** lies inferiorly at the tip of the heart.

2. **Internal anatomy**

–The right atrium receives blood from the systemic circulation through the **superior and inferior venae cavae.**

–**Coronary veins** return venous blood from the myocardium to the **coronary sinus,** which opens into the right atrium.

–Each atrium communicates with the ventricle on the same side by way of an **atrioventricular (AV) valve.** The **right AV valve** is a **tricuspid** valve; the **left AV valve** is a **bicuspid (mitral)** valve.

–Each cusp is braced by **chordae tendinae,** which are connected to **papillary muscles.**

–Unoxygenated blood leaving the right ventricle flows through the right semilunar valve (**pulmonic**) to the pulmonary artery.

–Oxygenated blood leaving the left ventricle flows through the left semilunar valve (aortic) to the aorta.

3. **Circulation through the heart**

–**Blood from the periphery** flows through the heart according to the following sequence: superior and inferior venae cavae, right atrium, tricuspid valve, right ventricle, pulmonic semilunar valve, pulmonary arteries, lungs.

–**Blood from the lungs** flows through the heart according to the following sequence: left pulmonary vein, left atrium, bicuspid valve, left ventricle, aortic semilunar valve, ascending aorta, systemic circulation.

B. **THE CIRCULATORY SYSTEM**

1. **Blood vessels**

a. **Arteries**

–are muscular-walled vessels that carry blood away from the heart.

–decrease progressively in size to become **arterioles** and then connect to capillaries.

b. **Capillaries**

–are vessels composed of one cell layer that functions to exchange nutrients and waste materials between the blood and tissues.

c. **Veins**

–are vessels that carry blood back to the heart.

–are classified according to size.

(1) **Venules** are small veins that carry blood from the capillaries to medium-sized veins.

(2) Medium-sized veins are larger in diameter and empty into large veins.

(3) Large veins include the two **venae cavae.**

2. **Blood flow**

–The heart circulates oxygenated blood through arteries to arterioles to capillaries.

–At the capillaries, blood delivers oxygen and nutrients to the tissues and carries waste products away.

–Unoxygenated blood returns to the capillaries and travels to venules, then veins, which return blood to the heart.

V. THE RESPIRATORY SYSTEM

A. **DIVISIONS**

1. The **upper respiratory tract** consists of the **nose** (including the nasal cavity) and paranasal sinuses, the **pharynx,** and the **larynx.**

2. The **lower respiratory tract** consists of the **trachea** and the **lungs,** which include the **bronchi, bronchioles,** and **alveoli.**

B. **THE LUNGS**

–are organs of respiration where oxygenation of blood occurs.

–occupy the **pleural cavities** and are covered by a **pleural membrane.**

1. The **right lung** has three distinct lobes: superior, middle, and inferior.

2. The **left lung** has two lobes: the superior and inferior.

3. The **apex** of each lung extends into the base of the neck above the first rib.

4. The **base** of each lung rests on the **diaphragm,** the respiratory muscle that separates the thoracic from the abdominopelvic cavities.

C. AIR FLOW AND GAS EXCHANGE

1. Air enters the respiratory system through two external **nares** and proceeds through the **nasal cavity** and **sinuses.**

   a. Air is **warmed, filtered, and moistened** prior to entry into the nasopharynx at the internal nares.

   b. **Cilia** line the nasal cavity and function to sweep mucus and trap microorganisms.

2. The incoming air then passes through the **pharynx.**

   –The pharynx extends between the internal nares and the entrances to the larynx and esophagus.

   –The pharynx is shared by the digestive and respiratory systems.

3. Incoming air leaving the pharynx passes through a narrow opening in the **larynx** called the **glottis.**

   –Air movement, which causes the vocal cords to vibrate, generates sound.

4. From the larynx, incoming air enters the **trachea.**

   a. The trachea extends from the larynx into the lungs.

   b. **C-shaped cartilages** of the trachea

–protect, support, and maintain an open airway.

–prevent overexpansion of the respiratory system.

–allow large masses of food to pass along the esophagus.

5. Air enters the **lungs** via the **tracheobronchial tree,** which consists of the **bronchi, bronchioles, and alveoli.**

   a. The trachea branches to form the right and left **primary bronchi.**

   b. Each primary bronchus enters a lung and branches into **secondary bronchi.**

   c. Further branching forms smaller, narrower passages that terminate in units called **bronchioles. Variation in the diameter of the bronchioles** controls the resistance to air flow and ventilation of the lungs.

   d. **Terminal bronchioles** are the smallest branches; they supply air to the **lobules** of the lung.

   e. The lobules consist of **alveolar ducts** and **alveoli,** where actual **gas exchange** occurs. **Alveoli** are one cell layer thick and have an abundance of capillaries on the outer surface.

VI. APPLIED ANATOMY

–Knowledge of basic anatomy is required for accurate anthropometric measurement, as well as for the assessment of pulse rate and blood pressure.

A. ASSESSMENT OF BODY COMPOSITION

1. **Skinfold thicknesses**

   –Skin and subcutaneous adipose tissue are measured at specific sites on the body to estimate body fat.

   –**Calipers** are generally used to assess thickness of various skinfold sites.

2. **Girth measurements**

   –assess the **circumferential dimensions** of various body parts.

   –provide an indication of **growth, nutritional status, and fat patterning.**

   –are determined using a **tape measure.**

   –Circumference measurement sites are listed and described in **Table 1-3.**

3. **Body breadth measurements**

   –provide information for determining **frame size and body type.**

–can be used **to estimate desirable weight** based on stature.

–are measured using **spreading calipers, sliding calipers, or an anthropometer.**

B. ASSESSMENT OF PULSE RATE

–**Pulse is a measurement of heart rate.**

–It can be palpated on any large or medium-sized artery by using a fingertip to compress the vessel and sense the pulse.

C. ASSESSMENT OF SYSTEMIC ARTERIAL BLOOD PRESSURE

–reflects hemodynamic factors such as cardiac output, peripheral vascular resistance, and blood flow.

–is **an indirect measurement of the pressure inside an artery** caused by the force exerted (by the blood) against the vessel wall.

–is usually measured in the arm over the brachial artery, medial to the biceps tendon, **using a sphygmomanometer and a stethoscope.**

Table 1-3. Standardized Description of Circumference Measurement Sites and Procedures

Circumference Site	Description
Abdomen	At the level of the umbilicus
Calf	At the maximum circumference between the knee and the ankle
Forearm	With the arms hanging downward but slightly away from the trunk and palms facing forward, at the maximal forearm circumference
Hips	At the maximal circumference of the hips or buttocks region, whichever is larger (above the gluteal fold)
Arm	With the arm to the side of the body, midway between the acromion and olecranon processes
Waist	At the narrowest part of the torso (above the umbilicus and below the xiphoid process)
Thigh	With the legs slightly apart, at the maximal circumference of the thigh (below the gluteal fold)

Procedures

- All limb measurements should be taken on the right side of the body using a tension-regulated tape

- The subject should stand erect but relaxed

- Place the tape perpendicular to the long axis of the body part in each case

- Pull the tape to proper tension without pinching skin

- Take duplicate measures at each site and retest if duplicate measurements are not within 7 mm or 0.25 in

(From American College of Sports Medicine: *ACSM's Guidelines for Exercise Testing and Prescription,* 5th edition, Reference Cards. Baltimore, Williams & Wilkins, 1995, Table 4-3.)

VII. PRINCIPLES OF BIOMECHANICS

A. PRINCIPLES OF BALANCE AND STABILITY

–Each segment of the body is acted upon by the **force of gravity** and has a **center of gravity.**

1. **Line of gravity (LOG)**

   –is the downward direction of the force of gravity on an object, i.e., vertically toward the center of the earth.

2. **Center of gravity (COG)**

   –is the **point of exact center around which the body freely rotates.**

   –is the **point around which the weight is equal on all sides.**

   –is the **point of intersection of the three cardinal body planes.**

   a. When all segments of the body are combined and the body is considered to be a single solid object (in **anatomic position**), the COG lies approximately anterior to the second sacral vertebrae.

   b. The COG changes as the segments of the body move away from anatomic position.

3. **Base of support**

   –is the area of contact between the body and the supporting surface.

4. **Balance and stability**

   a. **Balance** is maintained when the COG remains over the base of support.

   b. **Stability** is firmness of balance; the COG must fall within the base of support.

      –**Increased stability** occurs when COG is closer to the base of support.

      –For **maximum stability,** the COG should be placed over the center of the base of support.

B. APPLIED WEIGHTS AND RESISTANCES

1. The ability of any force to cause rotation of a lever is known as **torque.**

2. **Rotation** of a segment of the body is dependent on

   –the magnitude of force exerted by the **effort force** and the **resistance force.**

   –the **distance of these two forces from the axis of rotation.**

3. Moving the COG of segments alters resistive torque. **Changing the torque provides a method for altering the difficulty of an exercise when weight is applied** (Figure 1-7).

   a. Weight applied at the end of an extended arm changes the COG of the arm to a

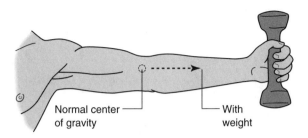

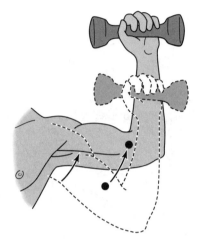

FIGURE 1-7 A change in center of gravity changes the torque.

more distal position, requiring greater muscular support to maintain the arm in a horizontal position. Conversely, by shifting the mass of the weight proximally, less muscular effort is required.

   b. Some externally applied forces, such as exercise pulleys, do not act in a vertical direction, and the **forces exert effects that vary according to the angle of application.**

   c. Weights applied to the extremities frequently exert traction (**distractive force**) on joint structures. A distractive force is sometimes used to promote normal joint movement in rehabilitation exercise, but distractive force can also be injurious or undesirable.

C. MOTION

1. **Translatory motion**

   –occurs when a freely movable object moves in a straight line when a force is applied on center of the object.

   –occurs when, regardless of where the force is applied, the object is free to move only in a linear path.

2. **Rotary motion**

   –occurs when a force is applied off-center to a freely movable object.

–occurs when, regardless of where the force is applied, the object is free to move only in a rotary path.

3. **Velocity**

   –represents the distance traveled in a period of time.

   a. **Acceleration** refers to increasing velocity.

   b. **Deceleration** refers to decreasing velocity.

4. **Momentum**

   –is the mathematical product of the mass and velocity of a moving object.

5. **Laws of motion (Newton's laws)**

   a. The **law of inertia** states that a body at rest tends to remain at rest, whereas a body in motion tends to continue in motion with consistent speed and in the same direction unless acted upon by an outside force.

   b. The **law of acceleration** states that the velocity of a body is changed only when acted upon by an additional force. The acceleration (or deceleration) is proportional to and in the same direction as the force.

   c. The **law of counterforce** states that the production of any force creates another force, opposite and equal to the first force.

D. LEVERS

–A lever is a rigid bar that **revolves around a fixed point** or axis (fulcrum).

–Levers are **used with force to overcome a resistance.**

1. **Parts of a lever**

   a. The **axis** is the pivot point between the force and the resistance.

   b. The **force arm** is the distance from the axis to the point of application of force.

   c. The **resistance arm** is the distance from the axis to the resistance.

2. **Classes of levers** (Figure 1-8)

   a. In a **first-class lever,** the axis is between the force and the resistance arm.

      –The force arm may be greater than, smaller than, or equal to the resistance arm.

   b. In a **second-class lever,** the resistance lies between the effort force and the axis of rotation; the force arm is greater than the resistance arm.

   c. In a **third-class lever,** the effort force lies closer to the axis of the lever than the resistance; the force arm is smaller than the resistance arm.

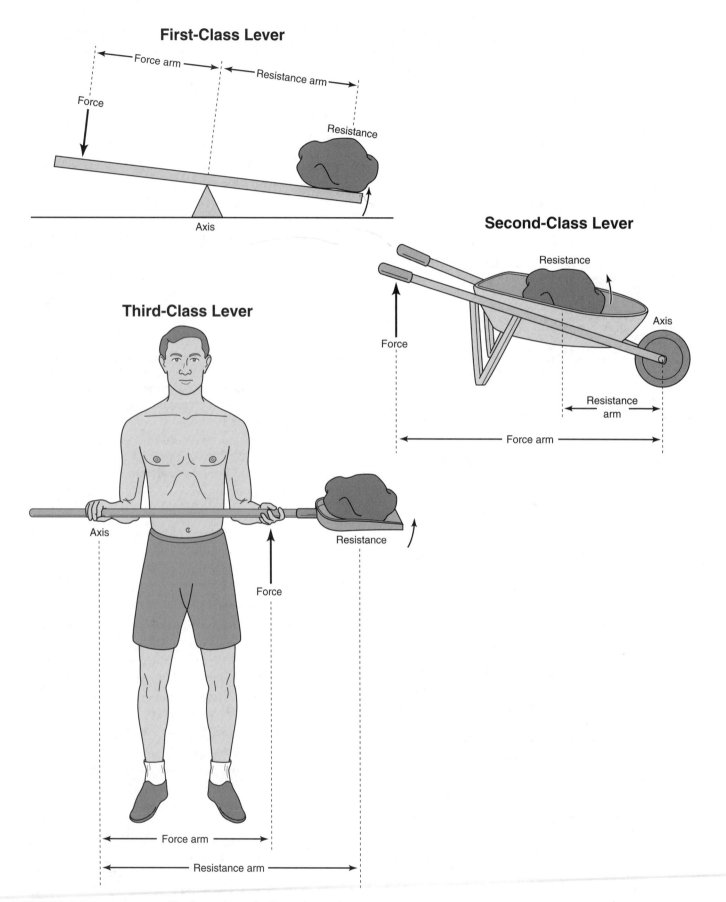

First-Class Lever

Force arm

Resistance arm

Force

Resistance

Axis

Second-Class Lever

Resistance

Force

Axis

Resistance arm

Force arm

Third-Class Lever

Axis

Force

Resistance

Force arm

Resistance arm

FIGURE 1-8 Lever systems. (F = force; A = axis; R = resistance.)

VIII. APPLICATION OF BIOMECHANICAL PRINCIPLES TO ACTIVITY

A. WALKING

1. Stride length

–is the distance covered with each stride.

–is measured from initial contact of one lower extremity to the point at which the same extremity contacts the ground again.

2. Stride frequency

–is the number of strides in a fixed time (e.g., 15 steps/minute).

3. Phases of the ambulation cycle

–During a single gait cycle, each extremity passes through two phases.

a. Stance phase

–begins when one extremity contacts the ground (heel strike).

–continues as long as some portion of the foot is in contact with the ground (toe off).

–**Subdivisions of the stance phase:**

(1) **Heel strike**

(2) **Foot flat**

(3) **Midstance**

(4) **Heel off**

(5) **Toe off**

b. Swing phase

–begins when the toe of one extremity leaves the ground.

–ends just before heel strike or contact of the same extremity.

–**Subdivisions of the swing phase:**

(1) **Initial swing (acceleration)**

(2) **Midswing**

(3) **Terminal swing (deceleration)**

B. RUNNING

–Running differs from walking in a number of ways.

1. Running requires greater balance because of the absence of a double support period and because of the presence of float periods when both feet are out of contact with the supporting surface.

2. Running requires greater muscle strength because many muscles are contracting more rapidly and with greater force.

3. Running requires greater range of motion because joint angles are greater at the extremes of the movement.

4. The **direction of the driving force is more horizontal,** and the **stride is longer.**

5. The body has a **greater forward incline.**

6. **Rotary actions** of the spine and pelvic regions **are increased.**

7. **Arm actions are higher and more vigorous.** (The arms should move in an anterior/posterior direction to improve efficiency.)

8. **Stride length and frequency are increased** with increasing speed.

C. SWIMMING

1. Buoyancy

–is the tendency of a body to float when submerged in a fluid.

–is **dependent upon the percentage of weight composed of bone and muscle** because these tissues are more dense (therefore, less buoyant) than other body tissues.

–According to **Archimedes' principle,** "a body immersed in fluid is buoyed up with a force equal to the weight of the displaced fluid."

2. Propelling forces

–in swimming result from the **stroke and kick.**

–should contribute to **forward progress,** not to vertical or lateral movement.

–During the propelling phase, the arms, hands, and feet should present a large surface to the water and should push against the water.

3. Resistive forces result from

–skin resistance (friction).

–wave-making resistance caused by up-and-down body movement.

–eddy current resistance.

D. LIFTING AND BODY MECHANICS

–In applying the laws of motion to lifting, reaching, pushing, pulling, and carrying of objects, the effects of gravity, friction, muscular forces, and external resistance are important.

–The **basic principles of good body mechanics** are:

1. Assume a position close to the object, or move the position of the object closer to the COG, allowing the use of upper extremities in a shortened position (short lever arms). Lower torque is required, thus allowing muscles to function more efficiently.

2. **Position COG as close to the object's COG as possible,** reducing torque and requiring less energy.

3. **Widen the base of support** by lowering the COG and maintaining the line of gravity within the base of support.

4. **Position the feet according to the direction of movement** required to perform the activity, thus increasing stability.

5. **Avoid twisting** when lifting.

6. When possible, **push, pull, roll or slide an object** rather than lift it.

7. **Use the "power position"** (Figure 1-9).

   –Knees slightly bent

   –Body bent forward from the hips

   –Back straight

   –Chest and head upright

E. LOW BACK PAIN: MECHANISMS, PREVENTION AND TREATMENT

–occurs most commonly in the lumbar region of the vertebral column.

–may be caused by traumatic injury, history of poor posture, faulty body mechanics, stressful living and working habits, lack of flexibility or strength, or a general lack of physical fitness.

1. **Mechanism of injury in disc herniation**

   –The **lumbar vertebrae** are the most massive, but least mobile, because they **support much of the body weight.**

   –The **lumbar discs** are the thickest of the vertebral discs and **are subject to the most pressure.**

   –As loading on the vertebral column increases, the intervertebral discs become more important as **shock absorbers.**

   –**Excessive or repetitive stresses** on the lumbar region due to slumped sitting, forward bending, lifting, or twisting may cause **herniation of the disc.**

   a. The **inner nucleus pulposus of the disc** breaks through the surrounding fibrocartilaginous annulus fibrosus and **protrudes** beyond the intervertebral space.

   b. The disc protrusion often occurs in a posterior direction. This causes **pressure on the nerves in the disc wall and nerve**

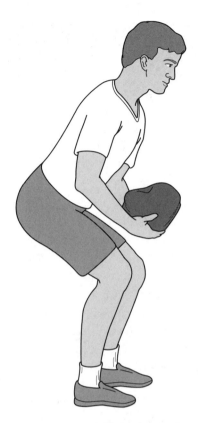

FIGURE 1-9 Power position of the body. The knees are slightly bent; the back is held in a neutral position (slightly arched); and the shoulders and head are up.

   roots, sending pain along the back and leg. This pain is referred to as **radiating symptoms** or **radiculopathy.**

2. **Prevention and treatment of low back pain**

   –Low back pain can occur due to various mechanisms of injury or overuse. Therefore, **people with low back pain should be evaluated by a physician.**

   –Knowledge of **proper body mechanics, adequate physical conditioning, and flexibility** may help prevent low back pain.

   a. **Disc protrusion with radiculopathy**

      –Backward bending of the spine, with avoidance of forward bending and slumped sitting postures, is often recommended to relieve pressure on the nerve root.

   b. **Pain due to muscle guarding and spasm** in the absence of signs of disc herniation is often treated with **muscle stretching.** Maintaining flexibility in the back is also helpful as a preventive method.

REVIEW TEST

DIRECTIONS: Carefully read all questions and select the BEST single answer.

1. The C-shaped cartilages of the trachea allow all of the following to occur EXCEPT
   (A) ciliated movement of mucus-secreting cells
   (B) distention of the esophagus
   (C) maintenance of open airway
   (D) prevention of tracheal collapse during pressure changes

2. Functions of bone include all of the following EXCEPT
   (A) support for the body
   (B) protection of organs and tissues
   (C) production of red blood cells
   (D) production of force

3. In the organization of skeletal muscle, the muscle cell contains the contractile proteins. Which of the following is a contractile protein?
   (A) Myosin
   (B) Muscle fascicle
   (C) Myofibril
   (D) Muscle fiber

4. A client in your exercise class has been complaining of back pain with no radicular symptoms. The person has been treated medically and is now joining the exercise program in order to improve flexibility in the low back. Which exercise would be most appropriate for this person to address the stated goal?
   (A) Hip flexor stretch
   (B) Knee-to-chest stretch
   (C) Gastrocnemius stretch
   (D) Lateral trunk stretch

5. All of the following are true regarding long bones EXCEPT
   (A) the diaphysis is composed of compact bone
   (B) the epiphysis consists of spongy bone
   (C) most bones of the axial skeleton are of this type
   (D) the central shaft encases the medullary canal

6. The arm is capable of performing all of the following motions EXCEPT
   (A) flexion
   (B) abduction
   (C) inversion
   (D) supination

7. The prime movers for extension of the knee are
   (A) biceps femoris
   (B) biceps brachii
   (C) quadriceps femoris
   (D) gastrocnemius

8. A baseball pitcher has been complaining of weakness in lateral rotation motions of the shoulder. You have been asked to evaluate him for a strengthening program. You would have him concentrate on strengthening which of the following muscles?
   (A) Subscapularis
   (B) Teres major
   (C) Latissimus dorsi
   (D) Teres minor

9. Cartilage is categorized as which of the following types of connective tissue?
   (A) Loose
   (B) Dense
   (C) Fluid
   (D) Supporting

10. Blood leaving the heart to be oxygenated in the lungs must first pass through the right atrium and ventricle by way of valves. Through which valve does blood flow when moving from the right atrium to the right ventricle?
    (A) Bicuspid valve
    (B) Tricuspid valve
    (C) Pulmonic valve
    (D) Aortic valve

11. An abnormal curve of the spine in which there is lateral deviation of the vertebral column is called
    (A) lordosis
    (B) scoliosis
    (C) kyphosis
    (D) primary curve

12. Which of the following is considered a "ball and socket" joint?
    (A) Ankle
    (B) Elbow
    (C) Knee
    (D) Hip

13. Which of the following is the ability of a force to cause rotation of a lever?
    (A) Center of gravity
    (B) Base of support
    (C) Torque
    (D) Stability

14. Standard sites for measurement of skinfolds include
    (A) medial thigh
    (B) biceps
    (C) infrailiac
    (D) forearm

15. A standard site for measurement of circumferences is the
    (A) abdomen
    (B) neck
    (C) wrist
    (D) ankle

16. The most common site used for measurement of the pulse during exercise is
    (A) popliteal
    (B) femoral
    (C) radial
    (D) dorsalis pedis

17. Blood from the peripheral anatomy flows to the heart through the superior and inferior venae cavae into the
    (A) right atrium
    (B) left atrium
    (C) right ventricle
    (D) left ventricle

18. Arteries are large-diameter vessels that carry blood away from the heart. As they course through the body they progressively decrease in size until they become
    (A) arterioles
    (B) anastomoses
    (C) venules
    (D) veins

19. The Law of Inertia
    (A) states that a body at rest tends to remain at rest, whereas a body in motion tends to continue to stay in motion with consistent speed and in the same direction unless acted upon by an outside force
    (B) states that the velocity of a body is changed only when acted upon by an additional force
    (C) states that the driving force of the body is doubled and the rate of acceleration is also doubled
    (D) states that the production of any force will create another force which will be opposite and equal to the first force

20. Running is a locomotor activity that is similar to walking, but with some differences. In comparison to walking, running requires greater
    (A) balance
    (B) muscle strength
    (C) range of motion
    (D) all of the above

21. "A body immersed in fluid is buoyed up with a force equal to the weight of the displaced fluid" was first described by
    (A) Einstein
    (B) Freud
    (C) Whitehead
    (D) Archimedes

22. Pain due to low back muscle guarding and spasm in the absence of signs of disc herniation is often treated with muscle stretching. Which of the following is (are) helpful stretching activities for the low back?
    (A) Knee to chest
    (B) Double knee to chest
    (C) Lower trunk rotation
    (D) All of the above

ANSWERS AND EXPLANATIONS

1–A. Cilia line the nasal cavity, not the trachea. The C-shaped cartilages of the trachea provide a certain rigidity to support the trachea and maintain an open airway so that collapse does not occur. In addition, the rigidity caused by these cartilages prevents overexpansion of the trachea when pressure changes occur in the respiratory system. The proximity of the trachea to the esophagus (the esophagus is posterior to the trachea) could cause obstruction to the airway if a large bolus of food is passed in the esophagus. This is remedied by the arrangement of the C-shaped cartilages of the trachea with the open end of the C being posterior. Distention of the esophagus can occur without compromise to the airway.

2–D. The bones of the skeletal system act as levers for changing the magnitude and direction of forces that are generated by the skeletal muscles attaching to the bones. The bones of the skeletal system provide structural support for the body through their arrangement in the axial and appendicular skeletal divisions. The axial skeleton forms the longitudinal axis of the body and supports and protects organs as well as provides attachment for muscles. The appendicular skeleton provides for attachment of the limbs to the trunk. It is in the marrow of bone that blood cells are formed.

3–A. The skeletal muscle consists of bundles of muscle fibers called muscle fascicles, or fasciculi. Each fasciculus contains the muscle cells. Within the muscle cells are cylinders, called myofibrils, which are responsible for the contraction of the muscle fiber. The myofibrils have this ability because they contain myofilaments, which are the contractile proteins actin and myosin. Actin is a thin filament twisted into a strand. Myosin is a thick filament having a tail and a head. During activation of the muscle, actin and mysosin interact, causing cross-bridging between the two filaments. Myosin pulls the actin, which shortens the muscle and causes tension development.

4–B. Treatment of a low back complaint depends upon the mechanism of injury or overuse. In the case of disc herniation, which is often accompanied by radiating symptoms into the leg, positioning of the spine is often able to alleviate painful symptoms because of reduced pressure on the spinal nerves. In the case of the individual addressed in the question, flexibility of the lumbar spine is prescribed to reduce symptoms. Performance of the knee-to-chest stretch exercise would be the most appropriate in this case, since it allows sustained stretch of the lumbar spinal musculature to increase muscular length and improve flexibility. The lateral trunk stretch is not sufficient to improve flexibility of muscles supporting the lumbar spine.

5–C. The majority of bones of the appendicular (rather than the axial) skeleton are long bones. Long bones have a central shaft (called the diaphysis) made of compact (dense) bone. The shaft forms a cylinder around a central cavity of the bone, which is called the medullary canal.

6–C. Inversion is a specialized movement that can be performed by the sole of the foot, but not by the arm. The arm is capable of angular and circular movements. Angular movements decrease or increase the joint angle and include flexion, extension, abduction, and adduction. Circular movements can occur at joints having a bone with a rounded surface that articulates with a cup or depression on another bone. Included in circular movements are circumduction and rotation, including the specialized rotational movements of supination and pronation.

7–C. The quadriceps femoris muscle is the major muscle responsible for knee extension, as dictated by its proximal and distal attachments. The muscle has four heads (quad), three of which originate from the anterior portion of the ilium and one originating on the shaft of the femur. All four heads converge and insert on the tibia via a common tendon (patellar). Contraction of the muscle causes the knee to extend. The biceps brachii is found in the upper body and is an elbow flexor. Although the biceps femoris and gastrocnemius muscles cross the knee joint, they do so posteriorly and are primarily active in knee flexion and ankle plantar flexion respectively.

8–D. The subscapularis, teres major, and latissimus dorsi are all medial rotators of the arm. They function as antagonists to the teres minor, which is a lateral rotator of the arm.

9–D. Connective tissues of the body are categorized according to specific characteristics of their ground substance. Connective tissue proper has many types of cells and fibers in a somewhat syrupy ground substance. Loose and dense connective tissue is of this type. Fluid connective tissue cells are suspended in a watery ground substance; included in this category are blood and lymph. Supporting connective tissues have a dense ground substance with very closely packed fibers. Cartilage and bone are found in the supporting connective tissue category.

10–B. Blood from the peripheral anatomy flows to the heart through the superior and inferior venae cavae into the right atrium. From the right atrium the blood passes through the tricuspid valve to the right ventricle and then out through the pulmonary semilunar valve to the pulmonary arteries and then to the lungs to be oxygenated. The tricuspid valve is so-named because of the three cusps, or flaps, of which it is made. The bicuspid valve is a similar valve, only with two cusps, and is found between the left atrium and left ventricle. Blood leaving the left ventricle will pass through the aortic semilunar valve to the ascending aorta and then out to the systemic circulation.

11–B. The vertebral column serves as the main axial support for the body. The adult vertebral column exhibits four major curvatures when viewed from the sagittal plane. Scoliosis is an abnormal lateral deviation of the vertebral column. Kyphosis is an abnormal increased posterior curvature, especially in the thoracic region. Lordosis is an abnormal, exaggerated anterior curvature in the lumbar region. A primary curve refers to the thoracic and sacral curvatures of the vertebral column that remain in the original fetal positions.

12–D. The ankle is a gliding joint and allows flexion, extension, inversion, and eversion motions. The shoulder and hip are both ball-and-socket joints, allowing circumduction, rotation, and angular motions. The knee is a hinge joint, allowing flexion and extension in only one plane.

13–C. The center of gravity is the point of exact center around which the body freely rotates, the point around which the weight is equal on all sides, and the point of intersection of the three cardinal planes of the body. Balance is maintained when the center of gravity stays over the base of support and stability is the firmness of balance. Torque is the ability of any force to cause rotation of the lever and is calculated as the product of the force and the perpendicular distance from the axis of rotation at which the force is applied.

14–B. The standard sites for measurement of skinfold thicknesses include the abdominal, triceps, biceps, chest, medial calf, midaxillary, subscapular, suprailiac, and thigh (a measurement taken on the anterior midline of the thigh).

15–A. The standard sites for measurement of body circumferences are the abdomen, calf, forearm, hips, arm, waist, and thigh.

16–C. The most common sites for measurement of the peripheral pulses during exercise are the carotid and radial pulses. They are more easily accessible during exercise than the femoral, popliteal, posterior tibial, or dorsalis pedis pulses.

17–A. Blood from the peripheral anatomy flows to the heart through the superior and inferior venae cavae into the right atrium. From the right atrium, blood passes through the tricuspid valve to the right ventricle and then out through the pulmonary semilunar valve to the pulmonary arteries and to the lungs to be oxygenated.

18–A. Arteries are large-diameter vessels that carry blood away from the heart. As they course through the body they progressively decrease in size until they become arterioles, the smallest vessels of the arterial system. From the arterioles, blood enters the capillaries, which are one layer thick. Venules and veins return blood back to the heart.

19–A. The Law of Inertia states that a body at rest tends to remain at rest, whereas a body in motion tends to continue to stay in motion with consistent speed and in the same direction unless acted upon by an outside force. The Law of Acceleration states that the velocity of a body is changed only when acted upon by an additional force and the driving force of the body is doubled and the rate of acceleration is also doubled. The Law of Counterforce states that the production of any force will create another force that will be opposite and equal to the first force.

20–D. Running is a locomotor activity that is similar to walking, but with some differences. In comparison with walking, running requires greater balance, muscle strength, and range of motion. Balance is necessary because of the absence of the double support period and the presence of float periods in which both feet are out of contact with the supporting surface. Muscle strength is necessary because many muscles are contracting more rapidly and with greater force during running as compared with walking. Joint angles are at greater extremes with the running gait.

21–D. Archimedes first described the principle of buoyancy. If a body displaces water weighing more than itself, the body will float. With the lungs filled with air, most individuals float in water. However, the ability to float is dependent upon the percentage of weight composed of bone and muscle because these tissues are denser than other body tissues.

22–D. Pain due to muscle guarding and spasm in the absence of signs of disc herniation is often treated with muscle stretching. Maintaining flexibility in the back is helpful as a preventative measure as well. All three of these exercises are good for stretching the lower back.

CHAPTER 2

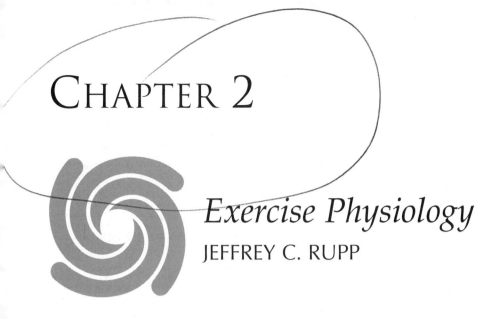

Exercise Physiology

JEFFREY C. RUPP

I. ENERGY SYSTEMS

A. ROLE OF ADENOSINE TRIPHOSPHATE (ATP)

–Energy used to fuel biological processes comes only from the breakdown of adenosine triphosphate (ATP), specifically from the chemical energy stored in the bonds of the last two phosphates of the ATP molecule. When work is performed, the bond between the last two phosphates is broken, **producing adenosine diphosphate (ADP),** a phosphate molecule, useful energy, and heat (**Figure 2-1**).

1. **ATP stores in skeletal muscle are limited.** These limited stores can fuel approximately 5–10 seconds of high-intensity work. Therefore, **ATP must be continuously resynthesized from ADP to allow exercise to continue.**

2. **Three energy systems are responsible for the resynthesis of ATP:**
   a. ATP–PC system (anaerobic—no oxygen required)
   b. Anaerobic glycolysis (lactic acid system)
   c. Oxygen system (aerobic—oxygen required)

3. **Muscular fatigue** begins when the exercise intensity demands ATP production at a higher rate than the energy systems can supply. **Steady state occurs** when ATP production and ATP demand are in balance.

4. The energy systems are described in terms of their power and their capacity to produce ATP.
   a. **Power** refers to the rate at which ATP can be produced.
   b. **Capacity** refers to how long the system can continue to produce ATP.

B. ADENOSINE TRIPHOSPHATE–PHOSPHOCREATINE (ATP–PC) SYSTEM

–When the limited stores of ATP are nearly depleted during high-intensity exercise (5–10 seconds), another high-energy source called **phosphocreatine (PC)** begins to break down. PC has only one high-energy phosphate bond (**Figure 2-2**). The energy from the breakdown of PC is used to resynthesize ATP, which then breaks down to provide energy for exercise.

1. **Power**
   –Because the number of reactions is small (only two), this system can provide ATP at a very rapid rate. The ATP–PC system is the most powerful energy system.

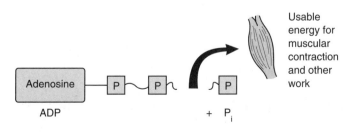

FIGURE 2-1 Schematic representation of an ATP molecule showing high-energy bonds and the splitting of an ATP molecule to release usable energy.

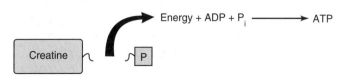

FIGURE 2-2 Schematic representation of phosphocreatine showing single high-energy bond.

2. Capacity

–There is enough PC stored in skeletal muscle for approximately 25 seconds of high-intensity work. Therefore, the ATP–PC system will last for about **30 seconds** (5 seconds for stored ATP, 25 seconds for PC). These activities include most sprint events, weight lifting, shotputt, etc.

C. ANAEROBIC GLYCOLYSIS (LACTIC ACID SYSTEM)

–The energy stored in the foods we eat is found in carbohydrates, fats, and protein. Anaerobic glycolysis uses only **carbohydrate,** primarily muscle glycogen, **as a fuel source.**

–Anaerobic glycolysis results in only a few ATPs, and the **metabolic end-product** is lactic acid (or **lactate**).

–The accumulation of excessive amounts of lactate in muscle tissue is associated with **fatigue.**

1. Power

–The lactic acid system is ranked second (among the energy systems) in terms of power.

2. Capacity

–The lactic acid system lasts for approximately **1–2 minutes,** until the accumulation of lactate and other metabolic by-products causes fatigue. These activities include middle distance sprints like 400-, 600-, and 800-meter runs. This system is ranked second in capacity among the energy systems.

D. OXYGEN (AEROBIC) SYSTEM

–The oxygen system can be **fueled by carbohydrate, fat, and protein,** although protein is not a significant fuel source during most types of exercise.

–**Fat, as a fuel source,** provides more energy (9 kcal per gram) than carbohydrate (4 kcal per gram) or protein (4 kcal per gram). However, fat produces less energy, per liter oxygen consumed, than carbohydrate. The use of fat as a fuel source is partially determined by the availability of oxygen to the muscle cell. Most body fat is **stored as**

triglyceride in adipose tissue. A small amount of triglyceride stored in skeletal muscle can be an important source of energy during exercise.

–The carbohydrates, fat, and small amounts of protein used by this energy system during exercise are **completely metabolized,** leaving only **carbon dioxide** (which is exhaled) **and water as metabolic by-products.**

1. Power

–The oxygen system is complicated and requires 2–3 minutes to adjust to a changing exercise intensity.

–The oxygen system ranks third among the energy systems in power production.

–**Maximal oxygen consumption,** also known as $\dot{V}_{O_2 \, max}$, is a measure of the power of the aerobic energy system and is generally regarded as the best indicator of aerobic fitness.

2. Capacity

–The capacity of the oxygen system to regenerate ATP is almost unlimited, and the only limitation is the amount of fuel and oxygen available to the cell. For this reason, it is ranked first in capacity among the energy systems.

E. FUEL UTILIZATION DURING EXERCISE

1. All of the energy-producing systems are active during most exercise; however, **different types of exercise place greater demands on different energy systems.** For example, middle distance events (e.g., the 1500-meter run) typically use all three energy systems. The ATP–PC system is used initially, then a combination of the oxygen system and anaerobic glycolysis during the middle, finally more emphasis is placed on anaerobic glycolysis at the end for the "kick."

2. Most aerobic exercise activities are fueled by a **mixture of carbohydrate and fat.** The ratio of fat to carbohydrate substrate utilization **is dependent on intensity and duration. Higher intensity exercise** utilizes predominantly **carbohydrates. Lower intensity, longer duration exercise** relies less on carbohydrates and more on **fat.**

II. MUSCLE PHYSIOLOGY

–There are **three types of muscle** in the human body: (1) skeletal, (2) smooth (found in some blood vessels and in the digestive system), and (3) cardiac muscle. Skeletal muscle physiology is discussed in this section; cardiac muscle physiology is discussed in the next section (III, Cardiovascular Physiology).

A. STRUCTURE OF SKELETAL MUSCLE

1. Motor units

–A motor unit consists of an **efferent (motor) nerve and all of the muscle fibers** supplied (or innervated) by that nerve.

–The total number of motor units varies among different muscles.

–The total number of fibers in each motor unit varies among muscles.

–A nerve impulse, regardless of its "strength," causes the muscle fiber it innervates to contract maximally or not at all. This is called the **all-or-none principle.**

–The major determinants of how much **force** is produced when a muscle contracts are the **number of motor units** that are recruited and the **number of muscle fibers** contained in each motor unit.

–A motor unit stimulated by a single nerve impulse responds by contracting one time and relaxing. This is called a **twitch.**

–When a motor unit receives a second impulse before repolarization occurs, the two impulses are added (or summated) and the tension developed is greater than each of the individual twitches. This is called **summation.**

–**Tetanus** occurs when a motor unit is repeatedly stimulated without adequate time for relaxation. Tetanus results in sustained tension within the motor unit until the stimulus is removed or fatigue occurs.

2. **Connective tissue**

   –Skeletal muscle consists primarily of contractile and connective tissue. Connective tissue gives contractile tissue an attachment to the bone and something upon which to exert force. There are three types of connective tissue:

   a. **Epimysium** surrounds the entire muscle.

   b. **Perimysium** surrounds a group or bundle of muscle fibers known as a **fasciculus.**

   c. **Endomysium** surrounds each individual muscle fiber.

3. **Microscopic structure of skeletal muscle** (Figure 2-3)

   a. Skeletal muscle is composed of **muscle fibers** or cells.

   b. Each muscle fiber consists of many **myofibrils.**

   c. Each myofibril is composed of **sarcomeres,** the smallest contractile unit of muscle.

   d. **Contractile proteins** are contained in the sarcomere.

      (1) **Actin** is a muscle protein (sometimes called the **thin filament**) that looks like a twisted strand of beads (see Figure 2-3). Actin contains two other proteins called **troponin** and **tropomyosin.**

         (a) Troponin is a specialized protein located on the actin filament.

      (b) Tropomyosin is a long string-like molecule that wraps around the actin filament.

      (2) **Myosin** is also known as the **thick filament** and contains many **cross-bridges.**

B. **CLASSIFICATION OF MUSCLE FIBERS**

   –Muscle fibers can be classified broadly as **fast-twitch** or **slow-twitch** with differing functional and metabolic characteristics.

   –The type of muscle fiber recruited to perform a specific activity depends on intensity and duration of exercise.

   –Most muscles contain both fast-twitch and slow-twitch muscle fibers, however the ratio of fast-twitch to slow-twitch muscle fibers varies in an individual. The ratio also differs within the same muscle from one individual to another.

   1. **Fast-twitch (type II) fibers**

      –Fast-twitch fibers are recruited when a person is performing high-intensity activities. These fibers can produce large amounts of tension in a very short time period, but the accumulation of lactic acid from anaerobic glycolysis causes them to fatigue quickly.

      a. Fast-twitch fibers are subdivided **into fast-twitch oxidative (type IIa)** and **fast-twitch glycolytic (type IIb).** The type IIa fiber is capable of some aerobic work.

      b. The motor nerve supplying fast-twitch muscle fibers is larger than that supplying slow-twitch muscle fibers, and the fast-twitch fiber is larger in diameter than the slow-twitch fiber.

   2. **Slow-twitch (type I) fibers**

      –Slow-twitch muscle fibers are recruited for lower intensity, longer duration activities.

   3. **Metabolic characteristics**

      –Table 2-1 shows the metabolic characteristics of both types of muscle fibers.

C. **SLIDING FILAMENT THEORY**

   –The **sliding filament theory** describes the events that occur during rest, stimulation, contraction, and relaxation of the muscle. These events are summarized in Table 2-2.

   1. **Rest**

      –There is no nerve activity (except normal resting tone). Calcium is stored in the **sarcoplasmic reticulum.** When calcium is not present, the **active sites** where the myosin cross-bridges attach are "covered" and the

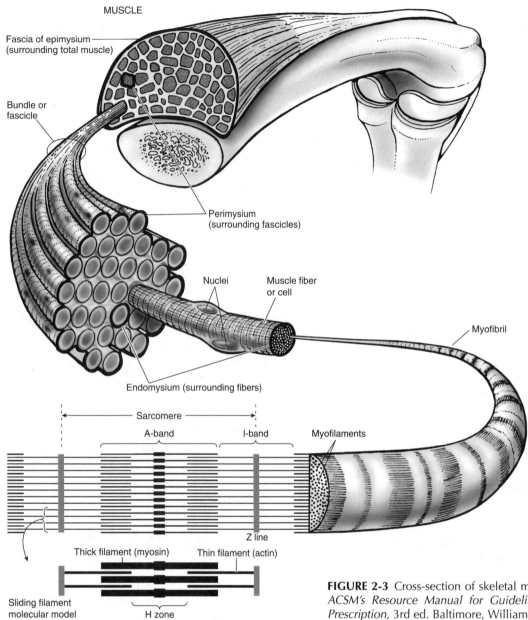

FIGURE 2-3 Cross-section of skeletal muscle. (With permission from *ACSM's Resource Manual for Guidelines for Exercise Testing and Prescription*, 3rd ed. Baltimore, Williams & Wilkins, 1998, p 80.)

Table 2-1. Characteristics of the Various Fiber Types

	Slow-Twitch	Fast-Twitch	
	Type I	Type IIa	Type IIb
Glycogen Stores	**High**	**High**	**High**
Anaerobic systems (ATP-PC, anaerobic glycolysis)	Low	High	High
Aerobic system	High	Moderate	Low
Force production	Low	High	High
Fatigability	Low	High	High
Fat (triglyceride) stores	High	Low	Low
Blood supply	High	Moderate	Low
Phosphocreatine (PC) stores	Low	High	High

Table 2-2. General Steps in the Sliding Filament Theory of Muscle Contraction

Rest	Stimulated	Contracted	Relaxed
1. No nerve impulse	1. Nerve impulse present	1. Cross-bridges pull actin filaments towards the center of the sarcomere	1. No impulse
2. Calcium stored in the muscle	2. Calcium released	2. Tension develops	2. No more calcium released, existing calcium pumped out of sarcomere
3. Active sites covered by tropomyosin	3. Calcium binds to troponin	3. ATP resynthesized	3. Active sites covered
4. ATPase inactive	4. Active sites uncovered	4. Cross-bridge releases active site and recoils to resting position	4. ATPase inactive
5. ATP available	5. Myosin cross-bridges bind active sites	5. If nerve impulse still present, process repeats	5. Muscle returns to rest by elastic recoil
	6. ATPase active		
	7. ATP breaks down		

enzyme that causes ATP to break down and release energy (ATPase) remains inactive.

2. **Stimulation**

–When a nerve impulse causes depolarization, calcium is released and binds to the troponin located on the actin filament and the active sites are "uncovered." The myosin cross-bridges bind to the active site and form **actomyosin.** The binding of the cross-bridges activates ATPase, and the ATP in the sarcomere breaks down to release energy.

3. **Contraction**

–The cross-bridges use the energy liberated from ATP to pull the actin filament towards the center

of the sarcomere and tension is created. When ATP is resynthesized (using one or more of the energy systems), the cross-bridges release the active site and it returns to its normal position. As long as a nerve impulse is present, the cross-bridges continue to bind to and release the actin filament and the contraction is maintained.

4. **Relaxation**

–When the impulse ceases, a "calcium pump" removes the calcium from the sarcomere and pumps it back to the sarcoplasmic reticulum. The removal of the calcium causes the active sites to become covered, which keeps ATPase inactive, and the muscle returns to resting length.

III. CARDIOVASCULAR PHYSIOLOGY

–The cardiovascular system consists of the heart and the blood vessels. The purpose of this system is to deliver nutrients to and remove waste products from the tissues.

A. PROPERTIES OF CARDIAC MUSCLE

–Cardiac muscle has several distinct features.

1. **Cardiac action potential**

–The action potential in cardiac muscle is longer than in skeletal muscle. This prevents heart muscle from being tetanized and allows for ventricular filling.

2. **Autorhythmicity**

–Cardiac muscle is capable of producing its own action potential.

3. **Cardiac muscle fibers**

–Cardiac muscle fibers are arranged end to end. The connecting point between two cardiac fibers is called an **intercalated disk.** This arrangement facilitates the complete depolarization of the myocardium.

B. ELECTRICAL CONDUCTION SYSTEM

–Cardiac muscle has a specialized conduction system.

1. Cardiac stimulation begins in the sinoatrial node.

2. The impulse spreads throughout the atrium, causing atrial depolarization and contraction. It proceeds to the **atrioventricular (AV) node,** which delays the transmission of the impulse

to the ventricles to prevent the atria and the ventricles from contracting simultaneously.

3. The AV node transmits the impulse to the ventricles via the **bundle of His,** the **right and left bundle branches** and, finally, the **Purkinje fibers** into the ventricular myocardium. The impulse propagates rapidly, causing ventricular depolarization and contraction.

C. CARDIAC FUNCTION

1. **Heart rate (HR)** is the total number of times the heart contracts in 1 minute.

    a. **Normal resting HR** is approximately 60–80 beats per minute. Resting HR can be measured by counting the number of pulses over a given time period (e.g., 15 seconds) and projecting that to one minute.

       (1) Avoid using your thumb when measuring HR by palpation because the prominent pulse of the thumb may cause measurement error.

       (2) Employ gentle pressure when measuring HR at the carotid artery because repeated or firm palpations of the carotid bodies may stimulate the **baroreceptor reflex,** resulting in a suddenly decreased HR, causing dizziness and/or syncope.

    b. **HR during maximal exercise** can exceed 200 beats per minute, depending on the person's age and training state. With the onset of dynamic exercise, HR increases in proportion to the relative workload.

       –Maximal HR (HR_{max}) can be estimated using the formula: $HR_{max} = 220 - Age$. There is considerable variability in this estimation.

2. **Stroke volume (SV)** is the amount of blood ejected from the left ventricle in a single beat.

    a. In an upright posture, SV is lower in untrained than trained persons.

    b. Males have greater SV than females.

    c. Body position affects SV. Supine or prone stroke volumes are near maximal.

    d. Static exercise may cause slightly decreased SV due to increased intrathoracic pressure.

    e. Dynamic upright exercise of increasing intensity (such as running, cycling, aerobics) causes increased SV in proportion to relative workload up to about 40–50% of $\dot{V}o_{2\,max}$. Thereafter, stroke volume plateaus and further increases in workload do not result in increased SV.

This is primarily due to reduced time for filling during diastole.

3. **Cardiac output ($\dot{Q}$)** is the amount of blood pumped by the heart each minute.

    –Cardiac output is calculated using the formula: $\dot{Q}$ **(l/min) = Heart Rate (beats/min) × Stroke Volume (ml/beat).**

    –**Resting $\dot{Q}$,** in both a trained and a sedentary individual, is approximately 4–5 liters per minute.

    –$\dot{Q}$ is maintained by HR and SV during exercise. Maximal $\dot{Q}$ is higher in trained than sedentary individuals.

    –$\dot{Q}$ may decrease during static exercise due to decreased venous return.

    –During dynamic exercise, cardiac output increases with increasing exercise intensity. Increases in $\dot{Q}$ beyond 40–50% of $\dot{V}o_{2\,max}$ are accounted for by increased heart rate.

4. **Blood pressure**—actually, mean arterial pressure (MAP)—is the driving force behind blood flow.

    –**Systolic blood pressure (SBP)** is the maximal force of the blood against the walls of the arteries when cardiac muscle is contracting (systole).

    –**Diastolic blood pressure (DBP)** is the force of the blood against the walls of the arteries when the heart is relaxing (diastole).

    a. **Normal resting SBP** is < 130 mm Hg, and **normal resting DBP** is < 85 mm Hg.

    b. **Effects of acute exercise**

       –SBP increases with increasing work intensity, whereas DBP remains unchanged or only slightly increases. DBP may also decrease in highly trained individuals **(Figure 2-4).**

       –Static exercise causes a greater rise in both SBP and DBP than dynamic exercise.

       –Failure of SBP to rise or decreased SBP with increasing work rates or a significant increase in DBP indicates exercise intolerance.

    c. **Effects of body position**

       –In the supine position, gravity has less effect on return of blood to the heart so that SBP is lower. When the body is upright, gravity works against the return of blood to the heart, so SBP increases. DBP does not change significantly with body position in healthy individuals.

    d. **Effects of arm versus leg exercise**

       –At similar oxygen consumptions, heart rate, SBP, and DBP are higher during arm

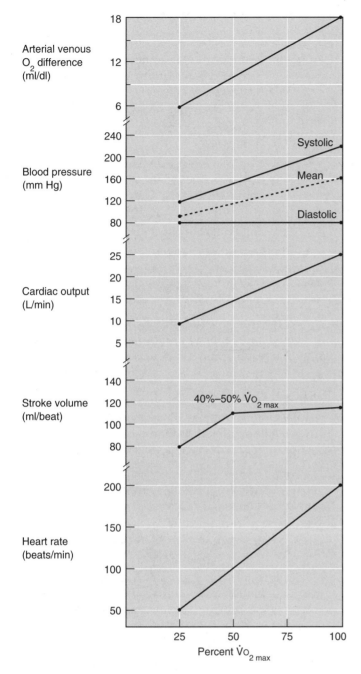

FIGURE 2-4 Effect of acute exercise at increasing exercise intensity on various cardiovascular variables.

(2) Place the center of the bladder (usually near the center of the cuff) directly over the brachial artery.

(3) Place the stethoscope head over the brachial artery and hold firmly with moderate pressure.

(4) Inflate the cuff to approximately 20 mm Hg above the point where the radial pulse disappears.

(5) Release pressure at a rate of approximately 2–3 mm Hg per second.

(6) The first sound **(Korotkoff sound)** is heard when the pressure in the cuff equals arterial blood pressure and a stream of blood flows through the forearm and strikes the static column of blood in the lower arm. This **"tapping noise"** is recorded as **the SBP.**

(7) As pressure in the cuff decreases, the sound eventually becomes muffled and disappears. **The point where the sound disappears is noted as the DBP.** In some situations, the sound may not disappear until the cuff pressure has reached zero. Under these conditions, DBP is usually reported as the point where the sound was muffled over zero (e.g., 120/70/0).

5. **Blood flow**

    –The initiation of exercise coincides with an increase in sympathetic nerve activity causing arteriolar constriction. In tissues with increasing metabolic rate (e.g., working skeletal muscle), this constriction is inhibited to provide active tissue with increased blood flow. Local control of circulation allows for the redistribution of blood from non-active tissue to active tissue.

    –**Venous return** is maintained and/or increased during exercise:

    a. Contracting skeletal muscle acts as a "pump" against the various structures that surround it, including deep veins, thus forcing blood back toward the heart. This process is known as the **muscle pump.**

    b. During exercise the smooth muscle around venules contracts, causing **venoconstriction.** The narrowing of the vein increases the pressure on the venous side, maintaining blood flow toward the heart.

    c. Diaphragmatic contraction during exercise creates lowered intrathoracic pressure, which facilitates blood flow from the abdominal area and lower extremities. This process is known as the **respiratory pump.**

work than during leg work. This is primarily because the total muscle mass in the arms is smaller and hence a greater percentage of the available mass is recruited to perform the work. In addition, arm work is less mechanically efficient than leg work.

e. **Blood pressure measurement**

    –Blood pressure is usually measured with a **sphygmomanometer** and a **stethoscope.**

    (1) Place a properly sized cuff around the upper arm, approximately 2 cm above the antecubital space.

IV. EFFECTS OF EXERCISE TRAINING

A. CARDIOVASCULAR SYSTEM CHANGES

–The effects of regular (chronic) exercise on the cardiovascular system can be grouped into changes that occur at rest, during submaximal exercise, and during maximal work.

1. **Resting changes**

   a. Resting **heart rate** decreases with regular exercise, probably because of the combined effects of decreased sympathetic tone, increased parasympathetic tone, and a decreased intrinsic firing rate of the SA node.

   b. **Stroke volume** increases at rest because of an increase in myocardial contractility.

   c. There is little or no change in **cardiac output** at rest because the decline in heart rate is compensated by increased stroke volume.

   d. Resting relative **oxygen consumption** does not change significantly after training.

2. **Changes during submaximal work**

   –Submaximal work is defined as a workload during which a steady state is achieved.

   a. **Heart rate** decreases at any given workload owing to the increase in stroke volume and decreased sympathetic drive or firing rate.

   b. **Stroke volume** increases owing to an increase in myocardial contractility.

   c. **Cardiac output** does not change significantly because the oxygen requirement for a fixed workload is similar irrespective of the level of fitness. However, after training, the same cardiac output is generated with lower heart rate and higher stroke volume.

   d. Submaximal **oxygen consumption** does not change significantly because the oxygen requirement for a fixed workload is similar for trained and untrained individuals.

   e. **Arteriovenous oxygen difference** ($a - \overline{v}O_2$ Diff) increases during submaximal exercise in trained persons.

   f. **Lactate levels** are decreased because of increased metabolic efficiency and also because of increased lactate clearance rates.

3. **Changes during maximal work**

   a. Maximal **heart rate** does not change significantly with exercise training.

   b. Maximal **stroke volume** increases due to increased contractility and/or increased heart size.

   c. Maximal **cardiac output** increases because maximum stroke volume increases.

   d. Maximal **oxygen consumption** ($\dot{V}o_{2\,max}$) increases due to increased stroke volume and a $- \overline{v}O_2$ Diff.

   e. $a - vO_2$ **Diff** increases due to improved ability of the mitochondria to use oxygen.

4. **Blood pressure changes**

   –In **normotensive individuals,** regular exercise does not appear to have a significant impact on resting or exercising blood pressure.

   –**Hypertensive individuals** may experience a moderate reduction in resting blood pressure as a result of regular exercise.

B. BLOOD LIPID CHANGES

–**Total cholesterol** may be decreased in hypercholesterolemic individuals.

–**High-density lipoprotein cholesterol (HDL-C)** increases with exercise training.

–**Low-density lipoprotein cholesterol (LDL-C)** is either unchanged or may decrease with training.

–Changes in **very low density lipoprotein cholesterol (VLDL-C)** are dependent upon changes in triglycerides (see later).

–**Triglycerides** (and therefore VLDL-C) may be decreased in those individuals who have elevated triglycerides initially. Changes are facilitated by weight loss.

C. BODY COMPOSITION CHANGES

–**Total body weight** usually decreases as a result of regular aerobic exercise.

–**Fat-free weight** does not normally change as a result of regular aerobic exercise.

–**Percentage of body fat** declines as a result of a regular exercise program.

D. BLOOD VOLUME CHANGES

–Total blood volume increases as a result of regular exercise because of an increased number of red blood cells and expansion of the plasma volume.

–Increased plasma volume is beneficial when working in hot, humid environments.

–The exact mechanism for increased red blood cell volume is not known.

E.   BIOCHEMICAL CHANGES

–**Stored muscle glycogen** increases as a result of aerobic exercise training. This increase also occurs with resistance training programs.

–The percentage of **fast- and slow-twitch fibers** does not change with exercise training. However, the cross-sectional area occupied by these fibers may change due to selective hypertrophy of either fast- or slow-twitch fibers.

F.   ENERGY SYSTEM CHANGES

–**Specificity of training** refers to the fact that the changes that occur are specific to the muscles and energy systems that are being used.

–Chronic anaerobic training using the **ATP–PC system** results in improved capacity and power of this system by enhancing enzyme activity and increasing the amount of ATP and PC stored in the muscle.

–**Anaerobic glycolysis** is improved if the training program utilizes this system, as a result of increased stores of muscle glycogen and improved ability of enzymes in the system.

–Regular aerobic training improves $\dot{V}o_{2\,max}$. Training also increases muscle glycogen stores, as well as intramuscular triglycerides, the rate at which carbohydrate (glucose) and fat are metabolized, and the ability to mobilize fat for fuel.

G.   EFFECTS OF DETRAINING

–The changes induced by regular exercise training generally are lost after 4–8 weeks of detraining.

–If training is re-established, the rate at which the training effects occur does not appear to be faster.

H.   EFFECTS OF OVERTRAINING

–Overtraining refers to a condition usually induced after prolonged heavy exercise over an extended period of time. **Symptoms of overtraining** may include any or all of the following:

1. Sudden decline in quality of work or exercise performance
2. Extreme fatigue
3. Elevated resting heart rate
4. Early onset of blood lactate accumulation
5. Altered mood states
6. Unexplained weight loss
7. Insomnia
8. Injuries related to overuse

–The occurrence of these symptoms as a result of overtraining may require complete rest up to weeks or months.

I.   EFFECTS ON OVERALL HEALTH

1. Improved cardiorespiratory endurance
2. Greater muscular strength
3. Improved muscular endurance
4. Greater flexibility
5. Improved body composition

J.   EFFECTS ON MOTOR FITNESS COMPONENTS

1. Increased agility
2. Greater speed
3. Improved balance
4. Greater power

REVIEW TEST

DIRECTIONS: Carefully read all questions and select the BEST single answer.

1. Which of the following is NOT a major food fuel during exercise?
   (A) Glucose
   (B) Fatty acids
   (C) Protein
   (D) Glycogen

2. The chemical energy that is directly converted to do work is
   (A) ATP
   (B) creatine phosphate
   (C) beta oxidation of fatty acids
   (D) all of the above

3. Which of the following is true when two people of different weights (80 and 70 kg) are exercising at 5 mph/5% grade on a treadmill?
   (A) $\dot{V}o_2$ will be different if expressed in ml/kg/min.
   (B) $\dot{V}o_2$ will be the same if expressed in L/min.
   (C) Cardiac output will be the same in L/min.
   (D) None of the above

4. Which of the following would provide the SMALLEST potential energy source in the body?
   (A) Fat
   (B) Protein
   (C) Phosphocreatine
   (D) ATP

5. Prior to and following 10 weeks of endurance training, an individual performs a submaximal exercise test at a constant work rate. Which of the following changes would most likely occur as a result of the endurance training?
   (A) A lower cardiac output
   (B) An increase in oxygen consumption
   (C) An increase in the blood flow to the exercising muscle
   (D) Lower blood lactate levels

6. When compared with leg exercise, arm exercise results in a relatively
   (A) increased heart rate at all intensities
   (B) lower systolic blood pressure at all intensities
   (C) increased venous return at all intensities
   (D) increased $\dot{V}o_{2\,max}$

7. During exercise of increasing intensity, the stroke volume of normal adults
   (A) continues to increase throughout the duration of exercise up to $\dot{V}o_{2\,max}$
   (B) remains relatively stable during submaximal exercise of greater than approximately 50% of $\dot{V}o_{2\,max}$
   (C) will continue to increase and then level off just prior to the achievement of $\dot{V}o_{2\,max}$
   (D) none of the above

8. The simplest and most rapid method to produce ATP during exercise is through
   (A) glycolysis
   (B) the ATP–PC system
   (C) aerobic metabolism
   (D) glycogenolysis

9. In general, the higher the intensity of the activity, the greater the contribution of
   (A) aerobic energy production
   (B) anaerobic energy production
   (C) the Krebs cycle to the production of ATP
   (D) the electron transport chain to the production of ATP

10. The energy to perform long-term exercise (i.e., > 15 minutes) comes primarily from
    (A) aerobic metabolism
    (B) a combination of aerobic and anaerobic metabolism, with anaerobic metabolism producing the bulk of the ATP
    (C) anaerobic metabolism
    (D) none of the above

11. In a rested, well-fed athlete, most of the carbohydrate used as a substrate during exercise comes from
    (A) muscle glycogen stores
    (B) blood glucose
    (C) liver glycogen stores
    (D) glycogen stored in fat cells

12. Fast-twitch muscle fibers have which of the following characteristics compared with a slow twitch?
    (A) Easily fatigued and well developed aerobic system
    (B) High force production and well developed blood supply
    (C) High phosphocreatine stores and high ATP-ase stores
    (D) None of the above

13. The motor neuron and all the muscle fibers it innervates are called a
    (A) motor junction
    (B) motor unit
    (C) motor end-plate
    (D) none of the above

14. The three principal mechanisms for increasing venous return during dynamic exercise are
    (A) a decrease in stroke volume, heart rate, and compliance of the vascular system
    (B) venoconstriction, pumping action of muscle, and the pumping action of the respiratory system
    (C) an increase in vascular resistance, an increase in heart rate, and a decrease in blood pressure
    (D) none of the above

15. Any physical activity whose performance time is approximately 30 seconds or less relies on which of the following energy systems?
    (A) ATP
    (B) PC
    (C) ATP–PC
    (D) Aerobic glycolysis

16. Which of the following is NOT a muscle type?
    (A) Skeletal
    (B) Smooth
    (C) Cardiac
    (D) Generic

17. When a motor unit is stimulated by a single nerve impulse, it responds by contracting one time and then relaxing. This is called a
    (A) twitch
    (B) summation
    (C) tetanus
    (D) summary

18. Which muscle protein contains many cross-bridges?
    (A) Myofibril
    (B) Sarcomere
    (C) Troponin
    (D) Myosin

19. Cardiac muscle action potentials are longer in duration than those of skeletal muscle. The longer action potential does not allow the muscle to
    (A) twitch
    (B) undergo summation
    (C) have tetanus
    (D) summarize

20. Which of the following cardiovascular variables does NOT increase as a result of chronic exercise while performing a single bout of maximal exercise?
    (A) Maximal heart rate
    (B) Maximal cardiac output
    (C) Maximal stroke volume
    (D) Maximal oxygen consumption

ANSWERS AND EXPLANATIONS

1–C. Glucose (and its storage form, glycogen) and fat are the primary sources of energy. For example, middle distance runners typically use carbohydrates and fats, whereas sprinters use ATP–PC as the energy substrate. Most aerobic exercise activities are fueled by a mixture of carbohydrate and fat. If the intensity is high, more ATP energy will come from carbohydrates. Protein (amino acids) are used only in severe energy deficit.

2–A. All energy for muscular contraction must come from the breakdown of a chemical compound called adenosine triphosphate (ATP). The energy is stored in the bonds between the last two phosphates; when work is performed, the last phosphate is split, forming adenosine diphosphate (ADP) and releasing heat. This release of heat contributes to the necessary mechanical energy.

3–D. During weight bearing exercise, when performing the same absolute workload, persons of different weights have the same relative $\dot{V}_{O_2}$ (ml/kg/min), different absolute $\dot{V}_{O_2}$ (L/min), and different cardiac output (because of different body mass).

4–D. The smallest potential energy source is ATP. The oxygen system is capable of using all three fuels: carbohydrate, fat, and protein. Significant amounts of protein are not used as a source of ATP energy during most types of exercise. Although all three can be used, the two most important are carbohydrates and fat. The carbohydrate, fat, and small amount of protein used by this energy system during exercise are completely metabolized, leaving only carbon dioxide and water (with small amounts of urea from protein).

5–D. Changes induced by training during submaximal work (defined as a workload where the individual can achieve a steady state) include a reduction in submaximal heart rate, an increase in stroke volume, and no change in cardiac output. Because the amount of work is less (expressed as a percentage of maximal work), the accumulated blood lactate will be less at the same relative submaximal amount of work.

6–A. The upper extremity is approximately two thirds of the muscle mass of the lower extremity. At the same relative workload, the upper extremity requires an increased heart rate to meet the metabolic demand. Systolic blood pressure is actually increased and venous return decreased due to an increase in intrathoracic pressure as a result of the upper extremity work.

7–B. During dynamic upright exercise of increasing intensity, stroke volume will increase with each increase in intensity until approximately 40% to 50% of $\dot{V}o_{2\,max.}$ Beyond this intensity, stroke volume will not increase because the time available for ventricular filling during diastole has become too short.

8–B. Because the number of reactions is very small (two), the ATP–PC system provides a very rapid source of energy followed by glycolysis.

9–B. Most aerobic exercise activities are fueled by a mixture of carbohydrate and fat. If the intensity of exercise is high, more ATP energy will come from carbohydrates (anaerobic energy production). If the intensity of exercise is lower (and long enough), less ATP energy comes from carbohydrates because some ATP energy can be derived from fat under these conditions.

10–A. Activities lasting longer than 2–3 minutes rely on aerobic metabolism to generate ATP.

11–A. The storage form of carbohydrates and those that are easily accessible for use as an energy substrate are muscle glycogen stores. Glycogen is the storage form of glucose and is found in the muscle and in the liver. Once the ATP–PC system has supplied energy within the first few seconds of physical activity, the glycogen stored in the muscle is next used to supply energy by breaking down to glucose and then creating ATP.

12–C. Fast-twitch muscle fibers are designed to deliver high power in a short period of time, as opposed to slow-twitch muscle fibers, which help deliver sustained power over a longer period of time. The fast-twitch muscle fiber, then, has a relatively small number of mitochondria but a high activity level of ATPase, the enzyme that splits ATP and produces energy.

13–B. A motor unit consists of the efferent (motor) nerve and all of the muscle fibers supplied (or innervated) by that nerve. The total number of fibers in each motor unit varies among and within muscles.

14–B. Stroke volume and heart rate increase in a healthy person with dynamic exercise. Vascular resistance also decreases with dynamic exercise. The primary mechanisms responsible for increasing venous return during dynamic exercise are the pumping action of the muscles on the deep veins, the increased ventilation that helps draw blood into the thorax from the abdominal cavity, and venoconstriction, which helps maintain cardiac filling pressure or flow back to the heart on the venous side.

15–C. There is enough phosphocreatine stored in skeletal muscle for approximately 25 seconds of high-intensity work. Therefore, the ATP–PC system has a capacity for about 30 seconds (5 seconds for stored ATP, 25 seconds for stored PC).

16–D. There are three types of muscle in the human body: skeletal, smooth (found in some blood vessels and in the digestive system), and cardiac (heart).

17–A. When a motor unit is stimulated by a single nerve impulse, it responds by contracting one time and then relaxing. This is called a twitch.

18–D. Myosin is also known as the thick filament and contains cross-bridges, which are very important during contraction.

19–C. The action potential in cardiac muscle is much longer in duration compared with skeletal muscle. This prevents the cardiac muscle from being tetanized. If cardiac muscle were tetanized, no relaxation (called diastole) of heart muscle would occur. This would prevent ventricular filling from occurring for the next contraction.

20–A. Maximal heart rate does not change significantly with exercise training. Maximal heart rate does decline with age.

CHAPTER 3

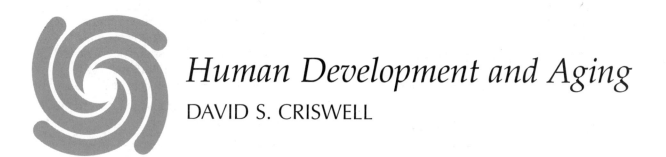

Human Development and Aging
DAVID S. CRISWELL

I. PHYSIOLOGIC CHANGES DURING DEVELOPMENT AND AGING

A. SKELETAL MUSCLE MASS AND STRENGTH

1. **Childhood**

   a. **The maximal number of skeletal muscle fibers** is established at an early age; however, large changes in muscle mass remain possible via the mechanisms of **muscle fiber hypertrophy.**

   b. **Strength development** in the growing child varies according to **body size.** **Strength measurements** can be standardized to any of **several indices of growth:**

      –The square of stature

      –The cross section of the active limb

      –The third power of height

      –Body mass

   c. Skeletal muscle mass, and therefore strength, does not differ between active preadolescent girls and boys.

2. **Adolescence: male and female differences**

   –In **males,** puberty initiates rapid hypertrophy of muscle fibers coincident with the adolescent growth spurt.

   –**Females** do not exhibit any disproportionate muscle growth during adolescence. Adolescent females have approximately 30% less muscle mass than males, due to both smaller stature (and thus smaller muscle dimensions) and a smaller average muscle fiber size.

3. **Early adulthood: male and female differences**

   –Muscular strength of the postadolescent female is approximately 30%–60% less than in the postadolescent male.

   –The discrepancy between muscle mass differences (about 30%) and strength differences (30%–60%) is more marked in the upper body. This may be due to the differences in androgen secretion and/or to socially conditioned differences in activity patterns between the sexes.

   –The **maximal level of muscle mass and strength** is reached in the early twenties for both sexes.

4. **Changes with aging**

   a. After age 30, skeletal muscle strength begins to decline (**Figure 3-1**). However, the loss of strength is not linear; most of the decline occurs after age 50. By age 80, loss of strength is usually in the range of 30%–40%.

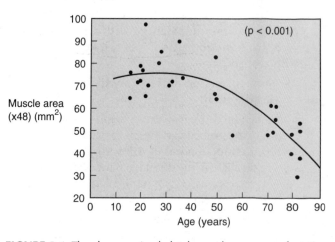

FIGURE 3-1 The decrease in skeletal muscle mass as a function of age in 43 previously healthy men aged 15–83 years. (Reprinted from Lexell J, Taylor C, Sjöström M: What is the cause of the aging atrophy? *J Neurol Sci* 84:275–294, 1988. With kind permission of Elsevier Science–NL, Sara Burgerhartstraat 25, 1055 KV Amsterdam, The Netherlands.)

b. The loss of strength with aging is due primarily to a **loss of muscle mass,** which in turn is caused by both the **loss of muscle fibers** and **atrophy** (decrease in size) of remaining fibers.

–It appears that most of the loss of muscle mass in aging humans is due to the loss of muscle fibers. As skeletal muscle fibers are lost, the force produced by a given cross-sectional area of muscle is reduced.

–**Fast-twitch fibers** (especially type IIb fibers) are particularly susceptible to atrophy in aging humans. This contributes to decreased contraction speeds and lower dynamic strength and power outputs in skeletal muscles of older adults.

c. Aging is also associated with **changes in the metabolic characteristics of skeletal muscle,** including reduced concentrations of adenosine triphosphate (ATP), phosophocreatine (PC), and glycogen. Further, the quantity and activity of enzymes involved in both anaerobic glycolysis and aerobic metabolism are reduced.

B. BONE STRUCTURE

–**Bone is specialized connective tissue** composed of cells embedded in an extracellular organic matrix impregnated with an inorganic component. This inorganic component, primarily calcium phosphate crystals called hydroxyapatite, makes up about 65% of the dry weight of bone.

–Mature bone continuously undergoes a process called **bone remodeling** in which bone matrix is reabsorbed and replaced by new matrix. This process **becomes unbalanced with advancing age** such that **bone formation does not keep pace with reabsorption.**

1. **Bone formation during growth and development**

    a. The human skeleton begins to develop in the embryo as the process of **endochondral ossification** gradually replaces the cartilage with bone tissue.

    b. In long bones, the ossification begins in the **diaphysis.** Secondary ossification occurs at the ends of the long bone or **epiphysis,** and remains separated from the primary ossification by **epiphyseal plates.**

    c. The epiphyseal plates are regions of cartilage that continue to produce chondrocytes that undergo ossification

and thereby add bone tissue to the shaft of the bone.

    d. Through this process, long bones continue to grow in length until **the epiphyseal plates close in response to hormonal changes** occurring **at about 16–18 years of age,** following the adolescent growth spurt. Bone mass reaches its peak for both men and women by 25–30 years of age.

2. **Bone loss during aging and the development of osteoporosis**

    –**Osteoporosis** is a condition characterized by a decrease in bone mass and density producing bone porosity and fragility. The efficiency of osteoblasts appears to decline with age, resulting in the inability of bone synthesis to keep pace with bone reabsorption.

    –Every population that has been studied exhibits a decline in bone mass with aging.

    a. **Sex-related differences in bone loss**

       –The age at which bone loss begins and the rate at which it occurs vary greatly between men and women.

       (1) Normally, men begin to lose bone mass by age 65; overall bone mineral content is about 10% lower than the peak value (**Figure 3-2**).

       (2) Bone loss in women may begin as early as 30–35 years of age, and the rate of bone loss is greatly accelerated following menopause. By age 65, overall bone mineral content in women is approximately 15%–20% lower than the peak value (see **Figure 3-2**).

       (3) Some studies suggest that the overall age-related loss of bone mineral content in men is proportional to the loss of lean body tissue with aging. Women, however, exhibit a disproportionate loss of bone tissue after menopause. **Estrogen replacement** has been shown effective in attenuating this bone loss in postmenopausal women.

    b. **Classification of osteoporosis**

       –With osteoporosis there is an increase in susceptibility to fracture from minor trauma. Osteoporotic conditions affecting older adults are classified as type I or type II osteoporosis.

       (1) Type I or **postmenopausal osteoporosis** is the most common and is associated with fractures of the vertebrae and distal radius.

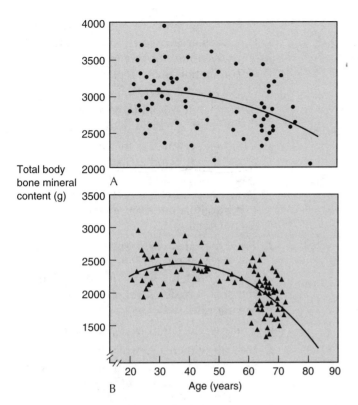

FIGURE 3-2 Changes in total body bone mineral content with aging in healthy men (*A*) and women (*B*). (From Holloszy JO, Kohrt WM: Exercise. In Masoro EJ [ed]: *Handbook of Physiology,* Section 11: *Aging.* New York: Oxford University Press, 1995, p 651.)

Approximately 90% of the cases of type I osteoporosis occur in women.

(2) Type II or **senile osteoporosis** is seen mostly in individuals older than 70 years of age and is manifested primarily by vertebral and hip fractures. The incidence of type II osteoporosis is also higher in women, with a ratio of approximately 2:1.

c. Risk factors

–Many of the risk factors for age-related bone loss, and hence the risk for developing osteoporosis, can be modified. The risk factors are:

(1) Being a **white** or **Asian female.**

(2) Being **thin boned** or petite.

(3) Having a **low peak bone mass** at maturity.

(4) A **family history** of osteoporosis.

(5) Premature or surgically induced **menopause.**

(6) Alcohol abuse.

(7) Cigarette smoking.

(8) Sedentary lifestyle.

(9) Inadequate dietary **calcium intake.**

C. REACTION TIME, MOVEMENT TIME, AND COORDINATION

1. **Childhood and adolescence**

   a. Performance of tasks requiring motor skills improves from the first years of life throughout the preadolescent and adolescent years. This improvement is due to growth and the associated increases in strength and endurance and to the progress of motor learning and the development of greater coordination.

   b. **By the age of 6 years,** most children have mastered basic skills such as throwing and jumping, and are beginning to refine more sophisticated skills such as those involved in sports and/or dance.

   c. **Reaction time** decreases (improves) with maturational development. There is an abrupt decrease in reaction time around 8 years of age, followed by a more progressive improvement throughout the remainder of childhood and adolescence.

   d. **Speed of movement** also improves with age.

   e. Although older children perform timed finger tapping tasks faster than younger children do, there are **no significant differences in accuracy between ages of 6 and 10 years.** This suggests that younger children are able to analyze feedback information but require more processing time to integrate discrete movements into a coordinated sequence.

   f. The **improvement of skill following a practice session** increases with age during childhood, indicating an increase in the capacity to integrate feedback during learning.

   g. **Gender differences** in skill performance

      –are minimal before adolescence.

      –During adolescence, the gap widens as girls' performance in skills requiring strength and gross motor patterns (e.g., running and jumping) plateaus whereas boys continue to improve.

      –Conversely, girls often outperform boys in skills requiring fine motor patterns.

      –It is important to note that there are wide individual variations in quantitative skill performances at all ages in both genders.

2. **Adulthood and changes with aging**

   a. Many **neurophysiologic changes** occur with aging **that affect motor performance,** including:

      –decreased **visual acuity.**

–**hearing loss.**

–deterioration of **short-term memory.**

–inability to handle several pieces of information simultaneously.

–decreased **reaction time.**

b. The ability to maintain performance of a motor skill at a given level throughout middle and older adulthood depends on the type of skill.

–**Skills requiring accuracy of movement** may be maintained at the level attained as a young adult.

–Performance of **skills requiring speed and/or strength of movement** declines with age.

c. **Movement patterns** of older adults are generally well maintained from younger adulthood. Decreases in performance during adulthood result from decreases in range-of-motion, reaction time, movement time, and coordination.

d. It is often difficult to separate the effects of aging from the effects of disease and/or deconditioning resulting from inactivity. Nevertheless, it is clear that individuals who remain active and continue to practice motor skills can minimize the decline in performance that occurs with aging.

D. TOLERANCE TO HOT AND COLD ENVIRONMENTS

1. **Temperature regulation in children**

   –Children are less efficient than adults at temperature regulation, owing to anthropometric and functional differences:

   a. The **surface area** of a child, relative to body mass, **is greater** than that of an adult, allowing a **greater rate of heat exchange** between skin and environment.

      (1) In neutral or warm climates, the increased surface area may facilitate heat dissipation.

      (2) In climatic extremes, however, this becomes a major handicap by increasing unwanted heat transfer from the body to the environment during cold exposure (e.g., swimming in an unheated pool), and vice versa during exposure to heat (e.g., exercising when the ambient temperature exceeds body temperature).

   b. **Sweating rate** for children is much lower than that in adults.

      (1) Although the number of sweat glands present in children equals that in the adult, the rate of sweat production for each gland is half that of the adult glands.

      (2) The threshold for sweating is higher in the child than the adult.

   c. Children **acclimatize** to hot environments less efficiently and **at a slower rate** than adults do. Children therefore require a longer and more gradual program of exposure to a hot environment for acclimatization.

   d. **Hypohydrated children** are at increased risk for heat-related illness because the rise in core temperature in proportion to the degree of dehydration occurs at a greater rate.

2. **Temperature regulation in older adults**

   a. In healthy men and women, aging does not appear to diminish the ability of the sweating mechanism to cope with heat stress during rest or moderate exercise.

   b. There is a general reduction in total cellular water with aging, predisposing the older adult to a more rapid dehydration.

   c. Elderly men exposed to prolonged heat stress exhibit lower subcutaneous blood flow values compared with young men.

   d. Heart rate, blood pressure, and oxygen consumption, expressed as a percentage of maximum, are higher in the older adult exercising at a submaximal workload in the heat.

   e. The **decreased tolerance for exercising in hot environments** with aging appears to be primarily related to decreases in **cardiovascular responses** to the heat stress, and to a **compromised aerobic capacity.**

E. MAXIMAL OXYGEN CONSUMPTION ($\dot{V}O_{2\,max}$)

–$\dot{V}O_{2\,max}$ may be expressed as an absolute value (liters of oxygen per minute), or may be standardized to an index of body size, such as mass.

– $\dot{V}O_{2\,max}$ is determined by the capacity of the cardiovascular system to **deliver oxygen** to the working muscles and the capacity of the muscles **to extract oxygen** for oxidative metabolism.

1. **Changes during growth and development**

   a. There is a **general increase in exercise capacity and absolute $\dot{V}O_{2\,max}$** (liters per minute) **during childhood.** This increase is dramatically accelerated during puberty, especially in boys, before leveling off after maturity.

b. The large increase in absolute $\dot{V}o_{2\,max}$ in adolescent boys corresponding to the growth spurt, which is due to androgen-induced hypertrophy of the heart and stimulation of red blood cell and hemoglobin production, facilitates oxygen delivery. Furthermore, increased skeletal muscle mass associated with male adolescence increases the capacity for oxygen extraction.

c. Despite the large increase in absolute $\dot{V}o_{2\,max}$, **relative $\dot{V}o_{2\,max}$ (ml/kg/min) shows a slight decline during puberty.** It is unclear whether this represents inadequate physical conditioning of this age group or some other physiologic factor.

2. **Changes with aging**

a. $\dot{V}o_{2\,max}$ reaches its peak value at about 20 years of age. For an average sedentary male of this age, relative $\dot{V}o_{2\,max}$ is approximately 50 ml/kg/min. Young adult females, because of their higher percentage of body fat and lower hemoglobin concentration, exhibit a relative $\dot{V}o_{2\,max}$ of 40 to 45 ml/kg/min.

b. The assessment of the effect of aging on $\dot{V}o_{2\,max}$ is complicated by extraneous factors such as physical inactivity, increases in fat mass, decreases in lean mass, and development of disease.

c. Nevertheless, it is clear **that there is a progressive decline in $\dot{V}o_{2\,max}$** and in the capacity for aerobic exercise **with aging,** beginning about age 25–30 years **(Figure 3-3).**

d. Physical activity can increase $\dot{V}o_{2\,max}$ at any age; however, there remains a 5%–10% decline in $\dot{V}o_{2\,max}$ per decade, even in active or exercising individuals.

F. FLEXIBILITY

–Joint stiffness and loss of flexibility are common in the elderly. It is difficult to separate the effects of aging on joint flexibility from the effects of injury and wear-and-tear that occur over the life span.

1. Aging is associated with **degradation and increased cross-linkage of collagen fibers,** which comprise much of the connective tissue in the joints of the body. This increases the stiffness and decreases the tensile strength of collagen fibers.

2. **Trauma to joint cartilage** causes the formation of scar tissue, which makes the connective tissue stiff and less responsive to stress.

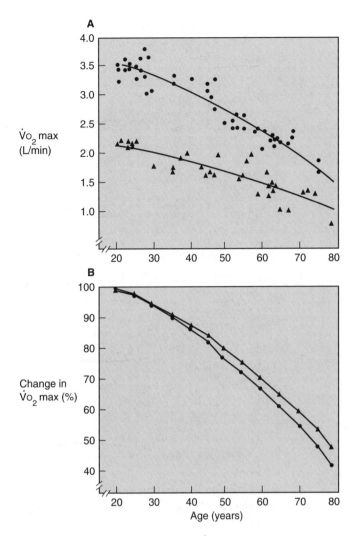

FIGURE 3-3 Age-related decline in $\dot{V}o_{2\,max}$ in healthy, sedentary men (*A*) and women (*B*). (From Holloszy JO, Kohrt WM: Exercise. In MasoroEJ [ed]: *Handbook of Physiology,* Section 11: *Aging.* New York: Oxford University Press, 1995, p 640.)

3. **Osteoarthritis** can severely restrict range of motion. This disease occurs primarily in areas of the body that receive the greatest mechanical stress, thereby suggesting that **it may be caused by repeated trauma** rather than by aging per se.

4. **Range-of-motion exercises and static stretching** may increase flexibility in subjects of all ages; however, it is unlikely that any exercise could undo the extensive degenerative damage that is sometimes seen with osteoarthritis in the elderly.

G. BODY COMPOSITION

1. **Childhood**

–Adipose tissue (a connective tissue consisting mostly of fat cells) accounts for about 16% of body mass in the full-term newborn infant.

–Absolute fat content progressively increases throughout childhood in proportion with growth in other body compartments.

–**Relative body fat** for boys and girls remains stable during preadolescence at **approximately 15% of body mass.**

2. **Adolescence**

–**In males, relative body fat decreases during puberty** to approximately 12%–13% of body mass as muscle mass increases. As postadolescence is approached, relative body fat increases in sedentary boys to an average of 16%–18% of body mass.

–**In females, relative body fat increases during puberty** to about 20%–25% of body mass owing to hormonally induced accumulation of fat in the breasts and around the hips.

3. **Adulthood and changes with aging**

–**Body mass continues to increase** at an average of 1–2 kg per decade throughout most of the adult life span for both men and women. However, **fat-free mass remains relatively constant.**

–After 70 years of age, body mass begins to decline, typically by 1–2 kg in the eighth decade and accelerating thereafter.

–This decline represents a **loss of fat-free mass,** which exceeds the continued rise in fat mass.

–The average change in percent body fat is linear between ages 25 and 75 years for both men and women.

–The **age-related increase in fat mass** accumulates primarily in central (i.e., **abdominal areas**) as opposed to peripheral areas.

–**Increased** measurements **of central-to-peripheral adiposity,** such as waist-to-hip circumference ratio, have been linked to an **increased risk for cardiovascular disease.**

–**Exercise training** can reduce the percent body fat at any age. However, longitudinal studies of highly competitive athletes suggest that exercise does not prevent the age-related increase in body fat.

H. CARDIOVASCULAR FUNCTION

1. **Childhood and adolescence**

   a. **Children exhibit hypokinetic circulation** at rest and during exercise, characterized by a small stroke volume and cardiac output relative to body size.

   b. **Hemoglobin concentration,** and therefore the oxygen-carrying capacity of the blood, **is lower in children** than in adults.

   (1) **In males,** average hemoglobin concentration increases during adolescence from 14 g/dl to an adult male value of 16.5 g/dl.

   (2) **In females,** increases in average hemoglobin concentration parallel that of males during preadolescence, but thereafter remain constant at 14–14.5 g/dl throughout adulthood.

   c. **Blood pressure** during submaximal and maximal exercise **is significantly lower** in preadolescents than in adolescents and adults.

   d. **Heart rate**

   (1) Factors that limit oxygen delivery to the periphery, along with a higher resting metabolism, cause heart rate (HR) in children to be **20–30 beats per minute higher** than in adults during both rest and submaximal exercise.

   –**Resting HR** for young children is often in the range of **80–100 beats** per minute.

   –This resting HR declines during childhood and adolescence to the adult value of 65 to 70 beats per minute.

   –A reasonable **estimate of maximal HR** in children and adults can be obtained by subtracting age in years from 220.

   (2) Although HR is higher, **cardiac output remains lower** than in the adult at any given submaximal $\dot{V}o_{2\ max}$. In compensation, **oxygen extraction from the blood is greater in children** than in adults. This is achieved through greater blood flow to the skeletal muscle in the child as compared with the adult.

2. **Older adulthood**

   a. **Resting HR** shows **little or no change** due to aging.

   b. **Maximal HR decreases** with increasing age, apparently due to an increase in stiffness of the heart muscle slowing the rate of ventricular filling and prolonging diastole.

   c. In older adults (≥ 65 years old) the formula for estimating maximal HR, 220 minus age in years, may underestimate the true maximal HR by 10–15 beats per minute.

   d. **Cardiac output** and **stroke volume** are **slightly reduced** during rest and submaximal exercise in the older adult. Significant differences may not be apparent except during high-intensity exercise.

–The decline in maximal stroke volume in the older adult distorts the linear relationship between HR and oxygen consumption. At submaximal work rates, the older adult must maintain a higher HR in order to provide adequate blood flow to the muscles.

e. The **elasticity of blood vessels decreases** with aging, resulting in increased peripheral resistance and increased blood pressure.

f. **Skeletal muscle capillary density** also **decreases** with aging, causing reduced muscle blood flow and oxygen extraction during exercise.

g. **Exercise training improves cardiovascular function** proportionally in the elderly, similar to effects seen in young adults.

II. SPECIAL CONSIDERATIONS FOR EXERCISE TRAINING IN CHILDREN AND ADOLESCENTS

A. BENEFITS AND RISKS

–Although children and adolescents tend to be more active than adults, many fail to meet health-related standards for physical fitness.

–Exercise programs for youths should increase physical fitness in the short term and lead to the adoption of a physically active lifestyle in the long term.

1. **Strength training**

–Strength training in preadolescents, as compared with adolescents and adults, probably results in smaller absolute strength gains but equal relative increases in strength.

–If proper technique instruction, exercise prescription, and supervision are provided, strength training in children and adolescents carries **no greater risk of injury** than comparable strength training programs for adults.

–**No detrimental cardiorespiratory effects** of strength training in children and adolescents have been reported.

2. **Cardiovascular considerations**

–Most children with cardiovascular disorders may participate in physical activities. Each child with known or suspected heart disease should be carefully evaluated and the limits of physical activity set by the health-care provider or exercise professional.

a. **Heart murmurs**

–are commonly heard in children.

–are usually **functional murmurs** and do not impair normal cardiovascular function.

–Children diagnosed with heart murmurs caused by **anatomic defects** are not necessarily excluded from physical activity, but rather should be considered

individually and an exercise prescription designed according to the primary physician's recommendations.

b. **Dysrhythmias**

(1) **Common symptoms** associated with dysrhythmias include sensation of skipped beats, headache, vomiting, loss of vision, syncope, or near syncope. **Suspected dysrhythmias should be referred to a physician.**

(2) Different types of dysrhythmias exist; **some are benign** whereas **others may preclude participation in physical activity.** The appropriate level of activity should be determined by a physician.

c. **Syncope**

–is the loss of muscle tone and consciousness caused by diminished cerebral blood flow.

(1) **Types of syncope include:**

–**vasopressor syncope,** caused by external stimuli, such as anxiety or emotion.

–**orthostatic syncope,** caused by pooling of blood in the lower parts of the body.

–**cardiovascular syncope,** caused by some form of heart disease.

(2) **Symptoms of presyncope** include dizziness, cold and clammy appearance, diaphoresis, and significantly decreased blood pressure.

(3) Following an episode of syncope or presyncope, children should be referred to a physician before participating in vigorous physical activity.

3. **Hot and cold environments**

   a. **Heat disorders**

     –Heat cramps, heat exhaustion, and heat stroke represent a continuum of progressive heat-related illness.

       (1) Heat cramps are characterized by painful involuntary spasms of skeletal muscle, and may be the first manifestation of hyperthermia during exercise. They are associated with **electrolyte imbalance** and **inadequate blood flow** to the active muscle.

       (2) Heat exhaustion is characterized by profuse sweating, headache, dizziness, and nausea or vomiting. It may develop quickly or over several days as a result of progressive dehydration.

       (3) Heat stroke is characterized by disorientation, confusion, lack of sweating, and pale, dry skin. Later stages are associated with adverse effects on cardiovascular, pulmonary, and renal function, and are life-threatening.

       (4) Treatment of any heat disorder **focuses on reducing body temperature and rehydration.** More severe illness (e.g., heat exhaustion or stroke) requires more drastic measures, such as water immersion and possibly administration of intravenous fluids.

       (5) Children at highest risk for heat-related illness include:

       –children with diseases affecting the sweating mechanism (e.g., cystic fibrosis, diabetes mellitus).

       –children with diseases affecting the cardiovascular system (e.g., congenital heart diseases, diabetes mellitus).

       –obese children.

       –children with a history of heat stroke.

       (6) Prevention of heat-related illness can be achieved by ensuring that children participating in physical activities, especially in hot, humid environments, are properly hydrated, acclimatized, and conditioned for the exercise.

   b. **Cold injuries**

     –are much less common than heat-related injuries.

     –may be superficial, such as frostbite, or systemic, such as hypothermia.

     –Little acclimatization occurs following repeated exposure to cold.

     –Physical fitness does not appear to decrease the risk of cold injury.

     –**Prevention** of cold-related injuries during exercise **is dependent upon proper clothing and limitation of exposure to cold.**

     –The greater body surface area–to–mass ratio of children results in a **greater heat loss in the cold, especially during swimming.** For this reason, it has been recommended that children exercising in cool water should exit and warm up at least every 15 minutes.

4. **Orthopedic considerations**

   a. **Bone mass**

     –During growth, overall **bone mass and bone mineral density increase** significantly. Weight-bearing physical activity during this time augments this process.

       (1) Animal studies show that growing animals have increased capacity to add bone in response to exercise.

       (2) Weight lifting and compressive exercises, such as gymnastics, have the greatest effect for enhancing bone mass in children.

       (3) It appears that the beneficial effects of exercise on bone mass do not occur if **dietary calcium intake** is inadequate.

   b. **Orthopedic injuries: overuse injuries**

     –result from repetitive microtrauma of articular cartilage, bone, muscle, and/or tendon.

     –are commonly seen in children and adolescent athletes, particularly those specializing in one organized sport that involves cyclic forces applied to an anatomic structure.

       (1) Overuse injuries of bone (stress fractures) commonly occur in the:

       –tibia, fibula, or foot in running sports.

       –femur, pelvis, or patella in jumping sports.

       –humerus, first rib, or elbow in overhand throwing and racquet sports.

       (2) Risk factors for overuse injuries

         (a) Training error

           (i) Increased total volume of training

           (ii) Increased rate of progression of training intensity beyond approximately 10% per week.

(b) Muscle-tendon imbalance

–Growth may cause changes in relative strength and flexibility across major joints, especially during the adolescent growth spurt. Repetitive techniques at this age may result in asymmetric stresses on bones and joints.

(c) Anatomic malalignments

–Malalignments, such as discrepancies of leg length or abnormalities of hip rotation, may result in excessive stress on skeletal units during repetitive exercise.

(d) High-impact forces during running and/or jumping sports

–These can be reduced by the use of proper footwear, but are exacerbated by hard playing surfaces.

(e) Growth

–Cartilage in growing children has been shown to be more susceptible to repetitive trauma.

5. **Onset of puberty in girls and amenorrhea**

–The age at which puberty begins in American girls varies from 9–14 years.

a. **Delayed onset of puberty and the abnormal absence or suppression of menses (amenorrhea) have been associated with chronic endurance training.**

–No single underlying cause has been identified.

–Young competitive athletes have a higher incidence of amenorrhea than either their nonathletic counterparts or older athletic women.

–Blood levels of estradiol, progesterone, and follicle-stimulating hormone are lower in adolescent and young adult women involved in intense exercise training.

–Recent evidence suggests that excessive training may interfere with the normal menstrual cycle in some women by inhibiting the release of gonadotropin-releasing hormone.

b. The **hormonal imbalances associated with long-term secondary amenorrhea** in young female athletes may have deleterious effects on the normal accumulation of bone tissue during growth, which, in turn, **may increase skeletal fragility later in life.**

6. **Exercise-induced asthma**

–Asthma is the most common chronic illness in childhood, affecting between 5% and 15% of children in the United States.

–Exercise-induced asthma (EIA) consists of cough, wheeze, chest tightness, chest pain, breathlessness, or any combination of these occurring during or more often immediately after exercise.

–EIA has been reported to occur in about 80% of patients with asthma, and in as many as 10%–15% of apparently healthy children and adolescents.

–The type of exercise affects the likelihood and severity of EIA episodes. Typically, **short and intense bouts of exercise are more likely to elicit EIA.**

–**Ambient conditions** such as cold, low humidity, and polluted air **can also exacerbate EIA.**

–Often, children suffering from EIA are physically unfit owing to restriction of activity, either self-imposed or imposed by parents or physicians.

–Control of EIA may be accomplished through pharmacologic intervention or through nonpharmacologic approaches, such as the use of a mask or scarf during exercise in cold weather. Once EIA symptoms are controlled, most children can engage in normal physical activity safely.

B. **UNIQUE RESPONSES OF CHILDREN DURING EXERCISE AND RECOVERY**

–The basic physiologic responses to exercise are similar in healthy individuals of any age. However, there are age-related quantitative differences during exercise and recovery.

1. **Metabolic responses**

a. **Submaximal, relative** $\dot{V}o_2$ at a given workload in children is similar to that in adults for cycling exercise, but 10%–20% higher for running or walking.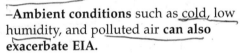

b. **Anaerobic capacity is lower in children** than in adults because of their lower concentration and rate of utilization of muscle glycogen and low levels of phosphofructokinase.

c. Upon initiation of exercise, **children reach metabolic steady state more quickly** than adults, resulting in lower oxygen deficit.

2. **Cardiovascular responses**

   a. **Cardiac output** at a given $\dot{V}o_2$ **is slightly lower** in children than in adults. Therefore, oxygen extraction from the blood is greater.

   b. **Heart rate** at a submaximal load **is higher** in children than in adults owing to their smaller heart size and stroke volume.

   c. **Maximal heart rate is higher in children** than in adults, but this does not fully compensate for the smaller heart size, **causing decreased maximal cardiac output.**

   d. **Arterial blood pressure,** especially systolic blood pressure, at submaximal and maximal workloads, **is lower** in exercising children than in adults.

3. **Pulmonary responses**

   a. **Absolute maximal minute ventilation** is lower in children than in adults because of body size.

   b. **Relative minute ventilation during maximal exercise** in children is similar to that in adults, but during submaximal exercise at a fixed $\dot{V}o_2$ is considerably higher than adults.

   c. Typically, children breathe at a higher frequency and have decreased ventilatory volume compared with adults during exercise.

4. Exercise at a given relative intensity (i.e., percentage of $\dot{V}o_{2\,max}$ or HR_{max}) is perceived to be easier by children.

C. **TRAINABILITY OF CHILDREN AND ADOLESCENTS**

1. **Skeletal muscle strength**

   a. **Resistance training** during preadolescence and adolescence **causes relative strength gains** (percentage improvements) similar to those found in young adults, with adequate intensity and volume of training.

   b. Strength gains associated with resistance training are consistently associated with **muscle hypertrophy in adolescents** and young adults. However, muscle hypertrophy is rarely reported following resistance training in preadolescent children, despite the increases in strength.

   c. **Neurologic adaptations** resulting in an increase in motor unit activation have been measured following strength training in preadolescents and adolescents. Increased motor unit activation has been inferred to mediate strength gains in young children.

2. **Functional capacity**

   –Children and adolescents respond to endurance training similarly to adults.

   –For **preadolescents,** the magnitude of change in relative $\dot{V}o_{2\,max}$ is lower than would be expected from changes in endurance performance. It appears that the cardiovascular system of preadolescents is trainable, but to a lesser extent than in adolescents and adults. Improvements in performance by endurance-trained children may be due in part to increases in biomechanical efficiency.

III. SPECIAL CONSIDERATIONS FOR EXERCISE TRAINING IN OLDER ADULTS

A. **BENEFITS AND PRECAUTIONS**

1. **Cardiovascular benefits and precautions**

   a. **Cardiovascular function**

      (1) Numerous studies have documented **increases in the $\dot{V}o_{2\,max}$** of older subjects ($\geq$ 60 years old) following programs of endurance exercise.

      (2) High-intensity exercise training **increases functional capacity** in the older adult, as much or more than percentage increase observed in young adults, depending on initial fitness levels. Improvements in $\dot{V}o_{2\,max}$ and endurance are due to increases in both maximal stroke volume and **arteriovenous oxygen difference.**

      (3) Moderate physical activity in older adults has been shown to augment tolerance for daily activities and is associated with **less fatigue and dyspnea** (shortness of breath), and lower ratings of perceived exertion.

   b. **Coronary artery disease and hypertension**

      (1) The prevalence of hypertension and coronary artery disease increases with advancing age. The **incidence** of these conditions and the **morbidity and mortality** associated with heart disease are greatly reduced in physically active individuals.

(2) Low-intensity endurance training:

–effectively **lowers systolic and diastolic blood pressure** by 8–10 mm Hg in normotensive and moderately hypertensive older adults.

–**reduces myocardial oxygen demand** as a result of peripheral adaptations (such as increased oxygen extraction, increased vagal tone, and decreased catecholamine release) and central changes (including decreased myocardial ischemia and improved left ventricular function).

c. **Cardiovascular events**

(1) Screening of exercise program participants is important because the incidence of cardiovascular disease (both diagnosed and undiagnosed) increases with aging.

(2) The **incidence of cardiac events during supervised adult fitness programs** for apparently healthy older adults **is very low,** with nonfatal cardiac events reported to be approximately 1 per 800,000 hours of supervised exercise and fatal events at about 1 per 1.1 million hours of supervised exercise.

(3) High-intensity exercise training increases risk for cardiac events.

2. **Benefits of strength training**

a. Men and women in the sixth decade of life gain strength in response to resistance exercise, but at a slower rate.

b. Muscle strength, power, and endurance begin to decline in middle adulthood.

(1) This decline accelerates after 50–60 years of age and is attributable to a number of changes, including:

–Decreased muscle fiber size

–Decreased muscle fiber number

–Decreased mitochondrial proteins and oxidative enzyme activities

–Decreased impulse conduction velocity

(2) Regular physical activity seems to slow this process. One exception is the loss of muscle fibers, which is due to age-related loss of motoneurons; this loss appears to be unaffected by exercise.

3. **Balance**

a. **Decreased balance** and an associated **increased occurrence of falls** in the elderly can be attributed to many factors, including:

–muscle weakness.

–inflexibility.

–degradation of neuromotor function.

–obesity.

–visual and vestibular deterioration.

b. Substantial evidence suggests that **physically active individuals maintain better balance during old age.**

–Regular exercise improves muscular strength and flexibility, which has a positive influence on speed and agility of walking, as well as on static balance.

–Regular exercise also appears to have positive effects on central nervous system functions, such as attention, short-term memory, and information processing speed, all of which commonly deteriorate with age and greatly impact balance and coordination.

4. **Preservation of bone mass**

a. Bone mass peaks in early adulthood and declines slowly thereafter.

b. **Regular weight-bearing exercise** can slow the loss of bone mass with aging.

–The stimulation of osteoblastic bone formation on the periosteal surface of long bones following a given load is greater in young animals than in old, but does occur in older adults if the stimulus is sufficient.

–The type of loading placed on the bone affects the degree of osteogenic stimulation. The **magnitude of the load** during an exercise session **seems to be of greater importance than the number of loading cycles.**

5. **Immune function**

–The immune system deteriorates significantly with advancing age. This is evidenced by the increased incidence of malignancy, infectious disease, and autoimmune disorders in the elderly.

–Numerous studies have indicated that lack of physical fitness and/or improper nutrition is also associated with compromised immune function. Although it remains unclear how much of the age-related loss of immune function is directly due to physical inactivity, available data suggest that immune function is better in active elderly compared with sedentary elderly.

6. **Obesity**

   –Longitudinal and cross-sectional studies have indicated that **weight gain** during adulthood is not due to aging but to an increasingly **sedentary lifestyle** in older adults.

   –**Physical activity plays an important role in the prevention and treatment of obesity as age progresses.** Programs of physical activity must be continued for months or even years to effectively reduce and control body mass.

7. **Insulin resistance**

   –**Insulin resistance,** a condition leading to **adult-onset diabetes,** is characterized by high levels of circulating insulin and reduced ability to maintain blood glucose concentration at a constant value.

   –Well-controlled studies indicate that physical inactivity and obesity, but not aging, are related to increased risk for insulin resistance.

   –**Regular exercise can decrease abdominal fat and increase insulin sensitivity, which may normalize glucose tolerance.**

8. **Psychological benefits**

   a. **Life satisfaction**

      –Older adults who exercise regularly have a more positive attitude toward work and are generally healthier than sedentary individuals.

   b. **Happiness**

      –Strong correlations have been reported between the activity level of older adults and self-reported happiness.

   c. **Self-efficacy**

      –"Self-efficacy" refers to the concept of or capability to perform a variety of tasks.

      –Older adults taking part in exercise programs commonly report that they are able to do daily tasks more easily than before they began exercising.

   d. **Self-concept**

      –Older adults improve their scores on self-concept questionnaires following participation in an exercise program.

   e. **Psychological stress**

      –Exercise has been shown to be effective in reducing psychological stress.

9. **Orthopedic injury**

   a. The **incidence of musculoskeletal injury among regularly exercising older adults**

is considerably **higher** than that found in younger populations.

   b. **Factors related to orthopedic injuries in older adults include:**

      –inadequate warm-up.

      –muscle weakness.

      –sudden violent movements.

      –rapid increases in exercise prescription.

10. **Thermoregulatory concerns**

    –Older adults have lower maximal cardiac output and compromised subcutaneous blood flow during exercise. Furthermore, total body water is reduced, which decreases maximal capacity for sweating.

    –**Exercise training improves thermoregulation** in older adults. Nevertheless, leaders of exercise programs involving older adults should ensure the **availability of fluids** for the participants, and they should **avoid exercising outdoors in hot and humid conditions.**

B. **UNIQUE RESPONSES OF OLDER ADULTS DURING EXERCISE AND RECOVERY (Table 3-1)**

1. **Cardiovascular and hemodynamic responses to exercise**

   a. The **increase in heart rate** in response to a given increase in relative exercise intensity **is blunted** in older adults.

   b. It appears that stroke volume and cardiac output at a fixed submaximal workload are similar in healthy young and old adults. However, **maximal stroke volume and cardiac output are decreased** in older adults because of decreased blood volume and maximal heart rate.

   c. Age-related **reductions in arterial compliance and left ventricular contractile reserve** combine to increase blood pressure and attenuate the increase in ejection fraction during exercise in the older adult.

   d. The response of arterial blood pressure to submaximal exercise appears unchanged with advancing age. Because blood volume is reduced, the **maintenance of blood pressure response** in the older subject **requires systemic vascular resistance to be elevated** above that found in young adults.

2. **Pulmonary regulation during exercise**

   a. **Expiratory flow limitation occurs at lower exercise intensities** with aging

Table 3-1. Exercise Responses Commonly Observed in Older Adults and Suggested Testing Modifications

Characteristic	Suggested Modification
1. Low aerobic capacity	Begin test at a low intensity (2–3 metabolic equivalents [METs]).
2. More time required to reach metabolic steady state	Increase length of warm-up (3+ min) and stages (2–3 min).
3. Poor balance	Bike preferred over treadmill or step test.
4. Poor leg strength	Treadmill preferred over bike or step test.
5. Difficulty holding mouthpiece with dentures	Add support or use face mask to measure $\dot{V}O_2$.
6. Impaired vision	Bike preferred over treadmill or step test.
7. Impaired hearing	Use electronic bike or treadmill to avoid the necessity of following a cadence.
8. Senile gait patterns or foot problems	Bike preferred; if treadmill is used, increase grade rather than speed.

Adapted with permission from Skinner JS. Chapter 5: Importance of aging for exercise testing and exercise prescription. In JS Skinner, Ed: *Exercise Testing and Exercise Prescription for Special Cases.* Malvern, PA: Lea & Febiger, 1993, p. 79.

owing to a loss of lung elastic recoil. This change can compromise inspiratory muscle function and increase ventilatory work. Older adults reach expiratory limitation at lower exercise intensities than younger adults.

b. **Dead space is increased** in the older adult from about 30% of tidal volume in the young to 40%–45% in the aged. This requires that total ventilatory response be elevated during exercise in the older adult to maintain alveolar ventilation and arterial PCO_2.

c. The reduction in pulmonary arteriolar compliance with aging causes **blood pressures in the pulmonary artery and capillaries to be elevated during exercise.** This may contribute to a **diffusion limitation of gas exchange** in the older adult during moderate to intense exercise.

C. TRAINABILITY OF OLDER ADULTS

–The precise decrements in trainability of older adults remain controversial because training programs for the elderly rarely employ the same absolute workloads as programs for young adults. Nevertheless, older adults can adapt to exercise training and significantly improve health and mobility. The following should be kept in mind when planning an exercise program for older adults:

1. Aging is associated with a **reduced adaptability to physiologic stimuli.**

2. Exercise programs for older adults require **more time to produce improvements** in variables such as muscle strength, $\dot{V}O_{2\,max}$, and muscle oxidative capacity.

3. The **goal** of most exercise programs for older adults should be to **increase self-sufficiency and ability to move with relative ease** and to perform activities of daily living.

IV. DEVELOPMENT OF EXERCISE PRESCRIPTIONS FOR CHILDREN AND ADOLESCENTS

A. EXERCISE TESTING

1. **Reasons** for exercise testing in children include:

   a. Assessment of physical working capacity **to identify deficiencies** in specific fitness components or **to establish baselines** before or after an exercise program.

   b. Identification of specific **pathophysiologic changes** that may be amplified during exercise.

   c. Evaluation of the functional **success of surgical corrections.**

   d. Assessment of the **adequacy of medication** (e.g., for asthma or diabetes).

   e. **Diagnosis of disease** (e.g., growth hormone deficiency or asthma).

   f. **To instill confidence** in the child and parents that the child is capable of physical exertion.

2. **Methodological considerations**

a. Most ergometers used in adult exercise testing can be used for children. However, because of relatively underdeveloped musculature of the legs and difficulty following the pace of a metronome, the treadmill is generally preferred over cycle ergometers and step tests.

b. Field tests provide a practical and efficient means of assessing physical fitness in children.

c. Protocols to measure **maximal aerobic power** should consist of a progressively increasing load. Because children reach steady state faster than adults, stages lasting 1–2 minutes seem to be adequate.

d. Testing protocols developed for adults can easily be modified for children by lowering the initial power output and subsequent incremental increases.

e. Protocols designed to predict **maximal aerobic capacity** from submaximal exercise should be interpreted cautiously because several congenital conditions and diseases can cause peak heart rate to be reduced, resulting in an overestimation of $\dot{V}o_{2\,max}$, if the tester assumes maximal heart rate is in the normal range. Nevertheless, a graded exercise test is generally not required when evaluating healthy, asymptomatic children.

B. **EXERCISE PRESCRIPTION**

–Most healthy children are habitually more active than adults and adolescents, and therefore often do not require a structured exercise prescription.

However, recent data have shown a **trend toward poorer physical fitness in school-age children** in the United States.

–The **goals** of exercise programs for young children should be **to increase energy expenditure** (especially for obese children) and **to establish an active lifestyle** that will continue into adulthood.

1. **Aerobic exercise programs**

a. **For older children and adolescents,** the recommended adult guidelines for frequency, duration, and intensity of exercise can be used.

b. **For prepubescent children,** exercise prescription should focus on keeping the child active and interested with various types of intermittent exercise and less emphasis on improving aerobic capacity.

2. **Strength training programs**

a. **Proper resistance training** in children and adolescents can enhance strength, muscle endurance, and muscle power.

–Proper resistance training exercise prescription for children and adolescents should focus on **proper lifting techniques** and on **increased repetitions and lower resistance** to improve flexibility and muscle tone.

b. **High-intensity or competitive weight-lifting or bodybuilding is inappropriate for preadolescent children.** These activities may pose a risk to developing muscles, bones, and connective tissue.

c. It is recommended that adolescents avoid high-intensity or competitive weight-lifting, also, until the epiphyseal growth plates have closed, following the adolescent growth spurt.

V. DEVELOPMENT OF EXERCISE PRESCRIPTIONS FOR OLDER ADULTS

A. **EXERCISE TESTING**

–In general, exercise tests for older adults (men aged 45 years or older; women aged 55 years or older) should focus on evaluation of factors important for health and well-being rather than on measurement of maximal exercise performance.

1. **Reasons** for exercise testing in the older adult include:

a. **To define the degree of risk** associated with exercise at different intensities.

b. **To establish the appropriate intensities** for exercise prescription.

2. **Who should be tested?**

a. Older adults with no signs of cardiovascular disease may not require an exercise test before beginning a program of moderate exercise such as walking.

b. Older adults who desire to engage in vigorous physical activities should be tested.

c. Older adults at high risk who desire to engage in moderate or vigorous physical activities should be tested.

3. **Medications** should be carefully considered when interpreting exercise test results.

Table 3-2. Typical Modifications of Exercise Prescription for Older Adults

Characteristic	Possible Modifications
1. Greater incidence of heart disease	Increase monitoring for safety.
	Avoid isometrics and Valsalva maneuver.
2. Lower cardiovascular ability	Start at lower workloads.
3. Less ability to perform high-intensity exercise	Decrease intensity and allow participants to select own work rate.
4. Less ability to recover from exercise	Use longer warm-up and cool-down periods.
5. Reduced adaptability to training	Use more gradual progression of frequency, duration, and intensity of exercise.
6. Muscle weakness	Moderate strength training.
7. Increased fatigability	Use short exercise intervals and more frequent rest periods.
8. Degenerative bone, joint, and tendon problems	Don't use activities with bodily contact.
9. Increased susceptibility to injury and soreness	Don't use fast turns or movements.
10. Poor flexibility	Emphasize stretching.
11. Poor coordination and balance	Have client exercise while seated or supine.
	Use exercise in water.
12. Impaired vision or hearing	Have client exercise on stationary bicycle.

Adapted with permission from Skinner J. S. Chapter 5: Importance of aging for exercise testing and exercise prescription. In: *Exercise Testing and Exercise Prescription for Special Cases.* J.S. Skinner, Ed: Malvern, PA: Lea & Febiger, 1993, p 84.

---

4. **Methodological considerations**
    a. **Submaximal tests** that estimate fitness and predict maximal values may be preferred over tests requiring maximal exercise for assessment of fitness and functional capacity, because physical function is usually more important to the older adult than maximal exercise performance.
    b. **Progressive exercise tests** should begin at a low initial workload (2–3 metabolic equivalents [METs]) and use small increases in intensity each stage (0.5–1.0 MET).
    c. **Older adults reach metabolic steady state more slowly** than young adults; therefore, exercise tests for the elderly should incorporate a long warm-up and stages lasting 3 minutes or more.
    d. The **type of ergometer** used for testing should be chosen based on the needs of the participant.
    e. **Increases in treadmill grade rather than speed** are easier and may be safer for older adults.
    f. The supervisor of the exercise test should be aware of **conditions that may require special attention** during a test such as

impaired vision, hearing loss, senile gait patterns, chronic foot problems, and dentures.

B. **EXERCISE PRESCRIPTION**
    –Exercise prescriptions for older adults follow the same general principles as those used for young adults. These guidelines are simply modified on an individual basis as age-related disabilities or clinical problems are encountered (**Table 3-2**).
    1. **Objectives** of exercise programs for older adults include:
        a. Improvement of general well-being and an increased independence of living.
        b. Reversal of the age-related losses in cardiovascular endurance, strength, and flexibility.
        c. Establishing enjoyable physical activity as a regular part of the lifestyle.
    2. **Age-related exercise modifications**
        –The longer an individual has been sedentary, the greater the modifications in exercise prescription.
        –Exercise programs should be more systematic and cautious because the incidence of disease is higher in older adults.

–Small, short-term goals with a high probability of success are appropriate.

–For elderly with extremely low functional abilities, simple activities such as housework or gardening may be used to increase habitual activity and improve endurance.

3. **Components of the exercise prescription**

   a. **Intensity**

   –**Intense exercise should be avoided** because deconditioned older adults may be easily fatigued and therefore more susceptible to injury.

    –Exercise training should **begin at a light intensity (20%–39% of HR reserve) and progress gradually** to 40%–85% HR reserve.

   b. **Duration**

   –Some older adults may have difficulty sustaining aerobic exercise for 20 minutes. Multiple 5- to 10-minute bouts spaced throughout the day may be indicated. Progression should aim at 20–30 minutes of continuous exercise daily.

–Increased duration, rather than intensity, is appropriate for older adults.

   c. A **frequency** of **at least three times per week** is recommended for exercise sessions.

   d. **Mode of exercise**

   –**Rhythmic, continuous exercise** involving large muscle groups should be used **for cardiovascular endurance.**

   –Exercise programs should include **stretching** of all major joints **to help improve or maintain flexibility and range of motion.**

   –**Strength training** using relatively low weights and high repetitions should be included **to improve muscle strength and neuromuscular coordination.** Lifting heavy weights, as well as isometric exercises, may be inappropriate for older adults because of possible adverse cardiovascular response.

   e. **Progression** of exercise frequency, duration, and intensity should be slow, allowing ample time for complete adaptation.

VI. LEADERSHIP TECHNIQUES FOR CHILDREN, ADOLESCENTS, AND OLDER ADULTS

A. PLANNING

–Fitness levels and goals vary greatly. Therefore, leadership of any exercise program begins with the proper planning to appeal to and address the needs of a specific population.

1. **Children**

   –**Preadolescent children** are usually primarily concerned with having fun. Planning exercise programs for this age group should **incorporate games** to hold the attention of the participants.

2. **Adolescents**

   –are typically more concerned about physical appearance and/or athletic performance than health issues. The potential for exercise to impact these areas should be stressed when designing the program and recruiting participants.

3. **Older adults**

   –Exercise programs for older adults require adequate **research to determine the specific exercise needs of the older population in the community.** Local government agencies may be able to provide information regarding age

demographics of a community, as well as provide lists of local organizations for senior citizens. Surveys and interviews with regional senior groups can provide data on the needs of this population and the level of interest in participating in an organized exercise program.

B. FACILITIES

1. **Children and adolescents**

   –Exercise programs often involve games and group exercises that are best performed **outdoors or in a large gymnasium.**

2. **Older adults**

   –The **facility should minimize the limitations** of the older participants as much as possible. The following take on greater importance when working with older adults:

   a. Adequate lighting

   b. Low background noise

   c. Resilient walking and/or jogging surface, and well-cushioned exercise mats

   d. Easy accessibility, preferably on ground floor

C.   MOTIVATIONAL TECHNIQUES

1. The exercise program should offer a **variety of activities** to help avoid boredom.

2. Activities should **encourage social interaction** to increase enjoyment of the exercise sessions and improve the likelihood that the participants will continue physical activity after the program is over.

3. Exercise professionals should be knowledgeable about the **specific goals and limitations of participants** and be willing to personally motivate and encourage members of the group.

D.   EMERGENCY READINESS

1. All staff involved in supervised exercise programs should be certified in **cardiopulmonary resuscitation and basic first aid.**

2. Exercise professionals who supervise exercise programs for children and/or older adults should have **knowledge of the exercise responses and limitations** common to those groups.

3. A **file card** should be kept for each participant in supervised exercise programs.

   a. **For children,** this card should have parents' names, telephone numbers, and the name and telephone number of the physician.

   b. **For older adults,** the file card should have emergency contacts, medications, and medical conditions.

REVIEW TEST

DIRECTIONS: Carefully read all questions and select the BEST single answer.

1. The decrease in maximal strength per cross-sectional area of skeletal muscle that accompanies aging is due, in part, to
   - (A) a loss of skeletal muscle fibers
   - (B) an increase in the concentration of fat and connective tissue
   - (C) a decrease in the activity of metabolic enzymes
   - (D) an atrophy of skeletal muscle fibers

2. During childhood and adolescence, the length of the long bones increases by the production and ossification of cartilage. In what portion of the bone does this process occur?
   - (A) The diaphysis
   - (B) The marrow
   - (C) The epiphysis
   - (D) The epiphyseal plates

3. Each of the following are characteristics of hypokinetic circulation in children EXCEPT
   - (A) lower heart rate
   - (B) small stroke volume relative to body size
   - (C) small cardiac output relative to body size
   - (D) lower hemoglobin concentration in the blood

4. Which of the following activities would be most effective in stimulating accumulation of bone mass in children?
   - (A) Jogging
   - (B) Swimming
   - (C) Gymnastics
   - (D) Cycling

5. Which of the following physiologic responses to exercise is NOT unique to children?
   - (A) Relative $\dot{V}o_{2\,max}$ at submaximal workloads is high.
   - (B) Metabolic steady state is reached very quickly after onset of exercise.
   - (C) A given physiologic strain is perceived to be easier by children than by adults.
   - (D) The capacity to perform anaerobic work is high.

6. Endurance exercise training produces improvements in $\dot{V}o_{2\,max}$ for older adults primarily through what mechanism(s)?
   - (A) Increases in maximal stroke volume and mean arterial blood pressure
   - (B) Increases in maximal heart rate and arteriovenous oxygen difference
   - (C) Increases in maximal stroke volume and arteriovenous oxygen difference
   - (D) An increase in maximal heart rate and a decrease in mean arterial blood pressure

7. Which one of the following cardiovascular and/or pulmonary responses to exercise is greater in older adults, compared with young adults?
   - (A) Stroke volume
   - (B) Heart rate
   - (C) Alveolar ventilation
   - (D) Total pulmonary ventilation

8. Strength training programs for preadolescent children should emphasize each of the following EXCEPT
   - (A) improving flexibility
   - (B) instruction in proper lifting technique
   - (C) increasing muscle tone
   - (D) competition as a form of motivation

9. Which of the following statements regarding exercise prescriptions for older adults is NOT true?
   - (A) One exercise session per day is preferred over two or more.
   - (B) Older people are capable of exercising at relative intensities (50%–70% $\dot{V}o_{2\,max}$) equal to those prescribed for younger adults.
   - (C) The progression of exercise intensity should be slower than that for young adults.
   - (D) Strength training programs should employ relatively low resistance and high repetitions.

10. The ratio of body surface area to body mass for a child differs from this ratio for adults. In which of the following circumstances would this difference aid thermoregulation in the child?
    - (A) Swimming in cool water
    - (B) Jogging in a mild climate
    - (C) Playing tennis in a cold climate
    - (D) Sitting outdoors when ambient temperature exceeds body temperature

11. Each of the following factors contribute to the large increase in absolute $\dot{V}O_{2\,max}$ occurring in boys during adolescence EXCEPT
    (A) androgen-induced hypertrophy of the heart
    (B) increased production of red blood cells
    (C) increases in skeletal muscle mass
    (D) increased oxygen consumption per unit of body mass

12. Each of the following contributes to the impairment of thermoregulation during exercise in older adults EXCEPT
    (A) decreased sensitivity of the sweating mechanism
    (B) decreased subcutaneous blood flow during exercise
    (C) decreased total body water
    (D) lower maximal cardiac output

13. Each of the following are reasonable expectations of an exercise program for older adults EXCEPT
    (A) prevention of age-related loss of muscular endurance
    (B) an increase in stroke volume and maximal cardiac output
    (C) prevention of the age-related increase in body fat
    (D) a decrease in percent body fat

14. Muscular strength in females
    (A) increases disproportionately to body mass during the adolescent growth spurt
    (B) equals that in males during postadolescence, if normalized to muscle mass
    (C) is 40%–60% less than that in males during preadolescence
    (D) does not differ from that in males during preadolescence

15. Which of the following statements about osteoporosis is NOT true?
    (A) A sedentary lifestyle is a risk factor for development of osteoporosis.
    (B) Estrogen replacement can be effective in attenuating bone loss in postmenopausal women.
    (C) Secondary amenorrhea in young athletes may contribute to osteoporosis later in life.
    (D) Bone loss in women begins at menopause.

16. Muscle strength, power, and endurance begin to decline in middle adulthood. This process accelerates after 50 to 60 years of age and is attributable to a number of changes including decreases in which of the following?
    (A) Muscle fiber size
    (B) Muscle fiber number
    (C) Mitochondrial proteins and oxidative enzyme activities
    (D) All of the above

17. Which of the following statements regarding aging, obesity, and insulin resistance is NOT true?
    (A) Carefully controlled studies have indicated that physical inactivity and obesity, but not aging itself, are related to an increased risk for insulin resistance.
    (B) Regular exercise is known to decrease abdominal fat and increase insulin sensitivity, which has the potential to completely normalize glucose tolerance in the aging individual.
    (C) The adverse changes in body composition and glucose tolerance commonly seen in aging individuals are not due to aging at all; rather they are the consequences of an increasingly sedentary lifestyle in older adults.
    (D) Insulin resistance, a condition leading to adult-onset diabetes, is not a common phenomenon in older adults and can be ignored except when the older person is taking insulin on a regular basis.

18. The risk of cardiovascular fatal events during supervised exercise training in older adults is approximately
    (A) 1 per 1,000 hours
    (B) 1 per 10,000 hours
    (C) 1 per 100,000 hours
    (D) 1 per 1,000,000 hours

19. Which of the following is NOT a good reason for exercise testing in children?
    (A) Assessment of physical working capacity to identify deficiencies in specific fitness components and/or establish baselines before or after an exercise program
    (B) Identification of specific pathophysiologic changes that may be amplified during exercise
    (C) Diagnosis of age-related diseases such as cancer, emphysema, and atherosclerosis
    (D) To instill confidence in the child and/or parents that the child is capable of physical exertion

20. Which of the following is NOT considered to be a contraindication to physical activity for older adults?
    (A) Hypertension
    (B) Peripheral vascular disease
    (C) Anemia
    (D) Cigarette smoking

21. The purpose of exercise testing in the older adult is to
    (A) define the degree of risk associated with exercise at different intensities
    (B) discover the severity of diseases such as cancer and its impact on the aerobic capacity
    (C) discourage the older adult from exercising at high intensities
    (D) limit exercise programming to 1 or 2 days a week

22. Each of the following are considered to be objectives of exercise programs for older adults, EXCEPT:
    (A) reduction of the incidence of coronary artery disease and hypertension.
    (B) reversal of the aging process.
    (C) improvement of general well-being and an increased independence of living
    (D) establishment of short-term goals with a high probability of success

23. For elderly people with extremely low functional abilities, which of the following physical activities might improve endurance?
    (A) Running 5 miles each day
    (B) Walking 7 miles 3 days a week
    (C) Housework or gardening
    (D) Cycling back and forth to the grocery store

24. The components of the exercise prescription for the elderly who are accustomed to exercise include
    (A) beginning at an intensity of 20%–39% of HR reserve, duration of 30 minutes each session, at least 3 days per week
    (B) beginning at an intensity of 60%–80% of HR reserve, duration of 20 minutes each session, at least 3 days per week
    (C) beginning at an intensity of 70%–90% of HR reserve, duration of 45 minutes each session, at least 3 days per week
    (D) beginning at an intensity of 20%–39% of HR reserve, duration of 10 minutes each session, at least 2 days per week

25. A decrease in size or the wasting away of a body part or tissue is called
    (A) hypertrophy
    (B) atrophy
    (C) endochondral ossification
    (D) osteoarthritis

ANSWERS AND EXPLANATIONS

1–B. An age-related increase in intramuscular fat and connective tissue effectively dilutes the concentration of force-generating myofibrils when an entire muscle from an older subject is considered in cross section. In other words, a greater proportion of the cross section of an old muscle is composed of non–force-generating material, when compared with a muscle from a young adult individual. It is true that there is a loss of skeletal muscle fibers and an atrophy of existing fibers with aging, which translates into a decrease in absolute maximal strength. However, the reduction in strength per cross-sectional area cannot be accounted for by these factors. Because of the anaerobic nature of a maximal muscular contraction, decreases in the activity of metabolic enzymes in the muscle would not contribute to a loss of maximal muscle force. Finally, skeletal muscle ATP concentration tends to be reduced with aging, not increased. Furthermore, the decrease in ATP observed by some investigators has not been shown to be related to a loss of muscle strength.

2–D. The long bones are divided into three main sections: the diaphysis or middle region of the bone, the epiphysis or ends of the bone, and the epiphyseal plates, which separate the diaphysis from the epiphysis. The skeleton takes shape very early in human development, with the structure being initially formed from chondrocytes and the cartilage they secrete. Through the process of endochondral ossification, bone gradually replaces the cartilage. Primary ossification in long bones (i.e., the first replacement of cartilage by bone) occurs in the diaphysis. Next, the epiphysis begins to ossify. When the child is born, most of the skeleton (including the epiphysis and diaphysis of long bones) is composed of bone. However, the epiphyseal plate regions retain active chondrocytes, which continue to add to the length of the bones during growth. Bone marrow is the spongy tissue located in the center of long bones that is involved in production of blood cells; the osteoclasts, on the other hand, are bone cells involved in bone resorption.

3–A. Hypokinetic circulation refers to a lower (hypo) movement (kinetic) of blood and oxygen to the tissues in children as compared to adults. This is a normal phenomenon in preadolescent children, resulting primarily from a smaller heart size in relation to body mass in this age group. The smaller relative heart size means that stroke volume and cardiac output will be reduced. Hemoglobin, which allows the oxygen delivery to the tissue, has a lower concentration in children. Finally, arterial blood pressure and the blood pressure response to exercise are lower in children than in adults. Therefore, the driving pressure to the capillaries is lower in children. All of these factors contribute to hypokinetic circulation in children. To compensate for this reduced stroke volume and oxygen-carrying capacity (and for other reasons), heart rate at rest and during exercise is elevated in children. Nevertheless, this does not completely compensate, and cardiac output per body mass remains somewhat lower than in adults. The hypokinetic circulation described above does not appear to significantly limit exercise capacity in children.

4–C. Weight-bearing physical activity has been shown to increase overall bone mass and bone mineral density at any age. However, during growth, bones are particularly susceptible to the positive effects of load-bearing activities. Therefore, weight-bearing activities during childhood can significantly increase peak bone mass during early adulthood. Although any weight-bearing activity will increase bone mass, weight lifting and compressive exercises, such as gymnastics, are the most effective. Non-weight-bearing activities, such as cycling and swimming, do not significantly stimulate bone mass accumulation.

5–D. Anaerobic capacity is lower in children compared with adults. Skeletal muscle of children has a smaller reserve of glycogen, the primary fuel for anaerobic exercise. Furthermore, the activities of the enzymes involved in glycolysis are lower than that in adult muscle. Together these factors limit the ability of children to perform anaerobic work. Relative $\dot{V}o_2$ at submaximal workloads is higher in children than adults owing to inefficient motor patterns in the child. Children reach a metabolic steady state very quickly following a change in activity level; this means that oxygen deficit at the onset of exercise and recovery time following cessation of exercise are much lower in children than in adults. Finally, for unknown reasons, a given intensity of exercise is perceived to be easier by children than by adults.

6–C. Older adults are capable of adapting to endurance training. As in younger adults, endurance exercise results in significant improvements in cardiorespiratory function. The chronic increase in preload on the heart during endurance exercise and a relaxation of sympathetic tone allows an expansion of cardiac volume, and, therefore, an increased stroke volume. Endurance muscular exercise also

results in an increase in capillarization and muscle mitochondrial volume. This allows for a more efficient extraction of oxygen and an increased arteriovenous oxygen difference. Endurance exercise effectively reduces resting systolic blood pressure and diastolic blood pressure at rest and during exercise. Therefore, mean arterial blood pressure is reduced compared with sedentary older adults. Maximal heart rate decreases with advancing age due to age-related changes in cardiac muscle compliance. This process is unaltered by endurance training.

7–D. Ventilatory dead space increases with age from about 30% of tidal volume in young adults to 40%–45% in older adults. This is due to a reduction in alveolar number and an increase in ventilation/perfusion mismatch. The result is that total ventilation at any given exercise intensity must be higher in the older adult compared with young adults in order to maintain alveolar ventilation and arterial Pco_2. Stroke volume and cardiac output responses are similar in older and younger adults during exercise; however, maximal values are somewhat lower in the elderly. The heart rate response to an increase in exercise intensity is typically lower in older subjects compared with younger.

8–D. Strength training programs for preadolescent children can effectively increase muscle strength and endurance. As with all exercise programs for young children, strength training programs should focus on the instruction of proper techniques and the establishment of proper exercise habits. Strength training can also improve flexibility and muscle tone by employing relatively low weights and high repetitions and moving through the entire range of motion. Weight lifting involving maximal weights may present a risk to developing bones, muscles, and connective tissue. Therefore, competition should not be used as a motivator for strength training in preadolescents.

9–A. The guidelines for prescribing exercise for older adults are essentially the same as those for younger adults. These guidelines are simply modified on an individual basis as outlined in **Table 3-2**. Generally, older adults are capable of the same physiologic adaptations as their younger counterparts, however, these changes occur more slowly with advancing age. Relative exercise intensity should be slower for the older adult. Because older adults typically do not desire to maximize strength performance, and are more susceptible to orthopedic injury, a frequency of exercise = 3 times per week is recommended for older adults. One exercise session per day is not preferred over two or more. Multiple exercise sessions can be very effective in achieving exercise duration and caloric expenditure goals while minimizing fatigue.

10–B. The surface area relative to body mass is greater for a child than for an adult. This allows a greater rate of heat exchange between skin and environment, which would aid thermoregulation only if heat needed to be dissipated from the skin to the environment. During exposure to cold, such as swimming in cool water and tennis or cycling in cold weather, the higher surface area relative to body mass in children would increase the rate of loss of body heat to the environment and therefore hinder thermoregulation. Conversely, when ambient temperature exceeds body temperature, the increased surface area would facilitate the acquisition of heat from the environment and, once again, hinder thermoregulation. Exercising (e.g., jogging) in a mild climate generates body heat that must be dissipated to the environment. Therefore, a larger surface area relative to body mass would facilitate thermoregulation in this situation.

11–D. There is a large increase in maximal oxygen consumption ($\dot{V}o_{2\,max}$) that accompanies the adolescent growth spurt. This increase is especially pronounced in boys. The rate of oxygen consumption is dependent upon two main factors: oxygen delivery to the tissues and oxygen extraction from the blood. Both of these factors are enhanced during male adolescence. Androgen-induced hypertrophy of the heart increases maximal stroke volume and cardiac output, whereas hormonally induced increases in skeletal muscle mass increase the overall rate of extraction of oxygen from the blood. In spite of these changes, the increase in body mass during male adolescence parallels the increase in absolute $\dot{V}o_{2\,max}$. Therefore, the maximal oxygen consumption per unit of body mass remains essentially unchanged.

12–A. In healthy older adults the sensitivity of the sweating mechanism remains intact. However, total body water is significantly reduced with aging. This predisposes the older adult to rapid dehydration once sweating begins. There is a direct relationship between body temperature and the degree of dehydration; therefore, the lower total body water in the elderly greatly contributes to impaired thermoregulation in warm environments. Additionally, the cardiovascular responses to a thermoregulatory challenge are diminished in older adults. A lower blood volume (due, in part, to the lower total

body water) contributes to a lower maximal cardiac output, which in turn compromises subcutaneous blood flow during exercise. These events also impair thermoregulation in older adults.

13–C. Exercise programs for older adults have proven to be very successful in many areas. Regular exercise can reduce body fat at any given age and minimize the accumulation of abdominal fat. However, longitudinal studies of master athletes indicate that the age-related increase in body fat cannot be prevented with exercise. In other words, the body fat of an individual who exercises regularly will increase at a rate essentially parallel, but below the rate of increase in body fat of a sedentary individual. Regular exercise causes many advantageous cardiovascular adaptations in older adults, including increases in maximal stroke volume and cardiac output. Bone mass typically declines throughout adulthood; however, bones continue to be sensitive to loading in old age. Therefore, chronic exercise can attenuate the loss of bone mass with aging. Finally, although the loss of muscle fiber number with aging appears to be irreversible, the decline in mitochondrial volume and oxidative enzyme activities is reversible by exercise. Therefore, regular exercise can prevent the age-related loss of muscular endurance.

14–D. Before adolescence, muscular strength does not differ between males and females. During adolescence, overall muscular strength increases in both sexes due to the increase in body mass. However, only the male has an increase in strength that is disproportionate to the increase in body mass. This is due to the disproportionate increase in muscle mass induced by the male hormones during puberty. Muscular strength reaches its peak following the growth spurt during early adulthood for both sexes. In postadolescence, muscular strength in females averages 30%–60% lower than males. However, muscle mass in postadolescent females averages about 30% lower than males. Therefore, a discrepancy between female and male muscular strength remains in postadolescence, particularly in the upper body, even when strength is normalized to muscle mass. This discrepancy may be due to hormonal differences or, perhaps, to sociological effects.

15–D. Bone loss in women may begin as early as age 30 to 35, but is accelerated following the hormonal changes of menopause. Estrogen replacement has been shown to be effective in minimizing bone loss in postmenopausal women. Weight-bearing activities stimulate the accumulation of bone mass. This "bone building" effect of exercise is pronounced during adolescence and early adulthood and diminishes during older adulthood. Therefore, physical activity, especially during youth, can effectively prevent or delay the onset of osteoporosis later in life. Finally, secondary amenorrhea, which is common among young female athletes, is associated with hormonal changes that predispose these women to osteoporosis later in life.

16–D. Decreases in muscle fiber size, muscle fiber number, mitochondrial proteins, oxidative enzyme activity, and impulse conduction velocity are all attributable to the aging process especially after the age of 50–60 years. Regular physical activity can attenuate the magnitude of most of these decrements. However, the loss of muscle fibers is due to an age-related loss of motoneurons, which does not appear to be affected by exercise. For this reason, exercise programs for older adults can be very successful in maintaining muscular strength.

17–D. Insulin resistance, a condition leading to adult-onset diabetes, is a common phenomenon in older adults and is characterized by high levels of circulating insulin and a reduced ability to maintain blood glucose concentrations at a constant value. Adult-onset diabetes should not be ignored under any set of circumstances.

18–D. The incidence of cardiac events during organized adult fitness programs for apparently healthy older adults is very low. The rate of occurrence of nonfatal cardiac events has been reported to be 1 per 800,000 hours of supervised exercise. Fatal events occurred at a rate of 1 per 1.1 million hours of supervised exercise.

19–C. Diagnosis of disease can be accomplished through exercise testing, but is usually not related to cancer, lung disease (except asthma), or cardiovascular disease. The exercise test can also provide for an assessment of the functional success of certain surgical corrections.

20–D. There are nine absolute contraindications to exercise in the elderly and 18 relative contraindications. Cigarette smoking is not considered to be a contraindication unless it has predisposed the individual to other chronic disease conditions.

21–A. The purpose of exercise testing in the older adult is to define the degree of risk associated with exercise at different intensities and to establish the appropriate intensities for the exercise prescription.

22–B. Objectives of exercise programs for older adults include the improvement of general well-being and an increased independence of living. Further, the incidence of coronary artery disease and hypertension is greatly reduced in physically active adults. Regular physical activity should be enjoyable and become a part of the older person's lifestyle. Goal setting is an important part of any exercise program. For older adults, many small short-term goals should be selected, each with a high probability of success. Although age-related losses in physical function can be slowed with regular physical activity, the aging process cannot be prevented.

23–C. For elderly people with extremely low functional abilities, simple activities such as housework or gardening can be prescribed to increase habitual activity and improve endurance.

24–A. Older individuals are often easily fatigued and, therefore, more susceptible to injury. For this reason, intense exercise should be avoided. Exercise training should begin at a low intensity of approximately 20%–39% and progress gradually to approximately 40%–85% of HR reserve. Once an individual is exercising regularly, each exercise session should last 20–30 minutes. If the prescribed duration of exercise exceeds 30 minutes per day, two shorter sessions can be used in place of one long session. This will minimize fatigue during the later stages of the exercise bout. A frequency of at least 3 days per week is recommended for exercise sessions. However, the need for older adults to be physically active every day should be emphasized.

25–B. A decrease in size or the wasting away of a body part or tissue is called atrophy. Hypertrophy refers to an increase in size of a body part or tissue. Endochondral ossification refers to the process of ossification that originates from centers arising in cartilage. Osteoarthritis is a condition characterized by degeneration of bone and cartilage of the joints.

CHAPTER 4

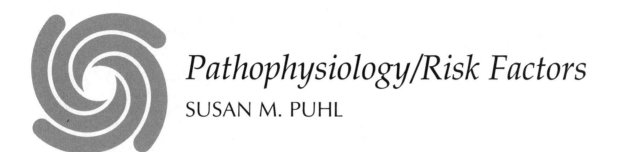

Pathophysiology/Risk Factors

SUSAN M. PUHL

I. PATHOPHYSIOLOGY OF CORONARY ARTERY DISEASE

A. THEORY OF DEVELOPMENT

–The development of coronary artery disease is often explained as a **response-to-injury.**

–The disease is a **chronic** (long-term), progressive response of the arterial walls to stress.

–The stress may be **acute** (sudden in onset, short-term), such as a viral infection, or **chronic,** such as hypertension.

B. INITIAL CAUSE

1. **Irritation of, or injury to, the tunica intima** (innermost of the three layers in the wall of a blood vessel, **Figure 4-1**)

2. **Sources of irritation/injury**

   a. **Dyslipidemia** (Table 4-1)

   –Elevated total blood cholesterol: > 200 mg/dl (5.2 mmol/L),

   –Lowered blood high-density lipoprotein (HDL): < 35 mg/dl (0.9 mmol/L),

   –Or elevated blood low-density lipoprotein (LDL): > 130 mg/dl (3.4 mmol/L)

   b. **Hypertension**—high blood pressure: ≥ 140/90 mm Hg measured on two separate occasions

   –An **elevation of either the systolic or diastolic pressure** is classified as hypertension.

   –The elevation must be measured on **2 different days,** preferably several days apart.

   c. **Immune responses,** such as may result from infections or chronic disease

   d. **Smoking** and other irritants from tobacco

   e. **Turbulence** (tumultuous, nonlaminar flow) in the **lumen** (center opening through which the blood flows) of the blood vessel

   f. **Vasoconstrictor substances** (chemicals that cause the smooth muscle cells in the walls of the vessel to contract, resulting in a reduction in the diameter of the lumen)

   g. **Viral or bacterial infection**

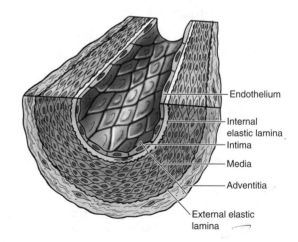

FIGURE 4-1 The normal coronary artery wall. (From Ross R, Glomset J: The pathogenesis of atherosclerosis. *N Engl J Med* 295:369, 1976.)

Table 4-1. Classifications of Serum Cholesterol

Classification	Definition	Comments/Criteria
Cholesterol	A fat synthesized by the liver or ingested in animal fat, carried in the blood in the form of *lipoproteins* (molecules composed of varying amounts of fats and proteins). It is essential in the formation of various digestive components and hormones, and as a component of cell membranes and nerve tissues.	A healthy diet includes: ≤ 30% total fat ≤ 10% saturated fat ≤ 300 mg cholesterol/day
Total cholesterol	The total of all the various subfractions (LDL, HDL, and VLDL) of cholesterol-carrying lipoproteins in the blood.	Adults (≥ 18 years): desirable < 200 mg/dl (5.2 mmol/l) borderline high 200–239 mg/dl (5.2–6.2 mmol/l) high ≥ 240 mg/dl (6.2 mmol/l) Children and youths: desirable < 170 mg/dl (4.4 mmol/l) borderline high 170–199 mg/dl (4.4–5.2 mmol/l) high ≥ 200 mg/dl (5.2 mmol/l)
High-density lipoprotein (HDL)	The smallest and most dense of the lipoproteins. It transports cholesterol out of the blood and into the liver.	Low HDL (< 35 mg/dl [0.9 mmol/l]) is a positive (bad) risk factor for coronary artery disease. HDL ≥ 60 mg/dl (1.6 mmol/l) is a negative (good) risk factor for coronary artery disease.
Low-density lipoprotein (LDL)	The principal carrier of cholesterol in the blood. The cholesterol in LDLs is used for various cell functions, but is also the source of the cholesterol that contributes to the atherogenic process.	Adults (≥ 18 years): desirable < 130 mg/dl (3.4 mmol/l) borderline high 130–159 mg/dl (3.4–4.1 mmol/l) high ≥ 160 mg/dl (4.1 mmol/l) Children and youths: desirable < 100 mg/dl (2.6 mmol/l) borderline high 110–129 mg/dl (2.6–3.4 mmol/l) high ≥ 130 mg/dl (3.4 mmol/l)
Total cholesterol–to–HDL ratio	The ratio between the total amount of cholesterol-transporting molecules circulating in the blood and the portion that removes cholesterol from the circulation. It is determined by dividing total cholesterol concentration by HDL concentration.	Optimal: 3.0 High risk: 5.0

Adapted from the Second Report of National Cholesterol Education Program (NCEP) Expert Panel on Detection, Evaluation, and Treatment of High Blood Cholesterol in Adults (Adult Treatment Panel II). 1993. NIH Publication No. 93.

C. DISEASE PROCESS

1. **Migration and proliferation** (increase in number and size) of cells

   –Smooth muscle cells and **fibroblasts** (nondifferentiated connective tissue cells) migrate from the **tunica media** into the tunica intima (**Figure 4-2**), which is lined by **endothelial cells.**

   –The migration of smooth muscle cells into the tunica intima is **abnormal.**

2. **Release of chemicals and growth factors**

   –**Platelets** and **monocytes** adhere to the irritated/injured site and release chemicals and growth factors that stimulate the **atherogenic** process.

3. **Collection and production of plaque components**

   –Smooth muscle cells and monocytes accumulate cholesterol, connective tissues, and proteins.

D. RESULTS OF ATHEROGENIC PROCESS

1. **Blood flow obstruction**

   –A developing atherosclerotic plaque bulges into the vessel lumen.

   –Blood flow is obstructed and consequently restricted.

2. **Clot lodging**

   –Plaque and a narrowed lumen increase the risk of clots at the site of the lesion.

   –The presence of plaque can make the membrane (endothelium) inherently unstable and subject to plaque disruption and rupture, causing the formation of a clot at the site.

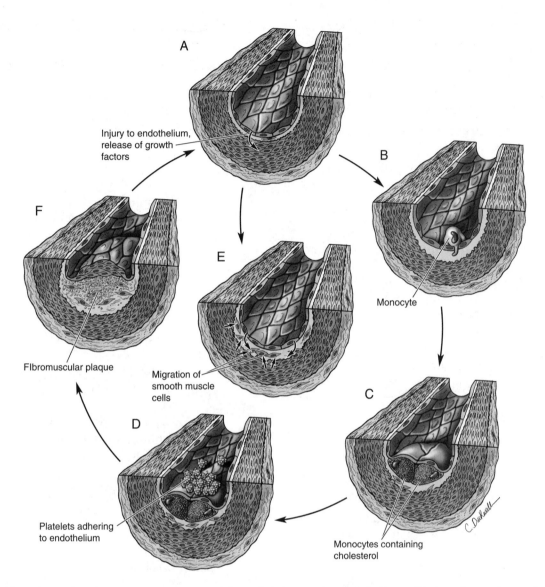

FIGURE 4-2 The atherosclerotic process—response to injury. *A,* Injury to the endothelium with the release of growth factors (*small arrow*). *B,* Monocytes attach to the endothelium. *C,* Monocytes migrate to the intima, take up cholesterol, and form fatty streaks. *D,* Platelets adhere to the endothelium and release growth factors. *F,* The result is a fibromuscular plaque. An alternative pathway is shown with arrows from *A* to *E* to *F,* with growth factor–mediated migration of smooth muscle cells from the media to the intima (*E*). (From Ross R. The pathogenesis of atherosclerosis—an update. *N Engl J Med* 314:496, 1986.)

II. RISK FACTOR IDENTIFICATION

A. RISK FACTORS FOR CORONARY ARTERY DISEASE

1. **Family history** of **myocardial infarction** (heart attack), **coronary revascularization** (bypass), or sudden death in your first-degree relatives (parent, sibling, child)

   a. Your male first-degree relatives (parent, sibling, child) < 55 years of age

   b. Your female first-degree relatives (parent, sibling, child) < 65 years of age

2. **Cigarette smoking**—current smoker or those who have quit within the previous 6 months

3. **Hypertension**

   a. Systolic blood pressure ≥ 140 mm Hg measured on two or more separate occasions **or**

   b. Diastolic blood pressure ≥ 90 mm Hg measured on two or more separate occasions **or**

   c. Current use of medication to treat hypertension

4. **Hypercholesterolemia**

   a. Total serum cholesterol of > 200 mg/dl (5.2 mmol/L). However, if low-density lipoprotein cholesterol (LDL) is known, use LDL > 130 mg/dl (3.4 mmol/L) rather than total cholesterol of > 200 mg/dl (5.2 mmol/L) **or**

b. High-density lipoprotein cholesterol (HDL) > 35 mg/dl (0.9 mmol/L) **or**

c. Current use of medication to treat high cholesterol **or**

d. HDL > 60 mg/dl (1.6 mmol/L) is a *negative* risk factor (good, thus reducing risk)

e. The relationship between the total amount of cholesterol-transporting molecules circulating in the blood and that portion of the total that functions to remove cholesterol from the circulation is known as the total cholesterol–to–HDL ratio. A lower ratio is favorable as it decreases the risk of CAD.

5. **Impaired fasting glucose**

–Fasting blood glucose of ≥ 110 mg/dl (6.1 mmol/L) measured on at least two separate occasions

6. **Obesity**

a. Body mass index (BMI) ≥ 30 kg/m² **or**

b. Waist girth > 100 cm

7. **Sedentary lifestyle/physical inactivity**

–Persons not participating in a regular exercise program or meeting the minimal physical activity recommendations from the U.S. Surgeon General's report

B. EFFECT OF EXERCISE ON CORONARY ARTERY DISEASE RISK FACTORS

1. Ongoing participation in an appropriate program of aerobic exercise can have a positive effect on risk factor status. Additionally, exercise may decrease the severity of risk associated with risk factors not directly affected by exercise.

2. The risk associated with increasing age is less for active than for inactive individuals.

3. The risk associated with cigarette smoking is less among chronically active adults compared with their sedentary counterparts.

C. ADDITIONAL EXERCISE RISK CONCERNS

–Presence of any of the following may require consultation with medical professionals prior to participation in physical activity or prior to any major increases in physical activities or habits.

1. **Signs and symptoms of cardiopulmonary disease**

a. Pain, discomfort (or other **anginal** [heart-related chest pain] equivalent) in chest, neck, jaws, and/or arms that may be due to **ischemia** (insufficient blood flow)

b. Shortness of breath at rest or with mild exertion

c. Dizziness or **syncope** (fainting)

d. **Orthopnea** (labored breathing in the recumbent position that is relieved by elevating the shoulders and head) or **paroxysmal nocturnal dyspnea** (labored breathing during sleep that often results in sudden panicky awakenings and is relieved by sitting upright)

e. Ankle **edema** (swelling)

f. **Palpitations** (unusually strong or rapid heart beats) or **tachycardia** (unusually fast heart beats)

g. Intermittent claudication (pain and decreased function of muscles due to decreased blood flow to the limbs resulting from obstructive peripheral vascular disease)

h. Known heart murmur

i. Unusual fatigue or shortness or breath with usual activities

2. **Cardiovascular abnormalities**

a. **Anemia** (low hemoglobin concentration, sometimes due to a low red blood cell concentration)

b. Inappropriate resting blood pressure or heart rate

   (1) Resting **hypertension** (≥ 140/90 mm Hg measured on two or more separate occasions)

   (2) Resting **bradycardia** (unusual slow heart rate, < 60 beats/min at rest) or tachycardia (heart rate > 100 beats/min)

c. Inappropriate exercising blood pressure or heart rate

   (1) Failure of heart rate to increase as exercise intensity increases

   (2) Excessively high (> 260 mm Hg) systolic blood pressure or no change or a significant drop (20 mm Hg) in systolic blood pressure as exercise intensity increases

   (3) Excessively high (> 115 mm Hg) diastolic blood pressure

Table 4-2. Effects of Medications on Heart Rate, Blood Pressure, the Electrocardiogram (ECG), and Exercise Capacity

Medications	Heart Rate	Blood Pressure	ECG	Exercise Capacity
I. Beta blockers (including labetalol)	↓*(R and E)	↓(R and E)	↓ HR*(R); ↓ ischemia†(E)	↑ In patients with angina; ↓ or ↔ in patients without angina
II. Nitrates	↑(R) ↑ or ↔ (E)	↓ (R) ↓ or ↔ (E)	↑ HR(R) ↑ or ↔ HR (E) ↓ ischemia†(E)	↑ in patients with angina; ↔ or ↔ in patients without angina; ↑ or ↔ in patients with congestive heart failure (CHF)
III. Calcium channel blockers				
Felodipine Isradipine Nicardipine Nifedipine	↑ or ↔ (R and E)	↓(R and E)	↑ or ↔ HR(R and E) ↓ ischemia†(E)	↑ in patients with angina; ↔ in patients without angina
Bepridil Diltiazem Verapamil	↓ (R and E)		↓ HR (R and E) ↓ ischemia†(E)	
IV. Digitalis	↓ in patients w/atrial fibrillation and possibly CHF Not significantly altered in patients w/sinus rhythm	↔	May produce nonspecific ST-T wave changes (R) May produce ST segment depression (E)	Improved only in patients with atrial fibrillation or in patients with (CHF)
V. Diuretics	↔	↔ or ↓ (R and E)	↔ (R) May cause PVCs and "false positive" test results if hypokalemia occurs. May cause PVCs if hypomagnesemia occurs (E)	↔, except possibly in patients with CHF
VI. Vasodilators, nonadrenergic	↑ or ↔ (R and E)	↓ (R and E)	↑ or ↔ HR (R and E)	↔, except ↑ or ↔ in patients with CHF
ACE inhibitors	↔	↓ (R and E)	↔	↔, except ↑ or ↔ in patients with CHF
Alpha-adrenergic blockers	↔	↓ (R and E)	↔	↔
Anti-adrenergic agents without selective blockade of peripheral receptors	↓ or ↔ (R and E)	↓ (R and E)	↓ or ↔ HR (R and E)	↔
VII. Antiarrhythmic agents		All antiarrhythmic agents may cause new or worsened arrhythmias (proarrhythmic effect)		
Class I Quinidine Disopyramide	↑ or ↔ (R and E)	↓ or ↔ (R) ↔ (E)	↑ or ↔ HR (R) May prolong QRS and QT intervals (R) Quinidine may result in "false negative" test results (E)	↔

Continued

Table 4-2. Effects of Medications on Heart Rate, Blood Pressure, the Electrocardiogram (ECG), and Exercise Capacity *Continued*

Medications	Heart Rate	Blood Pressure	ECG	Exercise Capacity
Procainamide	↔	↔	May prolong QRS and QT intervals (R) May result in "false positive" test results (E)	↔
Phenytoin Tocainide Mexiletine	↔	↔	↔	↔
Flecainide Moricizine	↔	↔	May prolong QRS and QT intervals(R) ↔ (E)	↔
Propafenone	↓ (R) ↓ or ↔ (E)	↔	↓ HR (R) ↓ or ↔ HR (E)	↔
Class II Beta blockers (see I.)				
Class III Amiodarone	↓(R and E)	↔	↓ HR (R) ↔ (E)	↔
Class IV Calcium channel blockers (see III.)				
VIII. Bronchodilators	↔	↔	↔	Bronchodilators ↑ exercise capacity in patients limited by bronchospasm
Anticholinergic agents Methylxanthines	↑ or ↔ (R and E)	↔	↑ or ↔ HR May produce PVCs (R and E)	
Sympathomimetic agents	↑ or ↔ (R and E)	↑, ↔, or ↓ (R and E)	↑ or ↔ HR (R and E)	↔
Cromolyn sodium	↔	↔	↔	↔
Corticosteroids	↔	↔	↔	↔
IX. Antihyperlipidemic agents		Clofibrate may provoke arrhythmias, angina in patients with prior myocardial infarction Nicotinic acid may ↓ BP Probucol may cause QT interval prolongation All other hyperlipidemic agents have no effect on HR, BP, and ECG		↔
X. Psychotropic medications Minor tranquilizers	↑ or ↔ (R and E)	May ↓ HR and BP by controlling anxiety. No other effects.		↔

Table 4-2. Effects of Medications on Heart Rate, Blood Pressure, the Electrocardiogram (ECG), and Exercise Capacity *Continued*

Medications	Heart Rate	Blood Pressure	ECG	Exercise Capacity
Antidepressants	↑ or ↔ (R and E)	↓ or ↔	Variable (R) May result in "false positive" test results (E)	↔
Major tranquilizers	↑ or ↔ (R and E)	↓ or ↔	Variable(R) May result in "false positive" or "false negative" test results (E)	↔
Lithium	↔	↔	May result in T wave changes and arrhythmias (R and E)	↔
XI. Nicotine	↑ or ↔ (R and E)	↑ (R and E)	↑ or ↔ HR, May provoke ischemia, arrhythmias (R and E)	↔, except ↓ or ↔ in patients with angina
XII. Antihistamines	↔	↔	↔	↔
XIII. Cold medications with sympathomimetic agents	Effects similar to those described in sympathomimetic agents, although magnitude of effects is usually smaller			↔
XIV. Thyroid medications Only levothyroxine	↑ (R and E)	↑ (R and E)	↑ HR May provoke arrhythmias ↑ ischemia (R and E)	↔, unless angina worsened
XV. Alcohol	↔	Chronic use may have role in ↑ BP (R and E)	May provoke arrhythmias (R and E)	↔
XVI. Hypoglycemic agents Insulin and oral agents	↔	↔	↔	↔
XVII. Dipyridamole	↔	↔	↔	↔
XVIII. Anticoagulants	↔	↔	↔	↔
XIX. Anti-gout medications	↔	↔	↔	↔
XX. Antiplatelet medications	↔	↔	↔	↔
XXI. Pentoxifylline	↔	↔	↔	↑ or ↔ in patients limited by intermittent claudication
XXII. Caffeine	Variable effects depending upon previous use		May provoke arrhythmias	Variable effects on exercise capacity
XXIII. Diet pills	↑ or ↔	↑ or ↔	↑ or ↔ HR	

Key: ↑ = increase, ↔ = no effect, ↓ = decrease.
*Beta-blockers with ISA lower resting HR only slightly.
† May prevent or delay myocardial ischemia.
R = rest; E = exercise.
From *ACSM's Guidelines for Exercise Testing and Prescription*, 6th ed. Philadelphia, Lippincott Williams & Wilkins, 2000.

d. Inappropriate recovery blood pressure or heart rate

    (1) Failure of heart rate to decrease during recovery

    (2) Failure of systolic blood pressure to decrease during recover

3. **Respiratory abnormalities**

  a. **Asthma** (acute constriction of the respiratory airways resulting from hypersensitivity of the smooth muscle lining of the bronchioles that produces difficulty in ventilating the lungs), including **exercise-induced asthma** (an increased irritability of the respiratory airways occurring during or following exercise)

  b. **Bronchitis** (obstructive pulmonary disease involving inflammation of the lining of the small respiratory airways)

  c. **Emphysema** (obstructive pulmonary disease involving overinflation of the lungs due to damage to the alveoli)

4. **Metabolic abnormalities**

  a. **High body weight** (> 120% of ideal weight)

  b. **Thyroid disease**

    (1) Hypothyroidism, resulting in decreased metabolic rate and accumulation of adipose tissue

    (2) Hyperthyroidism, resulting in increased metabolic rate and tissue wasting

  c. **Hypoglycemia** (chronic low blood glucose, < 50 mg/dl)

  d. **McArdle's syndrome** (defective enzyme activity in muscle, which results in limited ability to perform strenuous exercise because of painful muscle cramps)

5. **Musculoskeletal abnormalities**

  a. **Osteoarthritis** (erosion of the articular cartilage of a joint, resulting in painful, impaired movement. It usually affects weight-bearing joints and is more common in overweight and older adults.)

  b. **Rheumatoid arthritis** (a systemic disease affecting the connective tissue. It is characterized by a thickening of articular soft tissue over the joint cartilage, which may result in erosion of the cartilage. It often involves many joints including those of the hands and feet.)

  c. **Back pain**

  d. **Prosthesis** (artificial limb or limb segment) use

6. **Acute or chronic injuries or disorders**

  a. **Joint injury**

    (1) Sprain (acute injury to ligaments, ranging in severity from first degree, in which there is minimal tearing of the ligament, to third degree, in which there is a complete tear of the ligament)

    (2) Strain (acute injury to muscle resulting from stretching or tearing; the injury ranges in severity from first degree, in which there is minimal tearing of the muscle, to third degree, in which there is a marked muscle disruption)

  b. **Skin injury**

    (1) Blister

    (2) Contusion (bruise)

    (3) Rash

  c. **Inflammation of joint or tissue capsules**

    (1) Bursitis (inflammation of the fluid-filled sac that surrounds and cushions a joint)

    (2) Shin splints (an overuse injury with pain along the medial or lateral tibial border, resulting in inflammation of the muscle or tendon or stresses to the periosteal tissues)

    (3) Tendinitis (acute or chronic inflammation of a tendon)

    (4) Tennis elbow (tendinitis in the tendon at the lateral aspect of the elbow)

  d. **Bone or cartilage disorder**

    (1) Chondromalacia (deteriorating cartilage)

    (2) Osteoporosis (decreased bone mineral content)

    (3) Stress fracture (break due to a weakened mechanical structure resulting from repetitive overloading of bones, usually occurring in the tibia or metatarsals)

  e. **Sedentary lifestyle**

    (1) Muscular **atrophy** (decrease in size)

    (2) Deficiency in muscular strength and endurance

III. RISK ASSOCIATED WITH CARDIORESPIRATORY EXERCISE

A. INAPPROPRIATE CARDIOVASCULAR RESPONSE TO EXERCISE

1. **Inappropriate heart rate response**

   –Peripheral and central stimuli combine, causing an increase in exercise HR.

   –HR should therefore increase as the workload increases. Inappropriate HR responses to exercise include:

   a. **Failure to increase with increased workload**

   b. **Failure to decrease with decreased workload**

2. **Inappropriate systolic blood pressure response**

   –SBP is an indicator of **cardiac output** and should increase with increased workload.

   –Abnormal SBP responses to aerobic exercise include:

   a. **SBP > 260 mm Hg**

   b. **Decreasing SBP (≥ 20 mm Hg) during exercise**

   c. **Failure to increase with increasing workload**

   d. **Failure to decrease with decreasing workload**

3. **Inappropriate diastolic blood pressure response**

   –Both cardiac output and **total peripheral vascular resistance** affect DBP.

   –A **normal response to increased workload is no change or a small change** in DBP.

   –Inappropriate DBP responses include > 115 mm Hg during exercise.

4. **Angina pectoris** (chest pain caused by **myocardial ischemia**) or angina-like symptoms such as discomfort in the chest area, neck, shoulder, or arm

B. SAFETY OF PEAK OR SYMPTOM-LIMITED GRADED EXERCISE TESTING

1. The risk of death during or immediately after an exercise test is ≤ 0.01%.

2. The risk of acute myocardial infarction during or immediately after an exercise test is ≤ 0.04%.

3. The risk of a complication requiring hospitalization is ≤ 0.2%.

C. SAFETY OF SUBMAXIMAL EXERCISE TESTING

–The submaximal cycle ergometer test recommended by ACSM has resulted in no reported deaths, myocardial infarctions, or morbid events.

IV. PHARMACOLOGY

A. COMMON PRESCRIPTION MEDICATIONS

–Common prescription medications can have a great effect on the human body—its functions, symptoms, and capacity for exercise (see **Table 4-2**).

–These medications can alter commonly monitored exercise parameters such as HR and BP.

–Refer to the *ACSM's Guidelines for Exercise Testing and Prescription*, 6th ed., Table A-2 (pp. 277–283). A short list of common medications and their effects on the human body follows.

1. **Antianginals**

   a. Used to reduce chest pain associated with angina pectoris

   b. Classifications

      (1) Nitrates and nitroglycerin

      –promote vasodilation in large vessels.

      (2) Beta (β)-blockers

      –inhibit the action of adrenergic neurotransmitters at the β-receptors.

      –decrease cardiac output.

      –include drugs with generic names ending in "-olol" or "-olal" as well as other drugs.

      (3) Calcium channel blockers

      –inhibit the influx of extracellular calcium into vascular smooth muscle.

      –promote peripheral vasodilation, reducing afterload.

      –include drugs with generic names ending in "-dipine" as well as other drugs.

2. **Antihypertensives**

   a. Used to reduce BP

b. Classifications

(1) Alpha (α)-blockers

–inhibit the action of adrenergic neurotransmitters at the α-receptors.

–promote peripheral vasodilation.

–include drugs with generic names ending in "-azosin" as well as other drugs.

(2) Angiotensin converting enzyme inhibitors (ACE inhibitors)

–inhibit the conversion of angiotensin I to angiotensin II.

–promote peripheral vasodilation.

–decrease sodium (and consequently water) retention.

–include drugs with generic names ending in "-pril" as well as other drugs.

(3) β-blockers (see IV.A.1.b.[2] earlier)

(4) Calcium channel blockers (see IV.A.1.b.[3] earlier)

(5) Diuretics

–increase sodium and water excretion and decrease plasma volume.

–promote chronic reduction in peripheral resistance.

3. Antiarrhythmics

a. Used to reduce or prevent the development of cardiac arrhythmias

b. Classifications

–Antiarrhythmic drugs are classified by their action on cardiac tissue.

(1) Class I—affect fast sodium channels

(2) Class II—affect β-receptors

(3) Class III—affect potassium channels

(4) Class IV—affect slow calcium channels

4. Bronchodilators

–Used to relieve asthmatic events

5. Hypoglycemics

–Used to decrease blood glucose

6. Psychotropics and tranquilizers

–Used to control anxiety, depression, and psychosis

7. Nonadrenergic peripheral vasodilators

–Used to reduce vascular resistance

8. Antihyperlipidemics

–Used to lower blood lipids, especially cholesterol

–Include drugs with generic names ending in "-vastatin" as well as other drugs.

B. "OVER-THE-COUNTER" AND COMMON USE DRUGS

1. Alcohol
2. Antihistamines
3. Caffeine
4. Cold tablets
5. Diet pills
6. Nicotine
7. Tranquilizers

C. EFFECTS OF MEDICATIONS ON EXERCISE RESPONSES

–Determining the potential effects of a medication on response to exercise involves three stages:

1. Identify the **generic name or brand name** of the drug.

2. Determine the **classification** of the drug.

3. Determine any effects on exercise or response to exercise.

ACE - pril

Alpha Blocker - azosin

Beta Blocker - olol
        - olal

Calcium Channel Blocker
        dipine

REVIEW TEST

DIRECTIONS: Carefully read all questions and select the BEST single answer.

1. Coronary artery disease is a progressive response to
   (A) high amounts of cholesterol in the diet
   (B) injury or irritation of the tunica intima
   (C) production of platelets in the blood
   (D) smooth muscle cells in the tunica media

2. Which of the following is NOT an identified arterial irritant that may lead to coronary artery disease?
   (A) Dyslipidemia
   (B) Hypertension
   (C) Immune responses
   (D) Laminar blood flow

3. Your risk for coronary artery disease increases when
   (A) as a man, you reach 65 years of age.
   (B) as a woman, you reach 65 years of age.
   (C) your brother, who is younger than 65 years, has a heart attack.
   (D) your sister, who is younger than 65 years, has a heart attack.

4. The risk for coronary artery disease is increased in adults when the serum concentration of high-density lipoprotein is
   (A) less than 35 mg/dl (0.9 mmol/L).
   (B) less than 60 mg/dl (1.6 mmol/L).
   (C) greater than 60 mg/dl (1.6 mmol/L).
   (D) greater than 200 mg/dl (5.2 mmol/L).

5. Which of the following risk factors for coronary artery disease may be beneficially affected through participation in an appropriate program of aerobic exercise?
   (A) Age
   (B) Family history of cardiovascular disease
   (C) Hypertension
   (D) Smoking

6. The term "ischemia" refers to
   (A) blockage of blood flow.
   (B) insufficient blood flow to a tissue.
   (C) insufficient oxygen content in a tissue.
   (D) obstructed blood flow in a coronary vessel.

7. McArdle's syndrome is a condition in which the
   (A) ability to perform strenuous activity is limited.
   (B) airways of the lungs become overinflated.
   (C) joint surfaces become inflamed.
   (D) resting metabolic rate is increased.

8. Which of the following is an INAPPROPRIATE cardiovascular response to an increase in exercise intensity?
   (A) A decrease of 20 mm Hg in diastolic blood pressure
   (B) A decrease of 20 mm Hg in systolic blood pressure
   (C) An increase of 30 mm Hg in systolic blood pressure
   (D) An increase of 30 beats/min in heart rate

9. The risk of an acute cardiovascular event during aerobic exercise is
   (A) approximately one event in every 100,000 hours of exercise.
   (B) increased in men who are habitually active.
   (C) increased in men who have more than one risk factor for coronary artery disease.
   (D) less in women than in men.

10. Diuretics are commonly used in the treatment of
    (A) angina.
    (B) arrhythmias.
    (C) hypercholesterolemia.
    (D) hypertension.

11. An appropriate systolic blood pressure response to graded exercise includes
    (A) an increase of systolic blood pressure up to 260 mm Hg.
    (B) a decrease of systolic blood pressure of 20 mm Hg or more.
    (C) a decrease of systolic and diastolic blood pressures with exercise.
    (D) no change in systolic blood pressure with exercise.

12. An acute restriction of the respiratory airways can have a deleterious effect on the ability to transport oxygen into and out of the lungs. An example of acute restriction is
    (A) bronchitis.
    (B) emphysema.
    (C) hypoglycemia.
    (D) asthma.

13. Which of the following is an erosion of the articular cartilage of a joint resulting in painful, impaired movement, usually affecting weight-bearing joints, and more common in overweight and older adults?
    (A) Rheumatoid arthritis
    (B) Osteoarthritis
    (C) Prosthesis
    (D) Stress fracture

14. Which of the following antihypertensive medications initially increase sodium excretion and decrease plasma volume, followed by a reduction in peripheral resistance?
    (A) Alpha-blockers
    (B) Beta-blockers
    (C) Calcium channel blockers
    (D) Diuretics

15. Which of the following combinations of dietary intake is considered to be the best for reducing the risk of the development of coronary artery disease?
    (A) < 30% fat, < 10% saturated fat, = 300 mg/day of cholesterol
    (B) = 40% fat, < 20% saturated fat, = 400 mg/day of cholesterol
    (C) Between 30% and 40% fat, = 400 mg/day of cholesterol
    (D) = 50% fat, < 10% saturated fat, < 450 mg/day of cholesterol

16. Which of the following is the smallest and most dense lipoprotein, with the function of transporting cholesterol out of the blood and into the liver?
    (A) VLDL
    (B) IDL
    (C) LDL
    (D) HDL

17. If the total cholesterol is 240 mg/dl (6.2 mmol/L) of blood and the HDL is 60 mg/dl (1.6 mmol/L) of blood, what is the total cholesterol–to–HDL ratio?
    (A) 3
    (B) 4
    (C) 5
    (D) 6

18. Low-density lipoproteins are the principal carriers of cholesterol in the blood. The cholesterol in LDL is used for various cell functions, but is also the source of the cholesterol that contributes to the atherogenic process. What is the optimal (desirable) LDL in adults?
    (A) > 160 mg/dl (4.1 mmol/L) of blood
    (B) Between 130 and 150 mg/dl (3.4–4.1 mmol/L) of blood
    (C) < 130 mg/dl (3.4 mmol/L) of blood
    (D) There is no optimal level because it is age dependent.

19. On which combination of coronary artery disease risk factors does appropriate aerobic physical activity have the greatest effect?
    (A) Age, family history, smoking
    (B) Family history, smoking, hypertension
    (C) Smoking, hypertension, hypercholesterolemia
    (D) Hypertension, hypercholesterolemia, type 2 diabetes

20. Acebutolol (Sectral), atenolol (Tenormin), and metoprolol (Lopressor) are classified as what type of medication?
    (A) Alpha$_1$-blockers
    (B) Beta-blockers
    (C) Calcium channel blockers
    (D) Angiotensin-converting enzyme inhibitors

21. Which of the following classifications of drugs will decrease resting and exercise heart rate, decrease resting and exercise blood pressure, and increase exercise capacity in patients with angina?
    (A) Beta-blockers
    (B) Nitrates
    (C) Calcium channel blockers
    (D) Digitalis

22. Digitalis will
    (A) decrease heart rate in patients with atrial fibrillation.
    (B) increase the ventricular response in patients with third-degree atrioventricular block.
    (C) increase heart rate in patients with atrial fibrillation.
    (D) decrease exercise capacity in patients with atrial fibrillation.

23. Which of the following medications is not considered as "antiarrhythmic"?
    (A) Quinidine (Quinidex)
    (B) Procainamide (Pronestyl)
    (C) Beta-blockers
    (D) Nitrates

24. Nicotine is considered a drug because of its negative cardiovascular effects. Which of the following combinations of effects will nicotine have on the cardiovascular system at rest and during exercise?
    - (A) Decrease resting and exercise heart rate and blood pressure
    - (B) Increase resting and exercise capacity by increasing maximal heart rate
    - (C) Increase resting heart and increase resting and exercise blood pressure
    - (D) Increase resting heart rate but decrease exercise blood pressure

25. Some patients with asthma (or exercise-induced asthma) will take a sympathomimetic drug prior to engaging in exercise. These drugs may influence the interpretation of an exercise electrocardiogram because of the drugs' effect on
    - (A) exercise capacity.
    - (B) cardiac output.
    - (C) stroke volume.
    - (D) heart rate.

ANSWERS AND EXPLANATIONS

1–B. The tunica intima is the layer of a blood vessel that lies closest to the lumen. It is therefore the layer that is subjected to injurious/irritating stressors. The stressors initiate a sequence of events that result in migration of cells from the tunica media into the tunica intima and proliferation of these cells. The irritated intima is the site for an accumulation of platelets and white blood cells that release chemicals and growth factors to further increase the developing atherosclerotic lesion. The cells in the lesion accumulate cholesterol and make connective tissues and proteins that form a substantial portion of the atherosclerotic plaque.

2–D. Laminar blood flow is smooth blood flow. It is turbulent blood flow that may irritate the vessel wall. Dyslipidemia, hypertension, and immune responses are all potential sources of irritation to the vessel wall.

3–D. Age increases the risk for coronary artery disease. The risk increases when a man is older than 45 years of age or a woman is older than 55 years of age. Additionally, risk increases when a family history indicates a potential genetic/environmental propensity toward coronary artery disease. Thus, when a first-degree relative (e.g., parent, sibling, or child) has experienced a heart attack while relatively young (younger than 55 years of age for male relatives;

younger than 65 years of age for female relatives), an individual is at increased risk for coronary artery disease. A heart attack occurring in an older first-degree relative ($\geq$ 55 years of age for male relatives, $\geq$ 65 years of age for female relatives) does not increase an individual's risk for coronary artery disease.

4–A. High-density lipoproteins transport cholesterol out of the blood. Consequently, the lower the concentration, the lower will be the ability to remove cholesterol from the blood. Because the atherosclerotic process involves an accumulation of cholesterol by the smooth muscle cells and white blood cells in the developing plaque, the ability to remove cholesterol from the blood and transport it to the liver is important in reducing the risk for the development of plaque. Concentrations less than 35 mg/dl (0.9 mmol/L) are associated with this increased risk. Concentrations greater than 60 mg/dl (1.6 mmol/L) are associated with a decreased risk for coronary artery disease.

5–C. In many individuals, high blood pressure can be reduced through appropriate physical activity. The reduction can occur in either the systolic or the diastolic blood pressure, or both. Age and family history cannot be altered. The risk associated with smoking exists as long as the individual continues to smoke. However, the reduction in hypertension, as well as the improved lipid profile and reduction of a sedentary lifestyle that result from participation in appropriate physical activity, reduce an individual's overall risk for coronary artery disease, even though other risk factors exist.

6–B. Ischemia is an insufficient blood flow. The insufficiency may be caused by an obstructed or blocked blood flow, often resulting from an atherosclerotic plaque. The usual result of this insufficiency is a decrease in oxygen delivery to a tissue, as well as an insufficient removal of metabolic waste products.

7–A. McArdle's syndrome is a genetic condition that results in a deficiency of the enzyme phosphorylase. This enzyme is necessary for the utilization of glucose or glycogen in a muscle. Without the availability of these energy substrates, skeletal muscle is unable to perform high-intensity exercise. Thus, the ability to perform strenuous exercise is compromised. The medical condition involving overinflation of airways is emphysema, the condition involving inflamed joints is arthritis, and the condition increasing resting metabolic rate is hyperthyroidism.

8–B. As exercise intensity increases, there is an increase in both heart rate and stroke volume, which results in an increase in cardiac output. As cardiac output increases, systolic blood pressure increases. However, diastolic blood pressure normally stays about the same during aerobic exercise. Thus, there should be an increase in heart rate and systolic blood pressure but no large change in diastolic blood pressure with an increase in exercise intensity.

9–C. Aerobic exercise is safe for most adults. However, men who have more than one risk factor for coronary artery disease have an increased risk of a cardiovascular event during exercise compared with other men, whereas men who are habitually active have a decreased risk for cardiovascular events during exercise. There is currently no good information available on the risk for women of cardiovascular events during exercise.

10–D. Diuretics cause the body to excrete more water in the urine. The result is a decrease in body water, leading to a decrease in circulating blood volume and a consequent decrease in blood pressure.

11–A. Systolic blood pressure is an indicator of cardiac output. Cardiac output normally increases as workload increases, because the peripheral and central stimuli that control cardiac output normally increase with an increase in workload. Therefore, systolic blood pressure should increase with an increase in workload. Failure of systolic blood pressure to increase as workload increases indicates that cardiac output is not increasing.

12–D. Asthma is an acute restriction of the respiratory airways resulting from hypersensitivity of the smooth muscle lining of the bronchioles, making it difficult to ventilate the lungs. Bronchitis is an obstructive pulmonary disease involving an inflammation of the lining of the small respiratory airways. Emphysema is also an obstructive pulmonary disease involving overinflamation of the lungs as a result of damage to the alveoli. Hypoglycemia is low blood glucose.

13–B. Osteoarthritis is an erosion of the articular cartilage of a joint resulting in painful, impaired movement, usually affecting weight-bearing joints, and more common in overweight and older adults. Rheumatoid arthritis is a systemic disease affecting the connective tissue that is characterized by a thickening of articular soft tissue over the joint cartilage, which may result in erosion of the cartilage. A prosthesis is an

artificial limb, and a stress fracture is a break caused by a weakened mechanical structure resulting from repetitive overloading of bones, usually occurring in the tibia or metatarsals.

14–D. Alpha-blockers inhibit the action of adrenergic neurotransmitters at the alpha-receptors, thus promoting peripheral vasodilation. Beta-blockers inhibit the action of adrenergic neurotransmitters at the beta-receptors, thus decreasing cardiac output. Calcium channel blockers inhibit the influx of extracellular calcium into vascular smooth muscle, thereby promoting peripheral vasodilation. Diuretics initially increase sodium excretion and decrease plasma volume, followed by a reduction in peripheral resistance.

15–A. Cholesterol is a fat that is synthesized by the liver or ingested in animal fat and carried in the blood in the form of lipoproteins. It is essential in the formation of various digestive components and hormones. Cholesterol is also a component of cell membranes and nerve tissues. If taken in excess, however, it can increase the likelihood of atherosclerosis. The recommended dietary guidelines are < 30% fat, with only 10% coming from saturated sources. In addition, the diet should be limited to equal 300 mg/day of cholesterol.

16–D. High-density lipoproteins carry cholesterol away from the arteries and back to the liver for metabolism. The HDL is often referred to as the "good" cholesterol because of this function. It is a positive risk factor for the development of coronary artery disease if the HDL is less than 35 mg/dl (0.9 mmol/L) of blood and a negative risk factor for the development of coronary artery disease if the level of HDL is greater or equal to 60 mg/dl (1.6 mmol/L) of blood.

17–B. Divide 240 by 60 to determine the ratio of total cholesterol to HDL ($240 \div 60 = 4$).

18–C. As with total cholesterol, lower LDL reduces the risk of developing coronary artery disease. The most desirable level of LDL is less than 130 mg/dl (3.4 mmol/L) of blood.

19–D. Unfortunately, regular physical exercise has no influence on the aging process, family history, or smoking regardless of whether it is aerobic or anaerobic or any combination of aerobic and anaerobic. Regular exercise, however, decreases both systolic and diastolic blood pressure (hypertension), increases HDL (hypercholesterolemia), and improves glucose tolerance in type 2 diabetics.

20–B. Alpha$_1$-blockers include drugs such as prazosin (Minipress) and calcium channel blockers include diltiazem (Cardizem) and nifedipine (Procardia). Angiotensin-converting enzyme inhibitors include captopril (Capoten) and enalapril (Vasotec). Acebutolol (Sectral), atenolol (Tenormin), and metoprolol (Lopressor) are beta-blockers.

21–A. Beta-blockers increase exercise capacity in patients who have angina. They decrease or have no effect on exercise capacity in patients without angina. Beta-blockers will decrease both resting and exercise heart rate and decrease blood pressure. Nitrates increase resting heart rate, but decrease resting blood pressure and increase exercise capacity. Calcium channel blockers may decrease or increase heart rate at rest depending on the type of medication and improve exercise capacity in patients with angina. Digitalis will decrease the ventricular rate in patients with atrial fibrillation, but not significantly in patients with normal sinus rhythm and will improve exercise capacity in patients with atrial fibrillation.

22–A. Digitalis decreases the number of electrical impulses through the atrioventricular node in the presence of atrial fibrillation. By this action, the ventricular response to atrial depolarization is decreased, thus decreasing the rate. Digitalis also strengthens the vigor of ventricular contraction.

23–D. Quinidine (Quinidex) is a class I antiarrhythmic medication as is procainamide (Ponestyl). Beta-blockers are considered to be class II antiarrhythmic agents. Nitrates are vasodilators and have no effect on rhythm.

24–C. Nicotine will increase resting and submaximal exercise heart rate and blood pressure and will have no effect on exercise capacity. Some patients with angina may experience a decrease in exercise capacity.

25–D. Sympathomimetic agents such as ephedrine (Adrenalin), metaproterenol (Proventil), and albuterol (Bronkosol) may increase resting and exercise heart rate but will have no effect on exercise capacity. The exercise electrocardiogram is affected only by the heart rate, which may be caused only by the drug effect and not by the subject's exercise capacity.

CHAPTER 5

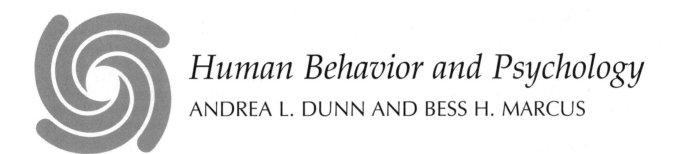

Human Behavior and Psychology
ANDREA L. DUNN AND BESS H. MARCUS

I. PSYCHOLOGICAL THEORIES: THE FOUNDATION FOR BEHAVIOR CHANGE

A. WHAT IS A THEORY?

—Within the field of behavior change, a **theory** is a set of assumptions that account for the relationships between certain variables and the behavior of interest.

—**Explanatory theories** have been developed to explain certain behaviors.

—**Other theories** have been developed to **guide interventions** (e.g., trying to create a change in some behavior, such as increasing physical activity).

B. HOW ARE PSYCHOLOGICAL THEORIES USED IN THE HEALTH AND FITNESS SETTING?

–Psychological theories provide the foundation for the effective use of the strategies and techniques of counseling and motivational skill-building for exercise adoption and maintenance.

–Psychological theories provide **a conceptual framework** for: (1) assessments, (2) development of programs or interventions, (3) application of cognitive-behavioral principles, and (4) evaluation of program effectiveness.

1. Assessments

–are performed **to establish baseline measures** of behavioral or psychological constructs and **to assess change.**

–help one **to understand where assistance might be required** (e.g., building confidence).

–Assessments **naturally lead to focusing on intervention strategies** (e.g., setting and achieving realistic fitness goals to build confidence).

2. Development of programs or interventions

–Interventions or programs can be designed to:

a. Build the skills of participants
b. Correct misunderstandings
c. Clarify relationships
d. Negotiate and solve problems
e. Establish a supportive relationship
f. Provide a target for follow-up

3. Application of cognitive-behavioral principles

–Cognitive-behavioral principles are the methods used within programs to improve motivational skills as suggested by the assessment.

–**Example:** Setting several small, short-term goals to attain a long-term goal is likely to increase self-efficacy (self-confidence, to be discussed in more detail later) as the person successfully reaches each short-term goal on the way to attaining the long-term goal.

4. Evaluation of program effectiveness

–The same cognitive-behavioral principles can be used to determine improvement.

–**Example:** If baseline self-efficacy for exercise was low, then appropriate application of behavioral tools should increase self-efficacy.

C. PSYCHOLOGICAL THEORIES HAVE LIMITATIONS.

–Most theories in psychology have been developed to explain the behaviors of individuals or small groups. They **cannot always explain the behavior of larger groups,** such as communities.

–Psychological theories **may leave out many important elements that may influence behavior,** such as sociocultural elements.

II. THEORIES USED TO ENCOURAGE EXERCISE ADOPTION AND MAINTENANCE AND TO IMPROVE ADHERENCE

–In 1996, The Surgeon General's Report on Physical Activity and Health cited studies of various psychological theories of behavior change.

A. LEARNING THEORIES

–propose that an overall **complex behavior arises from many small simple behaviors.**

–propose that by **reinforcing "partial behaviors"** and **modifying cues** in the environment, it is possible to **shape** the desired behavior.

1. **Reinforcing "partial" behaviors**

   –Reinforcement is **the positive or negative consequence** for performing or not performing a behavior.

   –**Reinforcement can be simple,** such as saying "Good job!" to participants who have performed an exercise correctly or achieved an exercise goal.

   –**Reinforcement can be more complex,** such as earning points to earn incentives (e.g., T-shirts for exercising 3 days or more a week over a period of a month).

   –**Positive consequences are rewards that motivate behavior.**

   a. **Intrinsic rewards** are the benefits gained because of the rewarding nature of the activity. For example, an intrinsic reward would be feeling good about being able to perform an activity or skill, such as finally being able to run one mile or to increase the speed of walking 1 mile.

   b. **Extrinsic or external rewards** are the positive outcomes received from others. This can include encouragement and praise or material reinforcements, such as T-shirts and money.

2. **Modifying cues in the environment**

   –**External or internal stimuli (cues)** can signal behaviors. For example, many traditional gym-based programs have participants keep gym clothes packed **(cues)** to remind them that they are ready to go to the gym.

   a. Behaviors can be **habitual** (e.g., coming home from work, turning on the television, and sitting down for the remainder of the evening).

   b. Behaviors can be **cued from the engineered environment** (e.g., the easy availability of elevators compared with stairways discourages stair-climbing).

   c. **Internal cues** such as fatigue or boredom can makes one feel "too tired" to exercise.

3. **Limitations of reinforcing behaviors and modifying cues**

   a. The techniques of modifying cues and providing reinforcement seem to be **more effective for helping people adopt a behavior than for maintaining a behavior.**

   b. For those who are not ready to start an exercise program or who need help maintaining exercise, **additional tools or strategies for change are required.**

B. THE HEALTH BELIEF MODEL ASSUMES THAT PEOPLE WILL ENGAGE IN A BEHAVIOR (I.E., EXERCISE) WHEN

–there is a perceived threat of disease.

–there is the belief of susceptibility to disease.

–the threat is severe.

1. Taking action depends on whether the **benefits outweigh the barriers.**

2. This model also incorporates **cues to action** as critical to adopting and maintaining behavior.

3. The concept of **self-efficacy** (self-confidence) has also been added to the Health Belief Model.

C. THE TRANSTHEORETICAL MODEL OF CHANGE (STAGES OF CHANGE OR STAGES OF MOTIVATIONAL READINESS)

–This model incorporates constructs from other theories including **intention to change** and **processes (or strategies) of change.**

1. The basic concepts of this model are as follows:

   a. People progress through five stages of change at varying rates.

   b. In the process of changing, people move back and forth along the stage continuum.

   c. People use different cognitive and behavioral processes or strategies.

2. **Stages of change** or **motivational readiness** describe five categories of readiness to change or maintain behavior. As applied to physical activity or exercise, they are as follows:

   a. **Stage 1: Precontemplation**

      –There is no physical activity or exercise occurring and there is **no intention to start** within the next 6 months.

   b. **Stage 2: Contemplation**

      –There is no physical activity or exercise, but there is **intention to start** within the next 6 months.

   c. **Stage 3: Preparation**

      –There is **participation in some physical activity** or exercise, but not at levels meeting the Centers for Disease Control and Prevention/American College of Sports Medicine (CDC/ACSM) 1995 recommendations or current ACSM exercise prescription guidelines.

   d. **Stage 4: Action**

      –The person is engaged in **physical activity or exercise that meets CDC/ACSM recommendations** for physical activity or the ACSM guidelines but has not maintained this program for 6 months or more.

   e. **Stage 5: Maintenance**

      –**Exercise or activity** has been occurring **for 6 months or longer.**

3. Other key components of the Transtheoretical Model are the **processes of behavior change.**

   –**Processes** are various behavioral or cognitive **skills or strategies** that are applied during the different stages of change.

   –There are numerous applications depending on the **stage of readiness.**

   –In general, **cognitive processes** are the most efficient strategies **for early stages** and **behavioral processes** are the most efficient strategies **for later stages.**

   a. The **five cognitive processes** include:

      (1) **Consciousness raising** (increasing knowledge)

      (2) **Dramatic relief** (warning of risks)

      (3) **Environmental reevaluation** (caring about consequences to oneself and others)

      (4) **Self-reevaluation** (comprehending benefits)

      (5) **Social liberation** (increasing healthy opportunities)

   b. The **five behavioral processes** include:

      (1) **Counterconditioning** (substituting alternatives)

      (2) **Helping relationships** (enlisting social support)

      (3) **Reinforcement management** (rewarding yourself)

      (4) **Self-liberation** (committing yourself)

      (5) **Stimulus control** (reminding yourself)

D. **THE RELAPSE PREVENTION MODEL**

   –incorporates **identifying high-risk situations** and **developing plans** for coping with high-risk situations.

   –An important element of this model is to learn how to **restructure thinking** in order to **distinguish between a lapse and a relapse** and to **develop flexibility** in the approach for attaining exercise and physical activity goals.

E. **THE THEORY OF REASONED ACTION AND ITS LATER EXTENSION, THE THEORY OF PLANNED BEHAVIOR**

   –postulate that **intention** is the most important determinant of behavior.

   –In turn, attitudes and subjective norms influence intention (**Figure 5-1**).

   1. **Attitudes** are determined by positive and negative beliefs about the **outcome** or about the **process of performing** the behavior.

   2. **Subjective norms** are influenced by the perceptions about what others think or believe (**normative beliefs).**

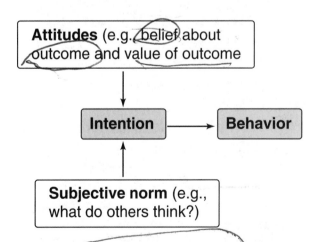

FIGURE 5-1 The Theory of Planned Behavior postulates that intentions influence behavior and that attitudes and subjective norms influence intentions. (Modified from Ajzen I, Fishbein M: *Understanding Attitudes and Predicting Social Behavior.* Upper Saddle River, NJ, Prentice Hall, © 1980, p 8. Adapted by permission of Prentice Hall.)

3. **The Theory of Planned Behavior** extends the Theory of Reasoned Action by incorporating **perceived behavioral control,** which is determined by **perceived power** and **control beliefs.**

F.　SOCIAL COGNITIVE THEORY

–is one of the most widely used and comprehensive theories of behavior change.

–This dynamic model asserts there are **three major interacting influences: behavior, personal,** and **environmental (Figure 5-2).**

–The theory contains **several different concepts or constructs** that are implicated in adoption and maintenance of healthy behavior and are used for purposes of increasing and maintaining physical activity or exercise:

1. **Observational learning** says that people can learn by watching others model a behavior and perceiving the rewards that another person receives for engaging in the behavior. This is sometimes called **vicarious reward.**

2. **Behavioral capability** means that the person has both the knowledge and the skill to perform the behavior.

3. **Outcome expectations and outcome expectancies** are the anticipated benefits from engaging in the behavior.

   –**Outcome expectations** are what the person **anticipates the outcome will be** for performing the behavior.

   –**Outcome expectancies** are the **values** of that outcome.

4. **Self-efficacy** is the confidence about performing a **specific behavior.** This construct has been **one of the strongest predictors of adopting a program of regular exercise** in many populations and in many settings.

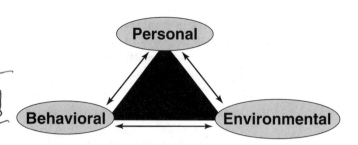

FIGURE 5-2 Social Cognitive Theory takes into account reciprocal relationships between the personal, behavioral, and environmental factors.

5. **Self-control of performance** refers to self-regulatory skills when directed toward a specific goal. This includes the concepts of **self-monitoring** and **goal setting.**

6. **Management of emotional arousal** is the ability to deal with emotions appropriately by:

   –**cognitive restructuring** (thinking about the problem in a more constructive manner).

   –**stress management techniques** for controlling symptoms of emotional distress.

   –**learning methods of effective problem solving.**

7. **Reinforcement** is derived from **operant learning theories,** which state that behavior is controlled by the consequences of the behavior and that behavior will increase if **positive reinforcement is applied** or if a **negative reinforcement is removed.** In social cognitive theory, there are **three types** of reinforcement:

   –**Direct reinforcement,** as described in operant conditioning

   –**Vicarious reinforcement,** as described in observational learning

   –**Self-reinforcement,** as one would apply as a self-control technique

III.　APPLYING CONCEPTS FROM THEORIES TO THE EXERCISE SETTING

A.　ASSESSING PARTICIPANTS AND DEVELOPING STRATEGIES TO INCREASE EXERCISE ADHERENCE

–Various assessments can be used to determine behavioral needs as well as strategies to encourage initiation, adherence, and return to participation if an individual has experienced a relapse.

1. **Assessing benefits and barriers** entails using a **decisional balance sheet.**

–All of the client's perceptions about exercise programs, both **negative** (lack of time) **and positive** (feeling more energetic), are written on a sheet of paper.

–Helping individuals see the **benefits of exercising** can increase the likelihood of participation in an exercise program.

–**Helping a client to problem-solve** by removing barriers to exercise, one by one, can help the client learn how to find time and enjoyment and can decrease the reasons for not being able to maintain a program of regular exercise.

–As a client finds more reasons to become active and reduces reasons for inactivity, the **decisional balance tips in the positive direction** and improves adherence.

2. **Assessing self-efficacy (confidence)** means determining the degree to which individuals believe that they can perform the desired behavior.

   a. Self-efficacy can be assessed by the use of **a paper-and-pencil questionnaire.** Using a 1-to-5 or a 1-to-10 scale, individuals rank how confident they are that they could exercise when it is raining or snowing, when they feel they don't have time, when they are tired, and so forth.

   b. **Four ways to increase self-efficacy:**

      (1) Performance accomplishments

      –**Example:** Setting a goal of walking 1 mile in 1 month by gradually increasing the weekly distance.

      –Assist by helping to set **realistic specific short- and long-term goals.**

      (2) Vicarious experience.

      –**Example:** "This person is like me; if she can do it, then I probably can."

      (3) Verbal persuasion

      –**Example:** Helping the person see how he or she might be able to understand the feasibility of a goal and a way to accomplish it.

      –Provide continuous reinforcement and feedback.

      (4) Physiologic states

      –Get the person to recognize and monitor the number of positive feelings that come from exercise.

      –Increase the use of **self-monitoring techniques** such as keeping an exercise log and counting steps using a mechanical step counter.

3. Techniques from learning theories, such as **shaping, reinforcement,** and **antecedent control,** have been used to increase adoption and maintenance of exercise.

   a. **Shaping** is setting a series of intermediate goals that lead to a long-term goal. Shaping is especially appropriate:

      –when applied to **increasing frequency, intensity, duration, or types** of activities.

–in initiating exercise programs where the **long-term goals may be too difficult for a novice.**

   b. **Reinforcement** should be scheduled to occur during and after exercise to offset any possible immediate negative consequences (e.g., feeling hot, sweaty, and out of breath). **Reinforcement** can take the form of:

      –**verbal encouragement.**

      –**material incentives** (based on **specific contingency contracts).**

      –**"natural" reinforcements** such as stress relief and self-praise.

   c. **Antecedent control** uses techniques that prompt the initiation of behavior, including such prompts as:

      –telephone reminders.

      –packing a gym bag for the next day before going to bed.

      –scheduling time for exercise in a daily schedule.

4. **Cognitive restructuring techniques** involve changing thought processes about a particular situation. These are particularly important for **adoption and maintenance of activity,** as well as for **relapse prevention.**

   a. **Relapse prevention strategies** include having the participant **identify high-risk situations** that may lead to a lapse. **Plans are then developed prior to a lapse.** If the lapse occurs, the plan is in place and a relapse is less likely.

   b. **Elimination of "all-or-none" thinking**

      –A momentary lapse in a regular exercise routine does not label a participant as a failure and subsequently lead to stopping exercising altogether.

      –This technique helps correctly label the lapse as a slight disruption and helps problem-solve the resumption of regular exercise. *Plan for LAPSES!*

B. **UNDERSTANDING CONFIDENCE LEVEL, PERCEIVED BENEFITS, AND BARRIERS**

   –This provides a focus for the exercise professional to **set realistic goals** and gradually shape and increase exercise behavior.

   –As the client progresses, it is important to continue to set goals **and plan for possible lapses.**

C. USING THE STAGES OF CHANGE MODEL TO INCREASE ADHERENCE (SEE ALSO II C)

1. Precontemplation

   –**Discussing benefits, what can be learned from previous attempts and the change process** may assist during this stage. For example, many people decide to become a regular exerciser and then have difficulty maintaining a regular program.

   a. Clients at this stage **may not be aware of the risks** associated with being sedentary or **may have become discouraged** by previous attempts to stay active and have feelings of failure. Multiple attempts may be required to succeed.

   b. The exercise professional should not assume that the participant in a precontemplation stage is ready for an exercise program.

   c. **Counseling should center on achievable goals** at which success is relatively certain (e.g., a 2-minute walk during the work week). This may not be the desired or long-term outcome, but using a gradual process of shaping, the exercise behavior can become more frequent and longer.

2. Contemplation

   –Contemplators believe the reasons for being inactive (e.g., I am too tired, exercise takes too much time) outweigh the benefits of initiating exercise. Useful approaches at this stage are as follows:

   –**Discuss the benefits of exercise** and **help the client problem-solve** to eliminate barriers. These techniques should increase the client's confidence level and self-efficacy.

   –**Encourage setting specific short-term goals** (e.g., exercise for 10 minutes on 1 to 7 specific days).

3. Preparation

   –**Irregular exercise behavior** is the hallmark of this stage.

   a. Discussing **further reductions of barriers** and **continued building of self-efficacy** is important.

   b. **Monitoring gains** and **rewarding achievement of goals** are two methods for increasing confidence.

   c. **Shaping by reinforcing small steps** toward action is also important. Gradually increasing time, intensity, and adherence to exercise will assist in achieving recommended levels of exercise behavior.

4. Action

   –People in the action stage are at the **greatest risk of relapse.**

   a. Instruction on **avoiding injury, exercise boredom, and burnout** is important to those who have recently begun an exercise program.

   b. Providing **social support** (e.g., asking how it is going) and praise are the most important contributors to maintained activity.

   c. **Planning for high-risk relapse situations** such as vacations, sickness, bad weather, and increased demands on time is important. The exercise professional can emphasize that a short lapse in activity can be a learning opportunity and is not failure. Planning can help to develop coping strategies and to eliminate "all-or-none" thinking sometimes typical of people who miss several exercise sessions and think that they need to give up.

5. Maintenance

   –After 6 months of regular activity, individuals are considered to be in the maintenance stage of exercise adoption.

   a. Some coping strategies have been developed, but **risk for dropping out remains present.**

   b. **Scheduling check-in appointments** can help the maintainer stay motivated.

   c. **Continued feedback** is important. If a maintainer is absent for several sessions, a **prompt such as a telephone call or letter noting the absence** can help to re-establish maintenance.

IV. EFFECTIVE COUNSELING TIPS

A. USING A THREE-FUNCTION MODEL OF PARTICIPANT-CENTERED EDUCATION AND COUNSELING

1. During **information gathering,** any or all of the following areas should be assessed for participants:

a. Current level of knowledge

b. The attitudinal beliefs, intentions, and readiness to change

c. Past experiences with exercise or physical activity skills

d. Behavioral skills

e. Available social support

2. In **developing a helping relationship,** it is important to **understand the process** and to **establish support.**

 a. An effective process is **interactive,** assesses information central to the issues, **asks questions** of the participant, **instructs,** and takes into account a willingness to **negotiate.**

 b. **To establish a supportive relationship:**

 (1) **Exhibit empathy** by restating expressed emotion (e.g., "This seems frustrating to you").

 (2) **Legitimize concerns** (e.g., "I can understand why you might be concerned with travel out of town").

 (3) **Respect abilities and positive efforts** (e.g., "You've worked hard to get this far").

 (4) **Support** by providing **reinforcement and follow-up** (e.g., "I'll be available to help you get on track and stay on track").

 (5) **Partner** by stating your willingness to work together (e.g., "You won't be alone, I will be there to help you").

3. **Participant education and counseling** is a multifactorial process that may involve various situations and issues. In order to effectively counsel about readiness to change, it is necessary to understand that **waning motivation to exercise is universal.** Effective counseling can assist a person who is experiencing a lapse (i.e., short break) to prevent it from turning into a relapse (i.e., longer period of inactivity) or a collapse (i.e., no plans for returning to exercise).

 a. During each counseling session, the **five A's** should be used:

 (1) **Address the agenda:** "I'd like to talk to you about. . ."

 (2) **Assess:** "What do you know about. . .?" "How do you feel?" "What are you considering. . .?"

 (3) **Advise:** "I'd advise. . ."

 (4) **Assist:** "How would you like for me to help you?" "What problems do you foresee?"

 (5) **Arrange follow-up:** "We will set up a time for you to let me know how you did. . ."

 b. Most sedentary people are not motivated to initiate exercise programs and, if exercise is initiated, it is likely to stop within 3–6 months.

 c. Participants in earlier stages benefit most from **cognitive strategies** such as listening to lectures and reading books without the expectation of actually engaging in exercise, whereas individuals in later stages depend more on **behavioral techniques** such as reminders to exercise and developing social support to help them establish a regular exercise habit and be able to maintain it.

B. RECOGNIZING AND ACKNOWLEDGING INDIVIDUAL DIFFERENCES

–There are **many ways to achieve a regular** exercise or physical activity routine. The recent Surgeon General's report on physical activity and health states that **moderate intensity lifestyle activity (e.g., brisk walking, gardening) performed for a total of 30 minutes at least five times a week** produces important health benefits. Some participants may feel more comfortable with this type of **home-based approach** rather than using an exercise facility where appearance and skill might be noticed by others. Other participants may not perceive that they can achieve 30 minutes continuously and may not be aware that activity benefits can be achieved by accumulating shorter bouts. **Intermittent activity prescriptions counteract the "all-or-none" thinking** (e.g., "I can't exercise for an hour so I might just as well not exercise at all") that leads to relapse.

C. DEALING WITH DIFFICULT CLIENTS

–Despite the best efforts, some clients are difficult to work with. Issues related to interaction with the exercise professional must be resolved before it is possible to achieve exercise goals. **Types of difficult clients and suggestions for dealing with them are as follows:**

1. The **dissatisfied client** is never pleased regardless of all efforts to please.

 a. The exercise professional must work hard at all times to remind the client that **the goal is to assist in achieving exercise adherence.**

 b. If dissatisfaction remains after developing all possible options, **state the options, acknowledge they may not be ideal,** and **ask the client for the preferred option.**

2. The **needy client** wants more support than can be given. A primary goal of needy individuals is often to gain attention. The exercise professional should:

–**establish specific expectations** of what is possible.

–**remain focused** on the exercise or physical activity issues and behavioral skills related to those issues.

–remind the participant that the goal is health education and exercise adherence.

–refer the client for additional help (e.g., professional counseling from a nutritionist or physician) if necessary.

3. The **hostile client** may try to elicit hostility in return. It is important to **maintain professionalism.**

–**Acknowledge** the anger.

–Try to **determine whether you should address the underlying issue** or ask the client what would make him or her feel less angry.

–If there is chronic hostility, **a different exercise leader** may help ameliorate the situation.

4. The **shy client** is usually pleasant, but not talkative. Try asking probing and **open-ended questions** instead of questions that just require yes/no answers.

V. PROBLEMS EXCEEDING YOUR LEVEL OF EXPERTISE

–Referrals to other resources may be required when participants have **health problems** that may limit the types of exercise that can be performed.

A. PARTICIPANTS WITH EXISTING HEALTH PROBLEMS OR PERCEIVED HEALTH LIMITATIONS MAY BE REFERRED TO A PRIMARY CARE PHYSICIAN FOR FURTHER EVALUATION OR REASSURANCE.

B. PARTICIPANTS WITH PSYCHOLOGICAL ISSUES (E.G., POOR COPING; DIFFICULTY MANAGING STRESS, DEPRESSION, OR ANXIETY; CHRONIC COMPLAINTS OF BEING OVERWHELMED) SHOULD BE REFERRED TO A PROFESSIONAL COUNSELOR OR A PHYSICIAN FOR EVALUATION.

1. **Symptoms of depression or anxiety** (Table 5-1) are serious; participants with these symptoms should be referred to a physician or professional counselor as soon as possible.

2. **Anxiousness prior to a fitness assessment** may be accompanied by high heart rate and rapid, shallow breathing. **Techniques for reducing pretest anxiety** include the following:

–Have the person sit quietly and do **deep breathing exercises.**

–**Give thorough explanations** and **allow practice** on unfamiliar equipment.

–**Schedule an additional practice session** on equipment to increase the participant's familiarity with staff, equipment, and setting.

3. **Persons with eating disorders** should be referred to a physician or mental health professional.

Table 5-1. Symptoms of Depression and Anxiety

Symptoms of Depression	Symptoms of Anxiety
• Feeling sad or "down in the dumps" for more than 2 weeks	• Panic attacks (sudden episodes of fear and physiologic arousal which occur for no apparent reason)
• Tearfulness	
• Withdrawal from social activities	• Increased nervousness associated with going into crowded places like the mall or a gym
• Excessive guilt	• Feeling "keyed up" or "on edge" most of the time
• Rapid weight loss or weight gain	
• Feelings of fatigue	
• Changing sleep patterns, e.g., early morning awakening	
• Expressions of wanting to be dead or wanting to die	

REVIEW TEST

DIRECTIONS: Carefully read all questions and select the BEST single answer.

1. Theories are used in programs for
   (A) giving individuals an exercise prescription.
   (B) perceiving rewards of certain behaviors.
   (C) self-reevaluation.
   (D) providing a conceptual framework for behavioral assessment.

2. Which stage of motivational readiness would a person who is an irregular exerciser be in?
   (A) Precontemplation
   (B) Contemplation
   (C) Preparation
   (D) Action

3. Setting several short-term goals to attain a long-term goal to increase self-efficacy is an example of
   (A) an application of cognitive-behavioral principles.
   (B) an evaluation.
   (C) a relationship to theory.
   (D) an explanatory theory.

4. A limitation of theories in psychology is
   (A) they do not reinforce behavior.
   (B) they leave out important elements such as sociocultural factors.
   (C) they make too many assumptions.
   (D) they cannot evaluate programs.

5. The idea that intention is the most important determinant of behavior is a central component of the
   (A) Relapse Prevention Model.
   (B) Social Cognitive Theory.
   (C) Theory of Planned Behavior.
   (D) Transtheoretical Model.

6. The Social Cognitive Theory postulates that which three major dynamic interacting influences determine behavior change?
   (A) Personal, behavioral, environmental
   (B) Reinforcement, commitment, social support
   (C) High-risk situations, social support, perceived control
   (D) Stage of readiness, processes of change, confidence

7. A decisional balance sheet is used to
   (A) assess barriers and benefits for physical activity or exercise.
   (B) determine a person's self-efficacy.
   (C) determine a person's readiness to change behavior.
   (D) all of the above

8. An individual would NOT increase self-efficacy by
   (A) performance accomplishments.
   (B) vicarious experience.
   (C) verbal persuasion.
   (D) using a decision balance sheet.

9. People in which stage are at the greatest risk of relapse?
   (A) Precontemplation
   (B) Contemplation
   (C) Preparation
   (D) Action

10. Which of the following strategies can help a person maintain his or her physical activity?
    (A) Schedule check-in appointments.
    (B) Reduce barriers.
    (C) Increase benefits.
    (D) All of the above educate them about different types of exercise.

11. Referrals to other sources may be required if someone
    (A) has health problems.
    (B) reports symptoms of depression.
    (C) has an eating disorder.
    (D) all of the above

12. Establishing specific expectations of what you are willing to do as a counselor and staying focused on exercise/physical activity issues and behavioral skills related to exercise are strategies for handling which type of client?
    (A) A dissatisfied client
    (B) A needy client
    (C) A hostile client
    (D) A shy client

13. Encouraging moderate-intensity activity and the accumulation of activity throughout the day are examples of
    (A) Relapse Prevention Counseling.
    (B) using the Stages of Change.
    (C) allowing for individuality in exercise choices.
    (D) addressing the individual's agenda.

14. Which of the following is an example of a behavioral process in the Transtheoretical Model?
    (A) Consciousness raising
    (B) Stimulus control
    (C) Dramatic relief
    (D) Environmental reevaluation

15. One mistake that health care providers and exercise promoters make is to
    (A) assume that most individuals are ready to change their behavior.
    (B) encourage the accumulation of moderate-intensity activity throughout the day.
    (C) legitimize a client's concerns.
    (D) use the five A's strategy for counseling (address the agenda, assess, advise, assist, arrange follow-up).

16. The concept of "shaping" refers to
    (A) using self-monitoring techniques such as exercise logs.
    (B) using visual prompts (e.g., packing a gym bag the night before) as reminders to exercise.
    (C) the process for establishing self-efficacy.
    (D) setting intermediate goals that lead to a long-term goal.

17. Verbal encouragement, material incentives, self-praise, and use of specific contingency contracts are examples of
    (A) shaping.
    (B) reinforcement.
    (C) antecedent control.
    (D) goal-setting.

18. The three functions of the "participant-centered education and counseling model" include
    (A) identifying high-risk situations, developing a plan for these situations, and eliminating all-or-none thinking.
    (B) information gathering, developing a helping relationship, and participant education and counseling.
    (C) exhibiting empathy, legitimizing a client's concerns, and forming a partnership.
    (D) assessing, asking questions, and establishing a supportive relationship.

19. The Transtheoretical Model assumes that individuals
    (A) move through the stages of behavioral change at a steady pace.
    (B) only progress forward through the stages.
    (C) move back and forth along the stage continuum.
    (D) tend to use behavioral processes in the earlier stages of change.

20. If an individual is in the Action stage, he or she
    (A) intends to start exercising in the next 6 months.
    (B) participates in some exercise, but does so irregularly.
    (C) has been regularly physically active for less than 6 months.
    (D) has been regularly physically active for more than 6 months.

21. Which does NOT help to establish a supportive relationship?
    (A) Exhibit empathy.
    (B) Legitimize concerns.
    (C) Respect the person's abilities and efforts.
    (D) Address the agenda.

22. The five A's of counseling are
    (A) Address, Assess, Act, Assist, Arrange follow-up
    (B) Address, Assess, Advise, Assist, Act
    (C) Address, Assess, Advise, Assist, Arrange follow-up
    (D) Act, Assess, Advise, Assist, Arrange follow-up

23. To assist anxious people prior to an exercise test, you could
    (A) ask them to sit quietly in a chair for a few minutes.
    (B) thoroughly explain the exercise test.
    (C) familiarize them with the exercise equipment by brief practice.
    (D) all of the above

24. Which of the following is (are) NOT symptoms of depression?
    (A) Hearing voices
    (B) Change in sleep patterns
    (C) Irritability
    (D) All of the above

25. Which of the following is (are) symptoms of anxiety?
    (A) Panic attacks
    (B) Increased nervousness
    (C) Feelings of being "on edge"
    (D) All of the above

ANSWERS AND EXPLANATIONS

1–D. Psychological theories are the foundation for effective use of strategies and techniques of effective counseling and motivational skill-building for exercise adoption and maintenance. Theories provide a conceptual framework for assessment, development of programs or interventions, application of cognitive-behavioral or motivational principles, and evaluation of program effectiveness. Within the field of behavior change, a theory is a set of assumptions that account for the relationships between certain variables and the behavior of interest.

2–C. The stages of motivational readiness describe five categories of readiness to change or maintain behavior. As applied to physical activity or exercise, they are Precontemplation (Stage 1, there is no physical activity or exercise occurring and there is no intention to start within the next 6 months); Contemplation (Stage 2, there is no physical activity or exercise, but there is intention to start within the next 6 months); Preparation (Stage 3, there is participation in some physical activity or exercise but not at levels meeting current and standard guidelines); Action (Stage 4, the person is engaged in physical activity or exercise that meets standard guidelines for physical activity but has not maintained this program for at least 6 months); and Maintenance (Stage 5, exercise or activity has been occurring for 6 months or longer).

3–A. Applications of cognitive-behavioral principles are the methods used within programs to improve motivational skills suggested by the assessment. For example, setting several small short-term goals to attain a long-term goal is likely to increase self-efficacy as the person successfully reaches each short-term goal on the way to attaining the long-term goal.

4–B. A limitation of most theories in psychology is that they have been developed to explain behaviors of individuals or small groups and, therefore, are limited in terms of understanding larger groups such as communities and may leave out many important elements that may influence behavior such as sociocultural elements. Despite these limitations, theories of behavior change provide important tools to help change exercise behavior.

5–C. The Theory of Planned Behavior postulates that intention is the most important determinant of behavior. In turn, attitudes and subjective norms influence intention. Attitudes are determined by positive and negative beliefs about the outcome or about the process of performing the behavior. Subjective norms are influenced by the perceptions about what others think or believe. The Theory of Planned Behavior extends the Theory of Reasoned Action by incorporating perceived behavioral control, which is determined by perceived power and control beliefs.

6–A. The Social Cognitive Theory is one of the most widely used and comprehensive theories of behavior change. This is a dynamic model that asserts that there are three major interacting influences: behavior, personal and environmental. Social Cognitive Theory contains a number of different concepts or constructs that are implicated in adoption and maintenance of healthy behavior and are used for purposes of increasing and maintaining physical activity or exercise. They include observational learning, behavioral capability, outcome expectations, self-efficacy, self-control of performance, management of emotional arousal, and reinforcement.

7–A. Various assessments can be utilized to determine behavioral needs and to determine strategies to encourage initiation, adherence, and return to participation if an individual has experienced a relapse. Assessing benefits and barriers entails using a decisional balance sheet. All of the perceived negative (e.g., lack of time) and positive (e.g., feeling more energetic) consequences for participating or not participating in exercise are written on a sheet of paper. This procedure can assist participants by reminding them of immediate and long-term positive consequences and helping to problem-solve negative consequences. Removing or resolving problem-solving barriers, one-by-one, can help with learning how to find time and enjoyment by decreasing the reasons for not being able to maintain a program of regular exercise. As a participant finds more reasons to become active and reduces reasons for inactivity, the decisional balance tips in the positive direction and improves adherence.

8–D. Self-efficacy (confidence) is the degree to which individuals believe they can perform the desired behavior. It is possible to increase self-efficacy in four ways: performance accomplishments (setting a goal of walking 1 mile in 1 month by gradually increasing the weekly distance), vicarious experience ("This person is like me, if she can do it then I probably can"), verbal persuasion (helping the person see how he or she might be able to understand the feasibility of a goal and a way to accomplish it), and physiologic states (getting the person to recognize and monitor the number of positive feelings that come from exercise). A decisional balance sheet would be used to assess benefits and barriers.

9–D.   People in the Action Stage are at the greatest risk of relapse. Instruction on avoiding injury, exercise boredom, and burnout is important to those who have recently begun an exercise program. Providing social support and praise are the most important contributors to maintained activity. Planning for high-risk, relapse situations such as vacations, sickness, bad weather, and increased demands on time is important. The exercise professional can emphasize that a short lapse in activity can be a learning opportunity and is not failure. Planning can help to develop coping strategies and to eliminate "all-or-none" thinking sometimes typical of people who have missed several exercise sessions and think they need to give it up.

10–A.   After 6 months of regular activity, individuals are considered to be in the maintenance stage of exercise adoption. Some coping strategies have been developed, but the risk of dropping out remains. Scheduling check-in appointments can help the maintainer to stay motivated. Continued feedback is also important. If a maintainer is absent for several sessions, a prompt such as a telephone call or letter noting the absence can help to reestablish maintenance.

11–D.   Referrals to other resources may be required when participants have health problems that may limit the types of exercise that can be performed. Existing health problems or perceived health limitations may be referred to a primary care physician for further evaluation and/or reassurance. Psychological issues such as poor coping; difficulty managing stress, depression, or anxiety; or chronic complaints of being overwhelmed should be referred for professional counseling and/or to a physician for evaluation. Symptoms of depression or anxiety are more serious and should be referred to a physician or professional counseling. Persons with eating disorders should be referred to a physician or mental health professional.

12–B.   Despite the best efforts, working with some clients is difficult. Issues related to interaction with the exercise professional must be resolved before it is possible to achieve exercise goals. The needy client wants more support than can be given. It is important, then, to establish specific

expectations of what is possible and remain focused on the exercise or physical activity issues and behavioral skills related to those issues. A primary goal of the needy individual is often to gain attention, and it is important to remember that the goal is health education and exercise adherence. It is also important to remember that the exercise professional is not a trained counselor and in some cases it may be appropriate to refer the client for additional help.

13–C.   Recognizing and acknowledging individual differences is an important component of effective counseling. There are many ways to achieve a regular exercise or physical activity routine. Many participants may not perceive that they can achieve 30 minutes of continuous physical activity and they may not be aware that activity benefits can be achieved by accumulating shorter bouts. Intermittent activity prescriptions counteract the "all-or-none" type of thinking that often leads to relapse.

14–B.   Key components of the Transtheoretical Model are the Processes of Behavior Change. These processes include five behavioral processes (counterconditioning, helping relationships, reinforcement management, self-liberation, and stimulus control) and five cognitive processes (consciousness raising, dramatic relief, environmental reevaluation, self-reevaluation, and social liberation).

15–A.   Participants progress through various stages of change at varying rates, and in the process of changing, move back and forth along the stage continuum. Different cognitive and behavioral processes or strategies are used during each stage. Discussing the benefits of physical activity and learning from previous attempts may assist those in the precontemplation stage. This group may not be aware of the risks associated with being sedentary or may have become discouraged by previous attempts to stay active and have feelings of failure. Multiple attempts may be required to succeed. The exercise professional should not assume that the participant in the precontemplation stage is ready for an exercise program.

16–D.   Shaping is setting a series of intermediate goals that lead to a long-term goal. This is especially appropriate when applied to increasing frequency, intensity, duration, or types of activities. When initiating exercise programs where the long-term goals may be too difficult for a novice, this strategy is particularly appropriate.

17–B. Reinforcement should be scheduled to occur during and after exercise to offset any possible immediate negative consequences. Reinforcement can take the form of verbal encouragement, material incentives (based on contingency contracts), and natural reinforcements such as stress relief and self-praise.

18–B. Effective counselors can use a three-function model of participant-centered education and counseling. The three functions of this model are information gathering, developing a helping relationship, and participant education and counseling.

19–C. The Transtheoretical Model of Change (Stages of Change or Stages of Motivational Readiness) incorporates constructs from other theories, including intention to change and processes (or strategies) of change. The basic concepts of this model are that people progress through five stages of change at varying rates and in the process of changing, they also move back and forth along the stage continuum. They also use different cognitive and behavioral processes or strategies.

20–C. Stages of motivational readiness describe five categories of readiness to change or maintain behavior. As applied to physical activity or exercise, they are Precontemplation (Stage 1), Contemplation (Stage 2), Preparation (Stage 3), Action (Stage 4), and Maintenance (Stage 5). The Action Stage is when the person is engaged in physical activity or exercise that meets the ACSM recommendations for physical activity but has not maintained this program for 6 months or more.

21–D. Effective counselors can use a three-function model of participant-centered education and counseling. The three functions of this model are information gathering, developing a helping relationship, and participant education and counseling. To establish a supportive relationship, exhibit empathy by restating expressed emotion, legitimize concerns, respect abilities and positive efforts, support by providing reinforcement and follow-up, and partner by stating your willingness to work together.

22–C. Participant education and counseling is a multifactorial process that may involve a variety of situations and issues. For example, in order to effectively counsel about readiness to change, it is necessary to understand that waning motivation to exercise is universal. Effective counseling can assist a person who is experiencing a lapse (i.e., short break) to prevent it from turning into a relapse or collapse. During each counseling session, the five A's should be used: Address the Agenda, Assess, Advise, Assist, and Arrange follow-up.

23–D. Anxiousness prior to a fitness assessment may be accompanied by high heart rate and rapid, shallow breathing. This may be alleviated by having the person sit quietly and using deep-breathing exercises. Thorough explanations and practice on unfamiliar equipment can also reduce anxiety prior to exercise testing. Scheduling an additional practice session on equipment to increase familiarity with staff, equipment, and setting may assist those unable to reduce pretest anxiety.

24–A. Symptoms of depression or anxiety are serious and should be referred to a physician or professional counselor. Symptoms of depression include feeling sad or "down in the dumps" for more than a few weeks, tearfulness, withdrawal from social activities, excessive guilt, rapid weight loss or weight gain, feelings of fatigue, changing sleep patterns (e.g., early morning awakening), or expressions of wanting to be dead or wanting to die.

25–D. Symptoms of anxiety include panic attacks (sudden episodes of fear and physiologic arousal that occur for no apparent reason), increased nervousness associated with going into crowded places like the mall or a gym, or feeling "keyed up" or "on edge" most of the time.

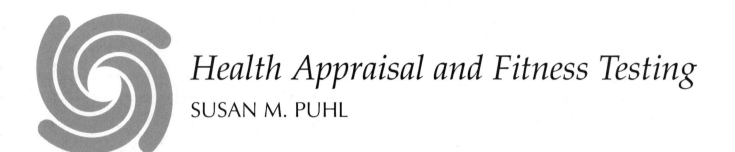

CHAPTER 6

Health Appraisal and Fitness Testing
SUSAN M. PUHL

I. PRETEST CONSIDERATIONS

A. HEALTH SCREENING

1. **Purpose**

   a. **Safety**

   –Provides health and fitness professionals with information that can lead to **identification of individuals for whom exercise is contraindicated.**

   b. **Risk factor identification**

   –Many medical conditions increase the health risk associated with physical activity or exercise testing.

   –Health screening allows the health/fitness professional to **determine who may participate** and **who should be referred to a physician** prior to participation in exercise testing or physical activity.

   c. **Exercise prescription and programming**

   –Information gathered allows health/fitness professional to **develop specific exercise programs appropriate to the individual needs** and goals of the client.

2. **Types**

   a. **General screening for participation in self-directed exercise**

   –Individuals who choose to begin a self-directed exercise program should be advised, at a minimum, to **complete a quick screening** of health status using such tools as the **PAR-Q.**

   b. **Screening for fitness assessment and exercise prescription**

   –In commercial settings, clients should be more extensively screened for potential health risks.

   –The information solicited should include the following:

   (1) Personal medical history

   (2) Current medical status

   (3) Medications

   (a) Prescription (type and dosage)

   (b) Over-the-counter (type and dosage)

   (4) Family history of medical conditions

   (5) Lifestyle considerations

   (a) Nutritional habits

   (b) Exercise habits

   (c) Stress

   (d) Smoking

   (e) Alcohol consumption

3. **Administration**

   a. **Timing**

   –Screening tools must be administered **prior to the** delivery of a fitness assessment or the initiation of an exercise program and **reviewed by the fitness professional before** any exercise testing/activity occurs.

   –**Contraindications** to exercise testing or activity **should stimulate referral** to the appropriate health care professional.

   b. **Setting**

–In order to solicit reliable information, the questionnaire should be completed in a **quiet, private area.**

–**Review the responses** with the client to confirm the accuracy of the information and to determine the health risk status.

B. INFORMED CONSENT

1. **Purpose**

   a. **Ethical considerations**

   –A well-designed consent form provides the client with sufficient information to enable an **informed decision** about participation.

   –It **details the expectations** of the client so that full participation is possible.

   b. **Legal concerns**

   –Although not a legal document, the use of a well-designed consent form provides written documentation that the client was made aware of the procedures, limitations, **risks** and **discomforts,** as well as the **benefits of exercise.**

2. **Limitations**

   –**Does not provide legal immunity** to a facility or individual in the event of injury to a client.

   –**Does provide evidence** that the client was made aware of the **purposes, procedures, and risks** associated with the test or exercise program.

   –Negligence, improper test administration, inadequate personnel qualifications, and insufficient safety procedures are **expressly not covered** by informed consent.

   –**Legal counsel** should be sought during the development of the document.

3. **Content**

   a. **Purpose**

   b. **Procedures** explained in lay terminology

   c. Potential **risks** and **discomforts**

   d. Expected **benefits**

      (1) To the participant

      (2) To society

   e. **Responsibilities** of the participant

   f. Provision of an **opportunity to ask questions** and have them answered

   g. **Confidentiality of results**

   h. **Right** of participant **to refuse or withdraw** from any aspect of the procedures

   i. **Signatures**

      (1) Participant

      (2) Test supervisor/administrator

      (3) Guardian for those younger than 18 years of age

      (4) Witness

   j. **Dates** of signatures

4. **Administration**

   –The consent form should be presented to the client in a **private, quiet setting.**

   –The order of activities associated with the completion of the document should be as follows:

   a. Private, quiet **reading** of the document

   b. Private, **verbal explanation** of the contents of the document with a verbally expressed **opportunity to ask questions** for which answers are provided

   c. **Signing and dating** the document

   d. **Presentation of a copy** of the signed document to the participant, for his or her keeping

II. RISK FACTOR IDENTIFICATION AND STRATIFICATION

A. PURPOSE

1. **Identification of high-risk individuals**

   a. Individuals with **contraindications** leading to potential exclusion from testing or exercise

      (1) **Absolute contraindications**— conditions that should result in **exclusion** from exercise testing or programming **until the conditions have stabilized**

      (2) **Relative contraindications**— conditions for which **careful evaluation of the risk/benefit ratio**

   should be made before proceeding with exercise testing or programming

   b. Individuals with **disease symptoms or risk factors that require medical evaluation** prior to testing or exercise

   c. Individuals with **clinically significant disease** who require medical supervision

   d. Individuals with **special testing or exercise needs**

2. **Selection of appropriate activities**

   a. **Assessments**

   b. **Exercise programming**

B. RISK STRATIFICATION

1. Low risk

–Men younger than 45 years of age and women younger than 55 years of age who are asymptomatic and meet no more than one risk factor threshold listed in Chapter 4, section II. A. (Risk Factors for Coronary Artery Disease)

2. Moderate risk

–Men age 45 years or older and women age 55 years or older or those who meet the threshold for two or more risk factors listed in Chapter 4, section II. A. (Risk Factors for Coronary Artery Disease)

3. High risk

a. Individuals with one or more of the symptoms listed in Chapter 4, section II. C. 1. (Signs and Symptoms of Cardiopulmonary Disease) **or**

b. Individuals with known cardiovascular disease (cardiac, peripheral vascular, cerebrovascular) **or**

c. Individuals with known pulmonary disease (chronic obstructive pulmonary disease, asthma, interstitial lung disease, cystic fibrosis) **or**

d. Individuals with known metabolic disease (diabetes mellitus types 1 and 2, thyroid disorders, renal disease, liver disease)

C. USING RISK STRATIFICATION

–Following identification of a client's risk status, the exercise leader or health/fitness instructor should make an informed decision as to whether or not the individual should be tested or permitted to exercise, according to the guidelines provided in Table 2-2 in the *Guidelines for Exercise Testing and Prescription,* 6th edition.

III. FITNESS ASSESSMENT: GENERAL CONSIDERATIONS

A. PURPOSE

1. Education

–A well-planned and implemented battery of fitness assessment provides information to current and potential clients about the various aspects of health-related fitness. The results of fitness assessment provide a client with information useful in making possible lifestyle decisions.

2. Exercise prescription

–Data collected via appropriate fitness assessments assists the health/fitness instructor to develop safe, effective programs of exercise based on the individual client's current fitness status.

3. Evaluation of progress

–Baseline and follow-up testing provides evidence of progression toward fitness goals.

4. Motivation

–Fitness assessment provides information needed to develop reasonable, attainable goals. Progress toward, or attainment of, a goal is strong motivation for continued participation in an exercise program.

5. Risk stratification

–Results of fitness assessment can sometimes detect the presence of risk factors, which may influence both the exercise prescription and subsequent assessment.

B. RISKS ASSOCIATED WITH EXERCISE TESTING

1. Peak or symptom limited testing

a. The risk of death during or immediately after an exercise test is $\leq 0.01\%$

b. The risk of acute myocardial infarction during or immediately after an exercise test is $\leq 0.04\%$.

c. The risk of a complication requiring hospitalization is $\leq 0.2\%$.

2. Submaximal exercise testing

–The submaximal cycle ergometer test recommended by the ACSM has resulted in no reported deaths, myocardial infarctions, or morbid events when care has been taken to ensure careful client screening, client compliance with appropriate pretest instructions, and appropriate supervision during the test.

C. SAFETY

–To maximize safety during the assessment, each of the following items should be assessed.

1. Site

a. **Emergency plans**

(1) Written, posted emergency **plans**

(2) Posted emergency **numbers**

(3) Regularly scheduled practices of responses to emergency situations,

including a minimum of one **announced** and one **unannounced** **drill**

   b. **Room layout**

      –The equipment and floor space should be arranged **to allow safe** exit from the facility in an emergency and **to prevent accidental upsetting of equipment.**

2. **Equipment**

   a. **Maintenance**

      –Develop a **written document that includes** procedures for all daily, weekly, and monthly activities **associated with maintaining** each piece of equipment.

   b. **Positioning**

      –The equipment used for testing should be **positioned to ensure maximal visual supervision** of the client.

   c. **Cleanliness**

      –Develop a **written document that includes procedures** for all daily, weekly, and monthly activities **associated with cleaning** each piece of equipment.

3. **Personnel**

   a. **Certifications** (cardiopulmonary resuscitation [CPR], American College of Sports Medicine Health/Fitness Instructor [ACSM H/FI])

   b. **Training**

D.   ACCURACY

–Can be affected by many external factors. Attempts should be made to control each of the following:

1. **Test environment**

   –The physical condition of the test area should **reduce anxiety and promote physical comfort.**

   –Care should be taken to ensure that each of the following elements of an appropriate testing site has been addressed fully:

   a. **Privacy**

   b. **Cleanliness**

   c. **Quiet**

   d. **Temperature** (70°F to 74°F, 21°C to 23°C) and **relative humidity** (≤60%)

   e. **Ventilation** (6–8 air exchanges per hour)

   f. **Comfortable** seat and table

   g. All necessary testing **equipment** and **supplies**

2. **Pretest preparation** of the client

   –The client should perform the test in an **optimal physical state** if possible.

–To ensure this, the following items should be expressly requested of the client:

   a. Appropriate, comfortable, **loose-fitting clothing**

   b. Adequate **hydration**

   c. **Avoidance of alcohol, tobacco, caffeine, and food** for an appropriate period of time before testing—usually at least **3 hours**

   d. **Avoidance of strenuous exercise** or physical activity on the day of the test

   e. **Adequate sleep** the night prior to the assessment

E.   OBJECTIVITY

–To ensure that the test administrator does not influence test results, the following elements should be addressed:

1. **Standardization** of:

   a. **Procedures**

   b. **Protocols**

2. **Checklists** for completion of:

   a. **Pretest**

   b. **Testing**

   c. **Debriefing**

F.   EASE OF ADMINISTRATION

–Both frequency of use and client satisfaction may be improved by using an assessment that is relatively easy to administer.

–Ease of administration can be affected by the following:

1. **Personnel**

   a. **Clarity of directions** for test performance and termination

   b. **Availability of equipment**

   c. **Manipulation of posttest data**

   d. **Availability of appropriate norms**

2. **Client**

   a. **Clarity of directions** for performance and termination

   b. **Familiarity with equipment**

   c. **Familiarity with testing mode** (e.g., walking, cycling)

G.   CONFIDENTIALITY

–Provisions for the confidential use and storage of client data should be made prior to any testing.

–Such provisions may include the following:

1. **Client ID numbers**

2. **Locked files** or computer

3. **Restricted access** to client data

H. TEST ORDER

–When a battery of fitness assessments is administered to a client in a single session, the following order of tests is recommended:

1. **Resting measurements** (e.g., heart rate, blood pressure, blood analysis)

2. **Body composition**

–Some methods of assessing body composition are sensitive to the hydration status. Because some tests of cardiorespiratory or muscular fitness may have an acute effect on hydration, it is inappropriate to conduct such assessments before the body composition assessment.

3. **Cardiorespiratory fitness**

–Assessments of cardiorespiratory fitness often use **heart rate** as a predictive measurement. Assessing muscular fitness or flexibility can produce an increase in heart rate. The cardiorespiratory assessment must therefore be conducted prior to any other assessment that may affect heart rate.

4. **Muscular fitness**

–When assessing both muscular and cardiorespiratory fitness in the same day, muscular fitness should be assessed after cardiorespiratory fitness.

–Strenuous assessments of cardiorespiratory fitness should be followed by an **appropriate recovery period** before tests of muscular fitness are attempted.

5. **Flexibility**

–Flexibility is most appropriately assessed when the body is **fully warmed.**

I. TEST TERMINATION

–Clearly written instructions and regular practice will help to ensure that an assessment is conducted in a manner that is both safe and provides valid, useful information.

1. **Criteria for stopping a test**

   a. **Attainment of desired performance**

   –The fitness professional must be familiar with the testing procedures to ensure **recognition of the desired endpoint** of the assessment.

   b. **Client or equipment complications**

   –Signs and symptoms consistent with guidelines for test cessation (see Box 5-3, p 104, in *ACSM's Guidelines for Exercise Testing and Prescription,* 6th edition.)

   –Equipment failure.

   –Subject asks to stop.

2. **Procedures**

   a. **Non–life-threatening situations**

   –An active cool-down should be completed.

   b. **Life-threatening situations**

   –The client should be removed from the testing equipment, and the site's emergency plan should be put into operation.

J. INTERPRETATION OF RESULTS

1. **Data reduction**

   –Equations used to predict a fitness score should be appropriate to both the tests conducted and the client.

2. **Normative data**

   a. **Selection**

   –The norms against which results are compared should meet the following criteria:

   (1) Appropriate to the test administered

   (2) Appropriate to the age, gender, and history of the client

   b. **Standard error of the estimate**

   –The standard error of the estimate is an indication of the error of the estimate compared with the actual measurement of the variable.

   –Knowledge of the standard error of the estimate associated with a test is critical to the appropriate interpretation of the results.

   –Reports to clients should clearly indicate the error associated with the testing.

3. **Repeated assessment**

   a. **Methods**

   –Follow-up assessment of any fitness component should **use the same test,** including procedures and protocols, as that used during the original assessment. It is therefore essential to keep precise records of all assessments.

   b. **Timing**

   –Repeat testing should be conducted only **after sufficient time for alteration in the fitness component is assessed.** The fitness professional should therefore be aware of the time course needed for physiologic adaptations.

   c. **Significance of any differences**

   –Care should be taken when interpreting small changes in fitness scores. Often, such changes are within the error of estimate of the procedures used.

IV. ASSESSING BODY COMPOSITION

A. DEFINITION

–The **relative proportions of fat vs. fat-free (lean) tissue** in the body

–Commonly reported as "**percent body fat**," thus identifying the proportion of the total body mass composed of fat

–**Fat-free mass** is then determined as the **balance of the total body mass.**

B. RATIONALE

1. Excess body fat

–Associated with **increased risk** for cardiovascular disease, pulmonary dysfunction, orthopedic difficulties, type 2 diabetes mellitus, and certain cancers

–Knowledge of a client's body composition **can assist in determining an appropriate program** of exercise and nutrition for optimal health status.

2. Insufficient body fat

–Some individuals lose too much body weight in an attempt to be eligible for participation in selected sports or to meet unrealistic societal preferences for physical appearance.

–These individuals often decrease body fat to unhealthy levels.

–Knowing the body composition of such clients can assist in working with them to set and reach realistic body composition goals.

C. METHODS

1. Hydrodensitometry (hydrostatic weighing, underwater weighing)

a. **Theoretical basis**

–The **standard** against which other methods of body composition estimation are based

–**Bone mineral is more dense than muscle tissue, which is more dense than fat.**

–Determining an overall measure of body density can thus be used to predict the proportion of the body that is composed of fat.

b. **Procedures**

–Measurement of dry body mass, submerged mass, and residual lung volume allows the calculation of body density and thus the estimation of body fat.

c. **Common sources of error**

(1) Measurement of **residual volume** of air in lungs

(2) Interindividual variability in the **amount of air in the gastrointestinal tract**

(3) Interindividual variability in the **density of individual lean tissue compartments**

d. **Accuracy when used appropriately**

–**Approximately 2% to 3% error** in the estimation of percent body fat

2. Skinfold measurement

a. **Theoretical basis**

–Based on the assumption that the amount of fat present in the subcutaneous regions of the body is proportional to overall body fatness

b. **Procedures**

(1) Locate the sites to be measured.

(2) Measure the skinfold thickness.

(3) Use the measurements of skinfold thickness in the appropriate estimation equation to predict body composition.

c. **Common sources of error**

(1) Incorrect site location

(2) Placement of thumb and forefinger on the site, rather than 1 cm away from the site

(3) Incorrect lifting of skinfold

(4) Inaccurate reading of the caliper

(5) Use of inappropriate equation

d. **Accuracy when used appropriately**

–Approximately **4% error** in the estimation of percent body fat

3. Anthropometry

a. **Theoretical basis**

–Measurements of height, weight, and/or girths provide information about the relative distribution of body mass compared with "standard" distributions.

–The addition of anthropometric measurements to skinfold measurements may be used to predict body fatness.

b. **Procedures**

–Height and weight should be measured, and appropriate sites for the anthropometric measures are required.

c. Common sources of error

(1) Inaccurate stance for assessing height

(2) Unfamiliarity with the use of balance scales

(3) Incorrect location of circumference site

(4) Incorrect placement of the tape measure around the body segment to be measured

(5) Inappropriate tension in the use of the tape measure

d. **Accuracy when used appropriately**

–Approximately 3%–8% error

e. **Special uses of anthropometry**

(1) **Body mass index (BMI)**

–The BMI, sometimes called the Quetelet index, is a common tool based on body mass and height.

(2) **Waist-to-hip ratio (W/H)**

–Individuals who deposit excess body fat over the trunk area appear to be at greater health risk than those who deposit it over the hips and thighs.

–W/H ratios **above 0.95 (for men) or 0.86 (for women)** are associated with greater risk for the development of such diseases as hypertension, type 2 diabetes, hyperlipidemia, and coronary artery disease.

4. **Bioelectrical impedance analysis (BIA)**

a. **Theoretical basis**

–The body is composed of two compartments: one rich in electrolytes, which conducts an electrical current readily (the fat-free mass), and one with few electrolytes and therefore resistant to the flow of electrical current (the fat mass).

–Measuring the resistance of the body to induced electrical current provides information that can be used to estimate body fatness.

b. **Procedures**

–Following appropriate skin preparation, electrodes are affixed, the current is applied, and the impedance to the current is measured. The impedance is then used to predict body fat.

c. **Common sources of error**

(1) Inappropriate skin preparation

(2) Inaccurate electrode placement

(3) Lack of adherence to pretest diet/exercise recommendations

(4) Use of inappropriate prediction equation

(5) Inadequate hydration

(6) Body temperature

d. **Accuracy when used appropriately**

–Approximately 3.5%–5% error

5. **Near-infrared spectrophotometry (NIR)**

a. **Theoretical basis**

–Different types of tissues in the body (e.g., fat versus muscle) have different optical properties.

–Introduction of a known light source, and subsequent measurement of its "reflection" from internal tissues, can be used to estimate overall body composition.

b. **Procedures**

–An emitter/sensor wand is placed over the site to be assessed (e.g., the belly of the biceps). An infrared light beam is emitted. The sensor in the wand detects the reflected beam.

–Variables associated with the reflected beam are entered into an equation along with gender, height, weight, body frame, and activity level to arrive at an estimate of body fatness.

c. **Common sources of error**

(1) Inaccurate placement of the wand

(2) Incorrect assessment of body frame or activity level

d. **Accuracy when used appropriately**

–**Unacceptably high** errors, ranging from 4%–11%

V. ASSESSING CARDIORESPIRATORY FITNESS (AEROBIC FITNESS)

A. DEFINITION

–The coordinated capacity of the heart, blood vessels, respiratory system, and tissue metabolic systems to take in, deliver, and use oxygen

B. RATIONALE

–Measurement of cardiorespiratory fitness provides information about the ability to engage in tasks that require repetitive use of most of the large muscles—activities such as walking and climbing stairs.

–The assessment serves as an indication of the types of tasks that the client can safely perform, and provides a basis for the development of safe, effective aerobic exercise programs.

C. METHODS

1. Types of tests

a. Maximal

–Direct measurement of maximal oxygen consumption ($\dot{V}O_{2\,max}$) is the **standard** for the determination of cardiorespiratory endurance.

–The client performs a graded exercise test, in which the workload is progressively increased until an increase in workload elicits no further increase in oxygen consumption.

b. Submaximal

–Because the actual measurement of $\dot{V}O_{2\,max}$ is technically demanding, **the use of submaximal tests to estimate actual $\dot{V}O_{2\,max}$ is common practice.**

–Submaximal tests are based on the correlation between the following:

(1) Actual $\dot{V}O_{2\,max}$ and such physiologic responses as heart rate during submaximal workloads. **Examples** are:

(a) Graded-intensity, multiple-stage tests on cycle ergometers, treadmills, or steps, (e.g., YMCA protocol cycle ergometer test)

(b) Single-stage tests on any type of quantifiable ergometer after which recovery heart rate is measured (e.g., 3-minute step test)

(2) Actual $\dot{V}O_{2\,max}$ and performance in quantifiable events. **Examples** are:

(a) Time to walk or run a fixed distance (e.g., Rockport One-Mile Fitness Test, or Cooper 1.5 mile run)

(b) Distance covered in a fixed time (e.g., Cooper 12-minute walk/run)

2. Basic skills needed to assess cardiorespiratory fitness

a. Heart rate determination

(1) Palpation

–Heart rate can be determined by counting the number of pulses in a given period of time (10–30 seconds).

–The most common sites at which the pulse may be palpated include:

(a) The radial pulse

(b) The carotid pulse

(2) Auscultation

–A stethoscope may be placed over the left aspect of the mid-sternum, or just under the pectoralis major.

–The heart rate may be counted as the number of heart beats in a given period of time (10–30 seconds).

(3) Electronic monitoring

(a) Radio frequency transmitters

–A chest strap with embedded electrodes is fastened around the chest just under the pectoral muscles. The electrodes sense the electrical current associated with the electrical activity of the heart to measure heart rate.

(b) Pulsatile blood flow monitors

–Sensors affixed to the ear lobe or finger sense the pulsing of blood. Some devices are currently not effective in monitoring exercise heart rate.

b. Blood pressure measurement

(1) Equipment

(a) Sphygmomanometer, with three important components:

–A cloth cuff placed around the upper arm. Encased in the cuff is a bladder made of rubber or similar material.

–A diaphragmatic bulb and valve used to increase or decrease the pressure in the cuff.

–A mercury column or aneroid (air pressure) manometer, used to indicate the pressure in the cuff.

(b) Stethoscope, with two important components:

–A diaphragm to focus sound waves

–Earpieces to direct the sound waves

c. Rating of perceived exertion (RPE) determination

–RPE provides the exercise professional with an indication of a subjective assessment of the relative intensity of the exercise.

–RPE correlates well with such physiologic measures as percent of maximal heart rate and percent $\dot{V}O_{2\,max}$.

Currently there are two widely used scales for assessing RPE:

(1) Original scale

(a) Ratings are from 6–20.

(b) The scale was developed largely on the basis of the linear response of $\dot{V}o_{2\,max}$ and heart rate to changing exercise intensity.

(2) Revised scale

(a) Ratings are from 0–10.

(b) The revised scale was based on not only the $\dot{V}o_{2\,max}$ and heart rate responses to exercise, but also lactate accumulation and ventilation during exercise.

3. **Timing of measurements during assessments**

–During most graded exercise tests, the following measurements are taken at the times indicated:

a. Heart rate

(1) During a 2-minute stage: every minute

(2) During a 3-minute stage: at minutes 2 and 3, and additionally at every subsequent minute until steady state is achieved

b. Blood pressure

–Measured once during each stage, toward the end of the stage

c. Rating of perceived exertion (RPE)

–Assessed once during each stage, toward the end of the stage

d. Sequence of measurements

–For most graded exercise tests (with 3-minute stages), it is practical to take the measurements according to the following schedule:

(1) Minute 2:00–heart rate

(2) Minute 2:15–rating of perceived exertion

(3) Minute 2:30–blood pressure

(4) Minute 3:00–heart rate

4. **Equipment calibration**

–Accuracy of instrumentation is essential for valid assessments of cardiorespiratory endurance as well as to all other areas of health-related fitness.

–All equipment should be calibrated at regular intervals.

–A regular schedule for equipment calibration should be established for all testing equipment.

a. Cycle ergometer

–**Workload** is determined by **resistance × distance flywheel traveled per revolution** × revolutions per minute.

(1) Resistance

(a) On most mechanically braked ergometers, calibration requires identification of the attachment of the resistance pendulum to the resistance belt.

(b) The zero mark on the resistance indicator is checked and adjusted as required.

(c) A known weight is hung from the point at which the resistance belt is attached to the pendulum.

(d) The resistance should be checked at each resistance that might be used during testing.

(e) Any discrepancies in the resistance markings are noted on a new scale fastened over the original resistance markings.

(2) Distance per revolution

–The distance the flywheel travels per revolution of the pedal must be accurately determined by measuring the circumference of the flywheel, then determining the number of flywheel revolutions per pedal revolution.

(3) Revolutions pedaled per minute (rpm)

–Because the workload on a cycle ergometer is expressed in $kg \cdot m/min$, it is necessary to check the accuracy of the device used to determine rpm.

–A mechanical or electronic metronome may be checked for accuracy using an accurate clock or stopwatch.

b. Treadmill calibration

(1) Speed

–Calibrating the speed of a motorized treadmill requires knowledge of both the length of the treadmill belt and the number of revolutions of the belt per minute.

(a) The length of the belt may be measured using a long cloth tape or a rolling measuring device.

(b) The treadmill rpm is determined by marking a fixed point on the belt, and a

[handwritten notes in margin:]
Flywheel
Distance
= Circumference
× #flywheel
Rev/pedal Rev

corresponding point on the treadmill frame or other fixed object and measuring the time needed for a fixed number of revolutions (e.g., 20 for slower speeds, 50 for higher speeds).

(2) Grade

(a) The grade of a treadmill is expressed as the relationship of rise to run.

–The run is the distance between two fixed points on the floor or other flat surface.

–The rise is the difference between two perpendicular distances measured from the belt surface to the floor.

(b) Treadmill grade is determined by dividing the rise by the run, and expressing the result as a percent.

VI. ASSESSING MUSCULAR STRENGTH AND ENDURANCE (MUSCULAR FITNESS)

A. DEFINITION

1. Muscular strength

–The maximal force that a muscle or muscle group can generate in a single effort

2. Muscular endurance

–The ability to sustain a held submaximal force, or to continue repeated submaximal contractions

B. RATIONALE

1. Adequate levels of muscular fitness are necessary to engage in daily activities such as lifting, transporting, and maintaining the position of the body, carrying packages, and performing sport-related activities.

2. Knowledge of current muscular fitness allows appropriate programming to ensure desirable functioning of the skeletal musculature.

3. Muscular fitness is unique to each muscle or muscle group, and there is no single test of overall muscular fitness. Various assessments, including tests of the upper, middle, and lower body, are recommended.

C. METHODS

1. Muscular strength

a. Types of assessments

(1) 1-repetition maximum (1-RM)

–In practice, this requires lifting successively heavier weights until a failure point is reached. The client should rest 2–3 minutes between lifts to allow some recovery. Fatigue resulting from the prior submaximal lifts may result in inaccurate assessment of true strength.

(2) Submaximal tests to estimate strength

–Submaximal lifts to fatigue are commonly used to estimate the 1-RM.

–The weight used for the submaximal assessment must be carefully selected so that the client performs from 2–14 repetitions before fatigue.

–**Table 6-1** provides an indication of the estimated 1-RM associated with the lifting of submaximal weight to fatigue.

b. Equipment

–Common equipment includes:

(1) Free weights, such as barbells and dumbbells, which require the lifter to determine the planes of movement

(2) Variable-resistance machines, for which the plane and range of movement are limited by the machine and the resistance is increased by adding additional plates of weight to the stack lifted

(3) Isokinetic machines, which limit movement to a constant velocity

(4) Isometric equipment (e.g., handgrip dynamometers), which measure strength at a constant joint angle

c. Safety

–To reduce the risk of injury during assessments of muscular strength, the following items should be addressed:

(1) One or more properly trained spotters should assist the lifter.

(2) Proper form should be demonstrated by the exercise professional and required of the lifter.

(3) The lifter should be coached to breathe during both concentric (exhale) and eccentric (inhale) movements.

(4) Adequate rest should be provided between lifting attempts.

Table 6-1. Estimating the Percentage of Repetition Maximum from Submaximal Lifts

Number of Repetitions to Fatigue	Estimated % of Maximal Force
2	95
4	90
6	85
8	80
10	75
12	70
14	65

2. **Muscular endurance**

    a. **Common assessments**

        (1) Bench press assessment of upper body endurance

        –The number of lifts performed correctly and in time with the cadence is counted. The weight lifted may be expressed either as absolute weight lifted or as a percentage of the body weight.

        (2) Push-up assessment of upper body endurance

        –The client assumes a standardized beginning position, with the body supported by the hands and toes for men, and hands and knees for women.

        –The straight body is lowered to the floor (or, for men, to a tucked fist held under the client's chest by the examiner), then pushed back up to the starting position.

        –The score is the total number of push-ups performed properly without a pause by the client. There is usually no time limit to this test.

        (3) Sit-up assessment of abdominal muscular endurance

        –The traditional test of abdominal muscular endurance has the client performing bent-knee (to an angle of approximately 90°) sit-ups with the feet held to the floor by the examiner.

        –The score is the number of properly performed sit-ups completed in the time allotted–usually 1 minute.

    b. **Common sources of potential error**

        (1) Inaccurate positioning of the client prior to or during the assessment

        (2) Inaccurate timing of the test

        (3) Counting improperly performed repetitions

        (4) Inaccurate count of properly completed repetitions

VII. ASSESSING FLEXIBILITY

A. DEFINITION

–The **functional range of motion about a joint**

–Flexibility is specific to each joint, and therefore can vary from one joint to another.

–The functional range of motion refers to **the ability to move the joint without incurring pain** or a limit to performance.

B. RATIONALE FOR ASSESSMENT

–Inadequate flexibility is associated with decreased performance of activities of independent living and decreased ability to engage in specific physical movements.

–Flexibility can decrease quickly with chronic disuse or can improve significantly with appropriate exercise intervention.

C. METHODS

1. **Joint specificity**

    –A variety of assessments of flexibility should be completed to provide the health/fitness instructor with a profile of an overall flexibility.

2. **Equipment**

    a. **Goniometers**

        –A goniometer is a mechanical or electronic device that has two arms attached to a common axis.

        –The axis incorporates a protractor or potentiometer that allows the assessment of arc angle based on the position of the arms of the goniometer.

        –The common axis is placed over the axis of rotation of a joint and the arms of the goniometer are held steady against the body segments proximal and distal to the axis.

–The difference between starting and ending angles is the range of motion about the joint.

b. Inclinometers

–Most inclinometers are gravity-dependent instruments composed of a freely rotating weight encased within a circular scale casing.

–The instrument is strapped to or held against a moveable body part.

–The device is zeroed at full flexion and the initial reading is taken.

–The joint is then moved through the full range of motion and the final reading taken.

–The difference between starting and ending angles is the range of motion about the joint.

c. Distance measures

–Measuring the distance between a starting point and an ending point as a client moves through a range of motion is a common method of assessing flexibility.

–For example, in the new sit-and-reach test, the distance moved along a measuring stick is determined and used as an indication of lower back/hamstring flexibility.

–Other such distance measures are used as indicators of shoulder flexibility, trunk rotary flexibility, and hip flexibility.

VIII. ASSESSING FITNESS IN SPECIAL POPULATIONS

A. CHILDREN

1. Purpose

a. Assessment of health status

b. Comparison with criterion-referenced standards

c. Determination of change resulting from exercise programs

2. Considerations

a. In performing laboratory assessments of cardiovascular function, a treadmill is preferable to a cycle ergometer.

for kids

–Inexperience, local muscle fatigue, inability to maintain cadence, and/or the short attention span of children makes it difficult for many children to complete a cycle ergometer test.

b. Closure of the epiphyseal plates is not complete until after puberty. Therefore, it is **not recommended that children perform maximal tests for muscular strength.**

3. Modifications

a. **Treadmill tests**

–Keep speed constant, adjusting only the grade.

b. **Cycle ergometer tests**

–Adjustments to the ergometer, including modifications to the handlebars, seat post, and pedal crank arms are often required to fit the smaller anatomy.

4. Protocols

–Recommended field tests for assessing health-related physical fitness in children include 1 mile or 1/2-mile run/walk, BMI, pull-ups, sit-ups, push-ups, and sit-and-reach test. (A referenced list of field tests for children may be found in Table 11-1, p 218, in *ACSM's Guidelines for Exercise Testing and Prescription,* 6th edition.)

B. OLDER ADULTS

1. Purpose

–Fitness testing is conducted in older adults for the same reasons as in younger adults, including exercise prescription, evaluation of progress, motivation, and education. See section III. A. for a discussion of these purposes.

2. General considerations

a. Adults of any specified age will vary widely in their physiologic response to exercise testing.

b. Deconditioning and disease often accompany aging. These factors must be taken into account in selecting appropriate fitness test protocols.

c. Adaptation to a specific workload is often prolonged in older adults. Therefore, a prolonged warm-up, followed by small increments in workload, is recommended.

3. **Modifications**

   –Test stages in graded exercise tests should be prolonged, lasting at least 3 minutes to allow the participant to reach steady state.

4. **Protocols**

   –The selection of a protocol for assessing the cardiorespiratory fitness of older adults is based on many factors, such as low $\dot{V}O_{2\,max}$, increased fatigability, poor ambulation, or poor balance. For more information, refer to pages 223–225 in *ACSM's Guidelines for Exercise Testing and Prescription*, 6th edition.

REVIEW TEST

DIRECTIONS: Carefully read all questions and select the BEST single answer.

1. A client's health screening should be administered prior to
   (A) any contact with the client.
   (B) any physical activity by the client at your facility.
   (C) fitness assessment or programming.
   (D) the initial "walk-through" showing of a facility.

2. A well-designed consent document developed in consultation with a qualified legal professional provides your facility with
   (A) documentation of good-faith effort to educate your clients.
   (B) legal documentation of a client's understanding of assessment procedures.
   (C) legal immunity against lawsuits.
   (D) no legal benefit.

3. Relative contraindications for exercise testing are conditions for which
   (A) a physician should be present during the testing procedures.
   (B) exercise testing should not be performed until the condition improves.
   (C) exercise testing will not provide accurate assessment of health-related fitness.
   (D) professional judgment about the risks and benefits of testing should determine whether to conduct an assessment.

4. A male client is 42 years old. His father died of a heart attack at age 62. He has a consistent resting blood pressure (measured over 6 weeks) of 132/86, and a total serum cholesterol of 5.4 mmol/l. Based on his coronary artery disease risk stratification, which of the following activities is appropriate?
   (A) Maximal assessment of cardiorespiratory fitness without a physician supervising
   (B) Submaximal assessment of cardiorespiratory fitness without a physician supervising
   (C) Vigorous exercise without a prior medical assessment
   (D) Vigorous exercise without a prior physician-supervised exercise test

5. Which of the following is a strategy to improve the accuracy of a fitness assessment?
   (A) Ensure appropriate pretest preparation of the client.
   (B) Ensure physician supervision of all assessments.
   (C) Use checklists of pretest procedures.
   (D) Use only certified staff.

6. When performing multiple assessments of health-related fitness in a single session, resting measurements should be followed in order by
   (A) body composition, cardiorespiratory fitness, muscular fitness, flexibility.
   (B) body composition, flexibility, muscular fitness, cardiorespiratory fitness.
   (C) cardiorespiratory fitness, flexibility, muscular fitness, body composition.
   (D) cardiorespiratory fitness, muscular fitness, body composition, flexibility.

7. Body composition is most accurately assessed via the determination of the body's
   (A) anthropometrics via measurements of circumferences.
   (B) bioelectrical impedance via appropriate electrode positioning.
   (C) density via skinfold measurements.
   (D) density via underwater weighing.

8. During calibration of a treadmill, the belt length was found to be 5.5 meters. It took 1 minute, 40 seconds for the belt to travel 20 revolutions. What is the treadmill speed?
   (A) 4 meters/min
   (B) 66 meters/min
   (C) 79 meters/min
   (D) 110 meters/min

9. Which of the following would most appropriately assess a previously sedentary 40-year-old female client's muscular strength?
   (A) Using a 30-lb (18-kg) barbell to perform biceps curls to fatigue
   (B) Holding a handgrip dynamometer at 15 lb (7 kg) to fatigue
   (C) Performing modified curl-ups to fatigue
   (D) Using a 5-lb (2.2-kg) dumbbell to perform multiple sets of biceps curls to fatigue

10. Flexibility is a measure of the
    (A) disease-free range of motion about a joint.
    (B) effort-free range of motion about a joint.
    (C) habitually used range of motion about a joint.
    (D) pain-free range of motion about a joint.

11. Individuals who choose to begin a self-directed exercise program on their own should be advised, at a minimum, to complete a quick screening of their health status. A typical screening instrument is the
    (A) PAR-Q.
    (B) Aerobics Center Longitudinal Study of Physical Activity Questionnaire.
    (C) Baecke Questionnaire of Habitual Physical Activity.
    (D) Modified Baecke Questionnaire for Older Adults.

12. Which of the following is NOT a lifestyle consideration when screening for fitness assessment and exercise prescription?
    (A) Nutritional habits
    (B) Exercise history
    (C) Stress
    (D) Family history of cardiovascular disease

13. Which of the following is a FALSE statement regarding an informed consent?
    (A) The informed consent is not a legal document.
    (B) The informed consent does not provide legal immunity to a facility or individual in the event of injury to a client.
    (C) Negligence, improper test administration, inadequate personnel qualifications, and insufficient safety procedures are all items that are expressly covered by the informed consent.
    (D) The consent form does not relieve the facility or individual of the responsibility to do everything possible to ensure the safety of the client.

14. The order of activities associated with the completion of the informed consent is in what order?
    1. Private, quiet reading of the document
    2. Signing and dating the document
    3. Private, verbal explanation of the contents of the document with a verbally expressed opportunity to ask questions for which answers are provided
    4. Presentation of a copy of the signed document to the participant
    (A) 1, 2, 3, 4
    (B) 1, 3, 2, 4
    (C) 1, 4, 3, 2
    (D) 1, 2, 4, 3

15. Which of the following criteria would NOT classify a client as having "increased risk"?
    (A) Signs and/or symptoms of cardiopulmonary disease
    (B) Signs and/or symptoms of metabolic disease
    (C) Two or more major risk factors for coronary artery disease
    (D) Male older than 40 years of age with a history of clinical depression

16. In order to maximize safety during a fitness assessment, the room layout should address which of the following issues?
    (A) The equipment and floor space should be arranged so that although exits are clearly marked, it is not essential for clients to be near the exit, and equipment can be moved from in front of exits in an emergency.
    (B) The equipment and floor space should be arranged to allow clients the opportunity to move equipment away from exits should an emergency develop.
    (C) The equipment and floor space should be arranged to allow safe exit from the facility in an emergency situation and to prevent accidental upsetting of equipment.
    (D) Annual drills announced early in the year allow the staff to properly prepare for any type of emergency.

17. The physical condition of a testing area should be designed to reduce anxiety and promote the physical comfort of the client. Which of the following is an INAPPROPRIATE element of a testing site?
    (A) The room is private.
    (B) The room is clean.
    (C) The room's temperature is between 70°F and 74°F (21°C and 23°C).
    (D) The room can be shared by several clients because they are there for the same purpose.

18. A client must be given specific instructions for the days preceding a fitness assessment. Which of the following is NOT a necessary instruction to a client for a fitness assessment?
    (A) Men and women should avoid liquids for 12 hours before the test.
    (B) Clients should be instructed to not drink alcohol, use tobacco products, or drink caffeine at least 3 hours before the test.
    (C) Clients should avoid strenuous exercise or physical activity on the day of the test.
    (D) Men and women should be instructed to get adequate sleep the night prior to the assessment.

19. Under which of the following conditions is a repeat test necessary?
    (A) Repeat testing should be conducted only after sufficient time for an alteration in the fitness component assessed to have occurred.
    (B) Repeat testing should be conducted at the request of the client even after 1 week.
    (C) Repeat testing should be conducted twice monthly.
    (D) Repeat testing should be conducted only when necessary because it is very costly and time consuming.

20. Body composition is determined by which of the following formulae?
    (A) Total weight – fat weight
    (B) Total weight – fat-free weight
    (C) Fat weight + fat-free weight
    (D) Fat-free mass + fat mass

21. Hydrodensitometry (hydrostatic weighing, underwater weighing) has several sources of error. Which of the following is NOT a common source of error when using this technique to determine body composition?
    (A) Measurement of vital capacity of the lungs
    (B) Interindividual variability in the amount of air in the gastrointestinal tract
    (C) Interindividual variability in the density of individual lean tissue compartment
    (D) Measurement of residual volume

22. Which of the following methods to determine body composition is accepted as the standard against which all other techniques are measured?
    (A) Skinfold measures
    (B) Anthropometry
    (C) Waist-to-hip ratio
    (D) Hydrostatic weighing

23. The definition of cardiorespiratory fitness is
    (A) the maximal force that a muscle or muscle group can generate in a single effort.
    (B) the coordinated capacity of the heart, blood vessels, respiratory system, and tissue metabolic systems to take in, deliver, and use oxygen.
    (C) the ability to sustain a held maximal force or to continue repeated submaximal contractions.
    (D) the functional range of motion about a joint.

24. Which of the following formulae is used for determining workload on a bicycle ergometer?
    (A) Belt length × resistance × grade
    (B) Belt length × resistance × revolutions pedaled per minute
    (C) Resistance × distance flywheel traveled per revolution × revolutions per minute
    (D) Resistance × distance flywheel traveled per revolution

25. Adults age physiologically at individual rates. Therefore, adults of any specified age will vary widely in their physiologic responses to exercise testing. Special consideration should be given to the older adult when giving a fitness test because
    (A) age is often accompanied by deconditioning and disease.
    (B) age predisposes the older adult to clinical depression and neurologic diseases.
    (C) the older adult cannot be physically stressed beyond 75% of age-adjusted maximum.
    (D) the older adult is not as motivated to exercise as a younger person.

ANSWERS AND EXPLANATIONS

1–B. A client should not be allowed to engage in any physical activity, including fitness assessment, at your facility before his or her health risk status has been determined. Informational meetings or "walk-throughs" of the facility that do not incorporate physical activity do not require health screening.

2–A. An appropriately prepared consent form is a written document that provides evidence that you made a good-faith effort to inform your client of the procedures, risks, and benefits of the activities in which he or she would participate. The document does not provide legal immunity against lawsuits.

3–D. Identification of risk conditions for exercise testing includes familiarization with those conditions that may increase risk but that may not necessarily preclude fitness assessment. Such conditions are called "relative" contraindications. Conditions that do preclude testing until they have stabilized are "absolute" contraindications.

4–B. The client has only one risk factor, hypercholesterolemia, with total serum cholesterol greater than 5.2 mmol/l (see section II. A. of Chapter 4, Pathophysiology/Risk Factors). He is, however, classified as "older" for exercise purposes because he is older than 40 years of age. Consequently, it is recommended that he should have medical clearance and an exercise test prior to engaging in vigorous exercise and that a physician should supervise any maximal assessment of cardiorespiratory fitness.

5–A. Accuracy requires that clients be tested while in an optimal physiologic state. Physician supervision may enhance safety, whereas checklists aid in objectivity. A "certified" staff member may not be certified through an organization such as ACSM and, therefore, may not know about test objectivity.

6–A. Body composition assessment may be influenced by hydration status, which may be affected by tests of cardiorespiratory and muscular fitness. Hence, body composition should be assessed immediately after resting measures are taken. Cardiorespiratory fitness assessment should precede any activity that might influence heart rate and should therefore precede tests of muscular fitness. Flexibility is best assessed when the body is fully warmed from activity and therefore should follow all assessments that may influence body temperature.

7–D. Underwater weighing (hydrodensitometry) is the standard against which other methods of body composition are validated. Consequently, other methods of assessing body composition rely on the accuracy of underwater weighing to accurately estimate body composition. Appropriate administration of a hydrodensitometric assessment results in an estimation of body composition with an error of 2%–3%, in contrast to the error associated with skinfold measurement of approximately 4% and bioelectrical impedance of approximately 3.5%–5%.

8–B. The belt length is 5.5. Twenty revolutions equals 110 meters total distance (20 revolutions × 5.5 meters per revolution). This distance was traveled in 100 seconds (60 + 40), resulting in a speed of 1.1 meters/sec (110 meters/100 sec). Converting this to meters/min (1 min = 60 sec) results in a treadmill speed of 66 meters/min.

9–A. Muscular strength is most appropriately assessed via either a determination of 1-RM, or through lifting a submaximal weight that a client can lift at most 2–14 times. A weight of 30 lb (18 kg) for a previously sedentary middle-aged woman is probably an adequate weight to allow 2 to 14 repetitions. The held handgrip exercise, the modified curl-ups, and the 5-lb dumbbell exercise meet the criteria for muscular endurance assessments.

10–D. Range of motion may be limited by pain. This decreases the function of the joint. Therefore, flexibility is limited by painful actions. Disease status and effort can affect the range of motion. The range of motion habitually used is not necessarily an indication of the complete range of motion through which an individual can move.

11-A. Although each of these questionnaires serves a specific purpose, the only questionnaire that is short, easy to understand, and can be self-administered is the PAR-Q.

12–D. Nutritional habits and exercise history as well as stress levels are all modifiable and are directly related to screening prior to a fitness assessment and exercise programming. Unfortunately, family history of cardiovascular disease is not a modifiable risk factor. Even though it must be considered as a program issue, it is not a lifestyle consideration.

13–C. Negligence, improper test administration, inadequate personnel qualifications, and insufficient safety procedures are all items that are expressly NOT covered by the informed consent. The informed consent is also not a legal document; it does not provide legal immunity to a facility or individual in the event of injury to a client and it does not relieve the facility or individual of the responsibility to do everything possible to ensure the safety of the client.

14–B. A private, quiet reading of the document is first; then, a private, verbal explanation of the contents of the document with a verbally expressed opportunity to ask questions for which answers are provided follows; third, signing and dating the document; and fourth, presentation of a copy of the signed document to the participant.

15–D. Signs and/or symptoms of cardiopulmonary disease, signs and/or symptoms of metabolic disease, and two or more major risk factors for coronary artery disease are all indications of an increased risk for the development of coronary artery disease. Known disease is the fourth condition that places a client into the increased risk category.

16–C. The equipment and floor space should be arranged so that exits are clearly marked and no equipment is standing in the way of clients' exit in the case of an emergency. Drills should be both announced and unannounced, and they should occur frequently.

17–D. The physical condition of the test area should be private, clean, at a comfortable temperature and humidity, well ventilated, and should have comfortable seating with all necessary supplies and equipment present. The area should also be private.

18–A. The client should wear appropriate, comfortable, loose-fitting clothing, be adequately hydrated, avoid alcohol, tobacco, caffeine, and food for at least 3 hours before the test, avoid strenuous exercise or physical activity on the day of the test, and get adequate sleep the night prior to the test.

19–A. Many clients want to be assessed even after the smallest change has occurred, with some requesting weekly assessments. However, although it is costly and time consuming, repeat testing should be conducted after a sufficient time has elapsed for the assessed fitness component to have occurred, which may be several weeks to months.

20–D. Body composition refers to the relative proportions of fat and fat-free (lean) tissue in the body. It is commonly reported as "percent body fat," thus identifying the proportion of the total body mass composed of fat. Fat-free mass is then determined as the balance of the total body mass.

21–A. It is the measurement of residual volume of air in the lungs and not the vital capacity of the lungs that is a source of error. Residual volume is difficult to directly measure and is often estimated using vital capacity.

22–D. Hydrodensitometry (hydrostatic weighing, underwater weighing) is still the standard against which all other measures are compared.

Other methods to determine body composition include bioelectrical impedance analysis, near-infrared interactance, and dual energy x-ray absorptiometry (DEXA).

23–B. The maximal force that a muscle or muscle group can generate in a single effort is the definition of muscular strength. The ability to sustain a held maximal force or to continue repeated submaximal contractions is the definition of muscular endurance. The functional range of motion about a joint is the definition of flexibility. The coordinated capacity of the heart, blood vessels, respiratory system, and tissue metabolic systems to take in, deliver, and use oxygen is the definition of cardiorespiratory fitness.

24–C. To determine the workload on a bicycle ergometer, you must know the resistance against the flywheel, the distance the flywheel travels per revolution, and the number of revolutions per minute.

25–A. Fitness testing is conducted in older adults for the same reasons as in younger adults, including exercise prescription, evaluation of progress, motivation, and education. Age is often accompanied by deconditioning and disease and these factors must be taken into consideration when selecting appropriate fitness test protocols. In addition, adaptation to a specific workload is often prolonged in older adults (a prolonged warm-up, followed by small increments in workload are recommended). Test stages in graded exercise tests should be prolonged, lasting at least 3 minutes, to allow the participant to reach a steady state. An appropriate test protocol should be selected to accommodate these special needs.

CHAPTER 7

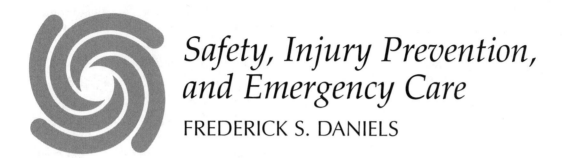

Safety, Injury Prevention, and Emergency Care
FREDERICK S. DANIELS

I. RISKS OF PARTICIPATION IN EXERCISE

A. PHYSICAL DEMANDS

–at higher intensities, the potential for either **injury** or an **emergency situation** requiring a correct and timely response

B. BENEFITS SHOULD OUTWEIGH RISKS

–The fitness instructor must create as safe an environment as possible by:

1. **Understanding the risks**
2. Being able to **implement preventive** measures
3. Having **knowledge of appropriate care of injuries**
4. **Creating, practicing, and implementing emergency plans** in the event of a medical emergency

C. POTENTIAL SOURCES OF RISK

1. **Exercise equipment**

   –can **malfunction**, be **used incorrectly** or be in **disrepair** or **poor condition.**

2. **Environment**

   –must be **clean and free of germs.**

   –must be properly **maintained.**

3. **Staff**

   –must be **properly trained** and act in a **responsible and safe** manner.

   –must **design safe exercise programs.**

4. **Medical history**

   –The exercise professional must **know the client's medical history, medication use, and restrictions.**

5. **Individual factors**

   –**Age**

   –**Level of exercise experience**

   –**Medical history**

   –**Lack of experience and familiarity** with equipment

   –**Lack of knowledge** about proper principles of exercise

D. PREVENTION STRATEGIES FOR STAFF AND CLIENTS

1. Think about safety.
2. Exercise intelligently.
3. Purchase good equipment and supplies.
4. Use proper technique.
5. Follow the rules.
6. Train staff on a regular basis.
7. In a group exercise setting, staff should understand the following:

   –exercise space for each client (size of the room and number of participants)

   –temperature and humidity of space

   –fitness level of participants and special needs considerations

   –proper flooring to match group activity

   –appropriate warm-up and cool-down

II. SAFETY IN THE FITNESS CENTER

A. AREAS OF SAFETY

–include the building design, physical plant, fixtures, furniture, equipment, program design, and staff training.

–The **Americans with Disabilities Act** (ADA) lists specific standards that enhance safety and access for both **disabled and nondisabled** exercisers. This Act is especially important for fitness facilities because of the **variety of individuals that may participate** in exercise programs.

B. CREATING A SAFE ENVIRONMENT

1. This is a primary responsibility in all fitness facilities.
2. Managers and staff must **meet a standard of care for safety** in developing and operating facilities and equipment by **looking beyond obvious safety parameters.**
3. Environmental factors such as temperature, humidity, altitude, and pollution must be monitored and controlled. Performance and health can be affected by these conditions.

   –High temperature can lead to dehydration, heat exhaustion, and even heat stroke. Low temperature can lead to dehydration, chills, and potentially frostbite.

   –High humidity can reduce the body's ability to control core temperature and lead to heat exhaustion.

   –Exposure to high altitude can lead to headaches, nausea, and altitude sickness.

   –In addition to negatively affecting performance, pollution can lead to wheezing, coughing, and irritation of the eyes and mouth.

C. EQUIPMENT

–includes pieces used for **testing, cardiovascular, strength, and flexibility** pieces.

–also includes that used for **rehabilitation** as well as the **pool, locker room,** and **emergency equipment.**

1. **Criteria for equipment selection include:**

   –Proper anatomic position

   –Ability to adjust to different body sizes

   –Quality of design and materials

   –Durability

   –Repair history

   –Cost

2. **Test the equipment** prior to purchase, and follow manufacturer's instructions for installation.
3. **Inspect equipment** regularly for cleanliness, disrepair, and proper functioning to allow early recognition of problems.
4. **Other safety considerations**

   a. Ensure that all **electrical plugs** are secured and grounded.

   b. Treadmills have **emergency cut-off** switches that are easily accessible.

   c. **Safety instructions should be mounted** on all equipment.

   d. Machines should **restrict joint movements beyond the normal range of motion.**

D. FURNITURE AND FIXTURES

–**Locker room and reception furniture** are used frequently and should be selected for **ergonomics and safety.**

–**Inspection, routine maintenance,** and **cleaning** are equally important with furniture.

–Lighting should be bright enough to see instructions and records clearly and should create a positive and motivating atmosphere.

E. SURFACES

1. Proper surfaces must be provided to **prevent slips and falls.**
2. Selection of surfaces **should meet minimal standards** for the activity being carried out and should **comply with the ADA.**
3. Maintenance includes:

   –proper cleaning and disinfecting.

   –removal of oil and dust.

   –inspection for cracks, holes, exposed seams, and warping.

F. SUPPLIES AND SMALL EQUIPMENT

–include heart rate (HR) monitors, blood pressure (BP) units, stopwatches, skinfold calipers, exercise gloves, etc.

1. **Must be in proper working order and be calibrated**
2. Devices that do not function correctly may provide incorrect information and precipitate an unsafe situation.

G. ROUTINE AND REQUIRED MAINTENANCE AND REPAIRS

–help ensure that equipment, furniture, and physical plant **function safely** and according to specifications.

–**increase the life of the equipment.**

–**reduce the risk of a mechanical problem.**

1. A **routine maintenance schedule** for exercise equipment should be in place.

2. A procedure for reporting problems and a repair process that reduces down-time include **documentation of the problem, repair history, and resolution of the problem (Figure 7-1).**

H. MAINTENANCE AND HOUSEKEEPING

–contribute to safety by presenting a clean environment.

–help to maintain proper equipment functioning.

1. Slippery surfaces, dirty equipment and furniture, poorly maintained ventilation, and equipment in disrepair **increase the risk of accidents.**

2. Equipment and fixtures must be **regularly cleaned and disinfected.**

   a. **Written standards** must clearly outline procedure for routine cleaning and maintenance.

   b. Solutions and materials must be **safe** for the skin and **hypoallergenic.**

   c. The professional staff should have a role in the cleaning and maintenance of exercise equipment. **Knowledge of procedures and chemical safety** is critical.

III. WEIGHT ROOM SAFETY

A. WEIGHTS

–The use of weights—machine or free weights (dumbbells and barbells)—increases risk of injury because of the **amount of weight used, improper technique, fatigue, and improper behavior.**

B. METHODS TO INCREASE SAFETY

1. **Spotting:** A second person assists in the initial lift, correcting technique, and lifting the weight to safety if the lifter is unable to handle the weight.

2. **Buddy system:** Exercise with a partner who can offer encouragement and motivation, knowledge of correct technique, and assistance if a problem develops.

3. **Speed of movement:** Movements should be controlled with a slow, smooth pace (4 seconds up and 4 seconds down).

4. **Replacing weights:** A safe environment requires returning weights to the proper place.

5. **Placement of equipment:** Adequate space between machines and weight benches is important for safety.

6. **Equipment inspection and routine maintenance**

IV. TESTING AND EVALUATION AREA

–must be safely organized and similarly prepared for emergencies.

–Equipment should include:

A. SPHYGMOMANOMETER, STETHOSCOPE, MOUTH GUARD FOR CARDIOPULMONARY RESUSCITATION (CPR), FIRST AID KIT

B. TELEPHONE TO ACTIVATE THE PUBLIC EMERGENCY MEDICAL SYSTEM

–Should have **posted, written procedures to activate the emergency medical system**—911

–Should include the following instructions:

1. **Identify** yourself, location, and phone number

2. **Provide** clear and succinct **explanation** of the problem

3. **Offer medical history and medications** (if known)

4. **Provide vital signs and state of consciousness**

5. **Explain the treatment actions** taken and results

C. BACK BOARD AND NECK BOARD

–not required in the testing area, but should be immediately accessible

D. ALL STAFF MUST HAVE CURRENT CPR CERTIFICATION

Fitness Equipment Repair Chart

Date	Equipment	Serial No.	Problem	Date repaired	Order No.	Cost

FIGURE 7-1 An example of a repair log for fitness equipment. (From *ACSM's Resource Manual for Guidelines for Exercise Testing and Prescription,* 3rd ed. Philadelphia, Lippincott Williams & Wilkins, 1998, p 630.)

V. SAFETY PLANS

–clearly outline procedures for maintaining a safe environment and reducing risk of accident.

–Appropriate safety plans include:

A. FIRE

1. Procedures for **evacuation**
2. Regular **inspection** of **fire extinguishers**

B. POWER FAILURE

1. Procedures that **reduce the risk of power outages** and **electrical malfunction**
2. Procedures for **evacuation** and **contacting the authorities**

C. FLOOD

1. Procedures to **reduce the risk of flooding** such areas as the pool, shower, and whirlpool
2. Procedures for **clean-up and salvage**

D. EARTHQUAKE

1. Procedures for **evacuation**

2. Procedures for **safety of equipment and persons** in the facility

E. BLOOD-BORNE PATHOGENS/ HAZARDOUS WASTE

1. The **Occupational Safety and Health Administration** (OSHA) has specific **standards** that must be **posted** and closely adhered to when applicable.
2. All staff must be familiar with and trained in these procedures.

F. STAFF CERTIFICATION IN FIRST AID AND CPR

G. POSTED INFORMATION

1. Clearly visible signs posted for fire extinguishers, first aid kits, CPR mouth shields, and for activating the emergency medical system (911)
2. Emergency procedures posted adjacent to all phones to assist in enacting the emergency plan

VI. PROPER DOCUMENTATION

–**records events.**

–includes **written policies** and procedures, **rules,** patient and client **rights,** as well as **benefits and risks** of exercise programs.

–offers important **protections for liability and negligence** for both facilities and professional staff.

–**Liability insurance and legal assistance** is recommended.

A. PARTICIPANT AGREEMENTS

–define the **risks** of an exercise program, the exact **type** of exercise program, exact **costs,** and **who shares the risk and responsibility** for the member's exercise (**Figure 7-2**).

–An **attorney** should assist in creating these forms.

B. INFORMED CONSENT

–provides **detailed explanation** of the test or exercise program, including:

1. Potential **benefits and risks**
2. **Purpose** of the test or exercise program

3. **Client responsibilities**
4. **Opportunity** for the member to **ask questions**

C. WAIVERS

–**allow clients to circumvent** a policy or rule, but **place the risk** for this directly **on the client.**

–offer a form of **protection** for both the **instructor** and the **facility.**

D. INCIDENT REPORT

–is a record of an incident or event that involves **unusual circumstances** such as a participant not following club policies or rules, or some other **unusual incident.**

–should include:

1. **Detailed documentation** of the entire incident
2. **Involved clients and witnesses**
3. All **actions of staff** to resolve the problem or emergency situation
4. **Follow-up action** required and/or taken

SAMPLE

PARTICIPANT'S RELEASE AND AGREEMENT

I, the undersigned, hereby agree to participate in an exercise class and/or program ("Program") offered by the XYZ Health Club. I understand that there are inherent risks in participating in a program of strenuous exercise. I warrant and represent that I am in acceptable health and that I may participate in the Program. I agree that I have been honest in my statements regarding my health and medical history and if there are any medical or health conditions or problems, I further agree to obtain a physician's clearance before participating in the Program. If restrictions exist, I will inform XYZ Health Club at the time and allow XYZ Health Club staff to contact my physician for additional information.

I agree that XYZ Health Club shall not be liable or responsible for any injuries to me or illnesses resulting from my participation in the Program and I expressly release and discharge XYZ Health Club and it employees, agents, and assigns, from all claims, actions or judgements which I or my heirs, executors, administrators or assigns may have or claim to have against XYZ Health Club, and/or its employees, agents or assigns for all injuries, illnesses or other damage which may occur in connection with my participtation in the Program. This release shall be binding upon my heirs, executors, administrators, and assigns.

I have read this release and agreement and I understand all of its terms. I execute it voluntarily and with full knowledge of its significance.

Signature: _____   Date: _____

Print name: _____

Witness: _____   Date: _____

FIGURE 7-2 A sample of a participant's release and agreement.

VII. EMERGENCY MANAGEMENT

–Safe and effective management of an emergency situation will ensure the best care and protection for clients, staff, and facility.

A. STAFF ROLE

–The professional staff role during an emergency should include:

1. **Control the situation** by implementing the emergency plan and taking charge.
2. **Maintain order and calm,** especially with the victim.
3. **Activate the emergency medical system,** if necessary.
4. Assure that proper **documentation** of the event occurs.

B. STAFF TRAINING

–Should include:

1. **In-services, safety plans,** and **emergency procedures**
2. **In-services with physicians, nurses,** and **paramedics** are recommended.
3. Review and update of **emergency plans** as necessary including regularly scheduled drills.
4. CPR and first aid **certification current** in all staff
5. Staff should be fully trained to recognize:

   –**absolute** and **relative contraindications** to exercise.

   –**absolute and relative reasons for terminating an exercise test or exercise session.**

Table 7-1. General Injury Classifications

Muscle Injuries	Major Signs and Symptoms
Acute	
Contusions	Soft tissue hemorrhage, hematoma, ecchymosis, movement restriction.
Strains	Hemorrhage, local tenderness, loss of strength/range of motion (ROM).
Tendon Injuries	Loss of strength/ROM; palpable defect.
Muscle cramps/spasms	Involuntary muscle contraction; muscle pain.
Acute-onset muscle soreness	Muscle pain, fatigue; resolves when exercise has ceased.
Delayed-onset muscle soreness	Muscle stiffness 24 to 48 hours after exercise; tenderness and pain.
Chronic	
Myositis/fasciitis	Local swelling and tenderness.
Tendinitis	Gradual onset, diffuse or localized tenderness and swelling, pain.
Tenosynovitis	Crepitus, diffuse swelling, pain.
Bursitis	Swelling, pain, some loss of function.
Joint Injuries	
Acute	
Sprains	Swelling, pain, joint instability, loss of function.
Acute joint synovitis	Pain during motion, swelling, pain.
Subluxation/dislocation	Loss of limb function, deformity, swelling, point tenderness.
Chronic	
Osteochondrosis	Joint locking, swelling, pain, disability.
Osteoarthritis	Pain, articular crepitus, stiffness, reduced ROM.
Capsulitis/synovitis	Joint edema, reduced ROM, joint crepitus.
Bone Injuries	
Periostitis	Pain over bone, especially under pressure.
Acute fracture	Deformity, bone point tenderness, swelling and ecchymosis.
Stress fracture	Vague pain that persists when attempting activity; local tenderness.

VIII. MUSCULOSKELETAL INJURIES

–The incidence of exercise-related injury has been reported to be as high as 80% in participants and instructors (**Table 7-1**).

A. THE RISK FACTORS INCLUDE:

1. Extrinsic factors

  a. Excessive load

  b. Training errors

    –Poor technique

    –Excessive stress on joints

    –Spine not in a neutral position

  c. Adverse environmental conditions

    –High or low temperature

    –High humidity

    –Altitude

    –Air pollution

  d. Faulty equipment

e. Overtraining (overuse) signs and symptoms include:
   – Chronic soreness
   – Fatigue
   – Changes in menstrual cycle
   – Lack of desire to rest

2. **Intrinsic factors**
   – Fitness level
   – Body composition
   – Anatomic abnormalities
   – Gender
   – Age
   – Past injury
   – Disease
   – Restricted range of motion
   – Muscle weakness and imbalance
   – Not performing warm-up and stretching exercises

B. **BASIC PRINCIPLES OF CARE**
   – Objectives are to **decrease pain, reduce swelling, and prevent further injury.**
   – Objectives can usually be met by:

   1. **"RICES":** Rest, Ice, Compression, Elevation, and Stabilization
      a. **Rest** prevents further injury and ensures the initiation of the healing process.
      b. **Ice** reduces swelling, bleeding, inflammation, and pain.
      c. **Compression** reduces swelling and bleeding.
      d. **Elevation** decreases blood flow and controls edema.
      e. **Stabilization** reduces muscle spasm in the injured area by assisting in relaxation of associated muscles.

   2. **Heat**
      – is used to relieve pain and muscle spasms.
      – should not be applied during the acute inflammatory phase.

   3. **Splints or casts**
      – may be used to immobilize the area and improve healing.
      – Immobilization is primarily used for fractures and severe sprains.

   4. **Medications**
      – may be used to reduce swelling and inflammation.
      – may be used to treat the pain associated with swelling.

   5. **Low back injury care**
      – neutral spine during exercise (pain free)
      – aerobic exercise
      – unloaded flexion/extension of spine (cat stretch)
      – hip and knee flexion and extension
      – lunges
      – single leg extension holds
      – abdominal curlups
      – horizontal isometric side support
      – low weight, high repetitions to emphasize endurance strength

IX. OTHER MEDICAL EMERGENCIES AND ASSOCIATED TREATMENT

– **Serious** complications rarely occur during an exercise session.

– When complications do occur, the exercise staff must be prepared to take appropriate action.

A. **HEAT EXHAUSTION/HEAT STROKE**
   – Replace fluids.
   – Have client lie down.
   – Elevate feet.
   – Remove excess clothing.
   – Cool with water (externally).
   – Seek immediate attention.

B. **FAINTING**
   – Place client in supine position with feet above head if possible.
   – Maintain an open airway.
   – Loosen tight clothing.
   – Take BP and HR if possible.
   – Seek medical attention if client remains unconscious.

C. **HYPOGLYCEMIA—EXTREMELY LOW BLOOD GLUCOSE LEVELS (MAY BE LIFE THREATENING)**

 1. **Symptoms include:**

 –Tremor

 –Tachycardia

 –Confusion

 –Fatigue

 –Slurred speech

 –Memory loss

 –Muscular weakness

 –Lightheadedness

 2. **Treatment includes:**

 –Ingestion of glucose (fruit juice, dextrose tablets, fruit, chocolate)

 –Maintenance of supervised control

 –Assessment of blood glucose

 –Seeking medical attention

D. **HYPERGLYCEMIA—EXTREMELY HIGH BLOOD GLUCOSE LEVELS (MAY BE LIFE THREATENING)**

 1. **Signs and symptoms include:**

 –Dehydration

 –Hypotension

 –Tachycardia

 –Nausea

 –Vomiting

 –Impaired consciousness

 –Hyperventilation

 –Odor of acetone on breath

 2. **Treatment includes:**

 –Immediate medical attention

 –Supervisory control of the individual until trained help arrives

E. **SIMPLE/COMPOUND FRACTURES**

 –Immobilize and splint the extremity.

 –Seek immediate medical attention.

F. **BRONCHOSPASM**

 –Maintain open airway.

–Give bronchodilator if prescribed.

–Seek immediate medical attention if spasm continues and medication is not available.

G. **HYPOTENSION/SHOCK (POTENTIALLY LIFE THREATENING)**

 –Place client in a supine position with feet elevated, if possible.

 –Maintain an open airway.

 –Monitor HR and BP.

 –Give fluids if client is conscious and not nauseated.

 –Seek immediate medical attention.

H. **SEIZURE**

 –Do not to touch the person during convulsions.

 –Attempt to assure safety by ensuring that the client does not injure herself or himself.

 –Seek medical attention.

I. **BLEEDING**

 –Follow blood-borne pathogen precautions.

 –Apply direct pressure over the site to stop the bleeding.

 –Protect the wound from contamination.

 –Elevate the injured area if bleeding is severe.

 –Seek medical attention if stitches may be required.

J. **CARDIAC CRISIS**

 1. **Symptoms of angina and myocardial infarction include:**

 –Pain, pressure, squeezing or discomfort in the chest, left shoulder, neck, or jaw that may radiate distally

 –Shortness of breath

 –Lightheadedness

 2. **Treatment includes:**

 –Terminate exercise immediately and monitor HR and BP.

 –Ensure client is at rest and comfortable, sitting or lying.

 –Initiate the emergency medical system (911).

 –Be prepared to begin CPR.

X. INJURY PREVENTION

A. **PREPARTICIPATION SCREENING**

 –may uncover medical and physical risks to exercise.

B. **IMPROVED FITNESS**

 1. **Musculoskeletal**

 –may reduce risk of injury.

2. **Physiologic**

   –may help prevent many chronic medical conditions.

3. All **four components of fitness** are important and should be a part of all fitness programs.

   a. **Conditioning should be well balanced among cardiovascular, flexibility, strength, and endurance,** as well as balanced throughout the muscle groups and major joints.

   b. The **progression** of exercise training should be gradual.

   c. **Flexibility** is an important component of fitness and may contribute to injury prevention.

   d. **Warm-up and cool-down** prepare the body for exercise and safely return the body to a resting state.

      –They may prevent complications (musculoskeletal injury, cardiac crisis, dizziness) that can result from immediate changes in exercise intensity.

   e. **Rest**

      –is an important part of conditioning.

      –can facilitate recovery from the stress of exercise.

   –can reduce risk of injury.

   –includes rest between exercises and exercise sessions, as well as rest prescribed for acute injury.

C. **PROPER INSTRUCTION**

   –assists in preventing injuries and avoiding emergency situations.

D. **EXERCISE CLOTHING AND EQUIPMENT**

   –Gloves, helmets, protective glasses, etc., are important to safety during certain modes of exercise.

   –Clothing should fit properly and be layered in order to maintain warmth (in cold environments), or be appropriate for hot/humid environments.

   –Shoes must be appropriate for the exercise or sport.

E. **HYDRATION**

   –is not always appropriately driven by thirst; hydrate regularly during exercise.

   –helps regulate body temperature and electrolyte balance.

REVIEW TEST

DIRECTIONS: Carefully read all questions and select the BEST single answer.

1. Serious complications during an exercise session
   (A) occur more often with women.
   (B) rarely occur.
   (C) occur at a rate of 1 in 3000 hours of exercise.
   (D) occur more often in the late hours due to client fatigue.

2. The exercise staff's role when an injury or emergency occurs should be to
   (A) control the situation by implementing the emergency plan and taking charge.
   (B) find someone to implement the plan.
   (C) get everyone out of the facility to avoid chaos.
   (D) hope that an emergency contact is available to help with the situation.

3. In preventing injuries, hydration is very important because
   (A) it controls breathing and the Valsalva maneuver.
   (B) it helps regulate carbohydrate utilization during cardiovascular exercise.
   (C) it helps regulate body temperature and electrolyte balance.
   (D) it helps prevent blood pooling during the cool-down.

4. What U.S. Government Act is critical for operators of fitness facilities to understand and adhere to regarding safety?
   (A) The Americans with Handicaps Act
   (B) The Civil Rights Act of 1966
   (C) The Health Portability Act of 1996
   (D) The Americans with Disabilities Act

5. What is the most appropriate action in assisting a person suffering from a seizure?
   (A) Hold the person down so that he or she does not hurt himself or herself.
   (B) Don't touch the person but be sure that he or she is in a safe area.
   (C) Place a wedge in the person's mouth so that he or she does not swallow the tongue.
   (D) Ignore the person and allow the seizure to pass.

6. One of the first actions that a fitness instructor should consider in preventing injury is to
   (A) teach the client how to warm-up and cool-down.
   (B) instruct the client on safety procedures when using the facility.
   (C) conduct a preparticipation screening.
   (D) instruct the client on how to use the exercise equipment safely.

7. How should a fitness instructor advise a client with regard to progression of the exercise program?
   (A) The progression should be gradual and slow.
   (B) The progression should be at specific increments based on a calendar schedule (e.g., add 10% every 2 weeks).
   (C) Be aggressive in increasing the program in order to increase fitness.
   (D) Progress the program only when the client feels ready.

8. How can exercise equipment add to the risk of participation?
   (A) Because it is expensive
   (B) Because it is hard to move
   (C) Because it is used incorrectly
   (D) Because of the time one waits to use it

9. Prevention strategies of staff and clients must include
   (A) following the rules.
   (B) keeping the facility clean.
   (C) hiring good front desk staff.
   (D) developing clever, unique programs.

10. An equipment maintenance plan should include
    (A) a floor plan.
    (B) a client advisory statement.
    (C) a document that records maintenance and repair history.
    (D) temperature and humidity readings.

11. In cleaning the facility and equipment, what must an operator be aware of?
    (A) That signs are written clearly
    (B) That surfaces are brightly colored
    (C) That solutions and cleaning materials are safe for the skin and hypoallergenic
    (D) That disinfectants smell pleasant

12. Which of the following are some of the symptoms of hypoglycemia?
    (A) Hypotension
    (B) Cold, clammy skin
    (C) Tachycardia and slurred speech
    (D) Bronchospasms and hyperventilation

13. RICES refers to
    (A) relaxation, ice, compression, energy, stabilization.
    (B) relaxation, incremental heat, care for injury, energy, standardization.
    (C) rest, ice, common sense, energy, standardization.
    (D) rest, ice, compression, elevation, stabilization.

14. Complaints of pain in the chest with associated pain radiating down the left arm may be signs of
    (A) a cardiac crisis.
    (B) hypotension.
    (C) a seizure.
    (D) heartburn.

15. Beyond the general safety parameters, such as equipment in good repair, a facility must create a safe environment for any individual, especially
    (A) guest clients.
    (B) staff.
    (C) health care providers.
    (D) special populations.

16. Weight room safety should include
    (A) a phone.
    (B) lifting gloves and back belts.
    (C) male trainers to help with spotting.
    (D) safe passageways and use of buddy system.

17. Fire, blood-borne pathogens, and power outage should all be included in
    (A) facility insurance.
    (B) safety plans.
    (C) maintenance plans.
    (D) testing by the facility and staff.

18. The potential benefits and risks of an exercise test should be written in what document?
    (A) Description of services
    (B) Safety plan
    (C) Informed consent
    (D) Exercise waivers

19. Documentation offers important
    (A) liability and negligence protection.
    (B) liability and risk protection.
    (C) safety and communication programs.
    (D) billing and classification tools.

20. Emergency procedures should be
    (A) given to all clients when they join.
    (B) put away in a safe place.
    (C) posted under each phone.
    (D) posted above each fire extinguisher.

21. Which of the following is NOT a principle of low back care?
    (A) Abdominal curlups
    (B) Unloaded flexion/extension of the spine
    (C) Neutral spine during all exercises
    (D) Controlled leg press or squat with light weights

22. What is the fitness instructor's primary responsibility in conducting an exercise test?
    (A) Maintaining a safe environment by not putting the client in danger
    (B) Making sure the data collected are accurate
    (C) Completing the test
    (D) Encouragement and support

23. What are some of the risks for musculoskeletal injury?
    (A) Poor signage in the facility
    (B) Extrinsic factors—intensity, terrain, equipment
    (C) Intrinsic factors—frequency, attitude, gender
    (D) Membership type

24. Chronic soreness and fatigue are symptoms of
    (A) hyperglycemia.
    (B) a strain.
    (C) an overuse injury.
    (D) hypoglycemia.

25. Exercise clothing
    (A) creates an important fashion statement.
    (B) should be bright, so you are easily seen in an aerobics class.
    (C) has only one rule: be comfortable.
    (D) must be safe and performs appropriately like the exercise equipment.

ANSWERS AND EXPLANATIONS

1–B. Medical complications and injury can and do occur in an exercise setting. Fortunately, serious complications rarely occur. There are no data to suggest that women suffer more serious complications with exercise than men. There are also no data to support the statement that serious complications occur late in the day, and the rate of serious complications occurs at a rate significantly lower than 1 in 3000 hours (it is closer to 1 in 3,000,000) hours of exercise.

2–A. One of the exercise staff's responsibilities when an injury or emergency occurs is to control the situation by implementing the emergency plan and taking charge. Staff should make sure the proper actions are taken to ensure the safety and care of the injured clients. One of those actions is to instruct the people around him/her in order to help implement the plan. It is inappropriate for the staff to sit back and let someone else implement the plan or hope that an emergency contact can take control of the situation. Controlling the situation and instructing those around you is the primary role and getting people out of the facility may only happen under certain situations.

3–C. Hydration is one of the most important principles of exercise. Two of the effects of hydration are regulating body temperature and electrolyte balance. If either of these is out of balance due to dehydration (lack of appropriate hydration), it can lead to nausea, lightheadedness, and heat exhaustion. Hydration does not affect breathing, carbohydrate utilization, or blood pooling.

4–D. The Americans with Disabilities Act protects individuals with any disability from discrimination or access. Fitness facilities must provide free and easy access to all disabled individuals throughout the facility. The Americans with Handicaps Act does not exist and the Civil Rights Act was enacted in 1964, not 1966. The Health Portability Act involves employees with health insurance and is not related to safety.

5–B. Most seizures display convulsing actions. With a convulsing seizure, the safest action is to not touch the person and let the convulsion pass. Any action can cause potential danger to you and the victim. It is not safe to hold the person down or try to wedge anything into the victim's mouth. Ignoring the person and not ensuring that the physical area is safe for the victim means you are acting irresponsibly.

6–C. Before starting a fitness program, it is important to understand the client's medical history and risk of a crisis during exercise. A preparticipation screening can help determine this understanding and help prevent injury or crisis. Teaching the warm-up and cool-down prevents injury, but it is not the first thing you do. The same argument applies to teaching the safety procedures and safe use of the equipment.

7–A. It is always safest to advise all clients to progress a fitness program gradually and slowly. This advice also increases the chance for program success and increased motivation. Using the calendar method does not take into account the individual effects in adjusting to exercise. Clients may not be ready to progress when the calendar indicates it is time to increase. Clients do not always know when to increase or may not be aggressive enough. Always taking an aggressive approach increases the risk of injury, because the increase may be too much too soon.

8–C. Using exercise equipment incorrectly can place excess stress on muscles and joints and increase the risk of injury, which adds to the risk of participation. The expense and ability to move exercise equipment have no bearing on the risk of participation. The time that one waits also does not add to the risk, unless the client uses the equipment incorrectly.

9–A. Prevention strategies refer to the risk of injury. One of the critical aspects in preventing injuries is to follow the rules, which are made to prevent problems. Keeping the facility clean and hiring good front desk staff are important and can help prevent problems, but are not considered prevention strategies. Unique programs are designed to attract clients, not to prevent risk.

10–C. The maintenance plan ensures that the exercise equipment is functioning properly and safely. Records that document maintenance and repairs are important in tracking when to maintain equipment and also to make sure that repairs are conducted and completed. A floor plan is not necessary in a maintenance plan. Temperature and humidity readings should be included in a program plan (where necessary), not a maintenance plan. A client advisory statement does not exist anywhere.

11–C. When cleaning a facility, it is very important that the solutions used do not cause skin problems or allergic reactions. A safe facility must avoid these problems. Cleaning a facility usually does not involve signs or require particular colors of surfaces. A pleasant smell is nice to have, but does not prevent problems or allergic reactions.

12–C. Hypoglycemia, or low blood sugar, has many symptoms, which include tachycardia and slurred speech. Hypoglycemia may increase blood pressure, but does not cause hypotension or low blood pressure. Bronchospasms and cold, clammy skin are not symptoms of hypoglycemia.

13–D. RICES refers to Rest (let the injury heal without stress), Ice (reduces swelling and promotes healing), Compression (reduces swelling), Elevation (reduces swelling), and Stabilization (reduces muscle spasm by assisting in relaxation of associated muscles). Energy, incremental heat, standardization, and common sense do not decrease swelling, promote healing, reduce muscle spasm, or reduce the stress to the injury.

14–A. Symptoms of a cardiac crisis such as heart failure or a heart attack include pain in the chest and pain radiating down the left arm. Hypertension, not hypotension, is a possible cause of a cardiac crisis. A seizure and heartburn are not associated with a cardiac crisis.

15–D. A safe environment is very important, and this fact is most important to many of the special populations that may have a difficulty negotiating around a facility because of injury, disability, or age. Health care providers, staff, and guest clients are important, but in most cases do not require special needs or attention regarding safety.

16–D. The weight room can be a dangerous place if safety is not a priority. Dumbbells, plates, and bars can fall or be thrown and cause injury. Safe passageways reduce the risk of a client getting hit by an exercising client. The buddy system helps with spotting and instruction, which reduces the risk of injury. A phone can cause distractions. Lifting gloves and belts may be helpful to clients in easing the burden of lifting, but are not critical for safety. Female trainers can be just as effective in spotting as males.

17–B. Safety plans help educate and guide staff in developing and maintaining a safe facility. The safety plan should include procedures for a fire, power outage, and the exposure to blood-borne pathogens. Facility insurance addresses fire and possibly power outages, but does not address blood-borne pathogens. Maintenance plans address the repair and maintenance of the equipment but do not address any of the three factors listed in the question. Testing by staff may involve blood-borne pathogens, but has no involvement in fires or power outages.

18–C. The informed consent is a document that a client reads, or is read by a staff member, that explains the exercise test to be conducted in detail along with potential benefits and risks, the purpose of the test, and the client's responsibilities. The informed consent does not explain the services. The safety plan is designed to create a safe exercise environment and does not discuss potential benefits or risks. Exercise waivers place the total responsibility of exercise on the client and may list the risks, but do not discuss the benefits.

19–A. Documentation provides a record of events and a written description of the rules, rights, and risks of the program. These documents are designed to ensure safety of clients and staff. They are also designed to protect the facility and staff from liability or negligence issues, because they promote safety and reduce the risk of injury. Documentation does not protect risk, but provides tools to help reduce it. While program design or policies are written into documents, they are not the programs. Documentation may be tools for billing and classification; it is not necessarily as important as computer software or the management of the data needed for both of these programs.

20–C. Emergency procedures should be easy to find, so the staff can act quickly to handle the emergency, not spend time looking for the procedures. It is recommended that the procedures be placed by the phones, because they are often used in an emergency to dial 911 and initiate emergency help. Emergency procedures should not be given to clients because they should not be involved in enacting them. Only the staff should implement the emergency procedures. Placing the procedures in a safe place does not make them easy to find when they are needed. The phone is a better place to put the emergency procedures than the fire extinguishers, because the phone is used in almost all emergencies, whereas fire extinguishers are not always used.

21–D. Leg press and squats with any type of weight adds compression to the spine, which can have significant adverse effects in the care of a low back injury. It is very important to increase flexibility and muscular strength without excessive load or compression. Abdominal curlups, unloaded flexion/extension of the spine (cat stretch), and maintaining a neutral spine during exercise are principles that do not place unnecessary load or compression on the spine and serve to increase flexibility and strength of supporting structures.

22–A. Safety is the most important responsibility for a fitness instructor. A fitness instructor must never endanger anyone. Safety is the top priority. Accurate data are good to obtain, but this is secondary to safety. Completing the test and encouragement are also goals of the fitness instructor, but not the top priority.

23–B. Included with the many risks for musculoskeletal injury are extrinsic or outside factors. If intensity is too high, one could over stress joints and muscles. Rough or uneven terrain can lead to falls. Poorly designed or maintained equipment can cause breakdowns or incorrect positioning, which can cause injury. Signage usually does not lead to injury, and membership type is not a factor in musculoskeletal injury. Although intrinsic factors are included in the risks, frequency is not an intrinsic factor, so this answer is incorrect.

24–C. Chronic soreness, fatigue, lack of desire to rest, and changes in menstrual cycle are all symptoms of an overuse injury. Overtraining is another term used for this condition and often occurs in individuals who are training for competition or become obsessed with fitness training. Hyperglycemia and hypoglycemia are related to blood glucose levels and do not exhibit chronic soreness. A strain may show as a symptom; however, fatigue is not usually associated with this condition.

25–D. Exercise clothing is also exercise equipment and like the exercise machines one uses, it is critical that it be safe and perform adequately. If not, then the risk of injury is increased. Fashion statements do not mean that the clothes are safe and perform appropriately. Bright clothing is not important in an aerobics class. Although comfort is important, safety and importance are more important and critical.

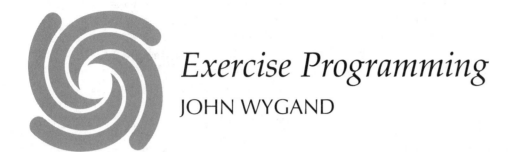

CHAPTER 8

Exercise Programming

JOHN WYGAND

I. INTRODUCTION

A. ESSENTIAL COMPONENTS OF AN EXERCISE PROGRAM

–Development of a systematic, individualized exercise prescription depends on the thoughtful, scientific integration of five essential components into a structured exercise program: **mode, frequency, intensity, duration, and progression.** These essential components are applied regardless of the participant's age, health status, or fitness level.

–Consideration of **limitations, needs,** and **goals** of each individual will result in a more individualized, safer, and effective exercise program.

–The following data obtained from a **graded exercise test** provide the **basis for the exercise prescription:**

1. **Heart rate (HR)**
2. **Blood pressure (BP)**
3. **Rating of perceived exertion (RPE)**
4. **Functional capacity**

B. PURPOSES OF EXERCISE PROGRAMS

–Enhancement of physical fitness for daily activities, recreation, or competitive athletic endeavors

–**Primary or secondary disease prevention**

II. COMPONENTS OF AN EXERCISE PRESCRIPTION

Five Essential Components of an Exercise Program
- Mode
- Intensity
- Duration
- Frequency
- Progression

A. MODE IS A PARTICULAR FORM OR TYPE OF EXERCISE.

1. Selection of mode should be **based on the desired outcomes,** focusing on exercises that are most likely **to sustain participation** (adherence and compliance) and **enjoyment.**

2. **Cardiovascular endurance exercise** requires the involvement of **large muscle group activity** performed in **rhythmic** fashion over **prolonged duration.**

3. **Resistance training** (e.g., circuit training) should be part of a comprehensive exercise program.

   –It **improves muscular strength and endurance.**

   –Some techniques can also be used to provide **cardiovascular benefits.**

B. INTENSITY IS THE RELATIVE PHYSIOLOGIC DIFFICULTY OF THE EXERCISE.

1. **Intensity and duration of exercise interact and are inversely related.**

   –Improvements in aerobic fitness from **low-intensity, longer duration exercise** are similar to those with higher intensity, short-duration exercise. This is an important consideration when developing an exercise prescription for individuals who do not enjoy high-intensity physical activity.

2. **Risk** of orthopedic and perhaps cardiovascular complications **increases with higher intensity activity.**

3. **Factors to consider when determining intensity** for a particular client include:

   –level of fitness.

   –medications that may influence exercise performance.

   –risk of cardiovascular or orthopedic injury.

   –individual preference.

   –program objectives.

C.   DURATION IS THE LENGTH OF AN EXERCISE SESSION.

1. **High-intensity/short-duration exercise** programs are associated with **increased potential for injury.**

2. Programs of **excessive duration** are associated with **decreased compliance.**

3. **Increases in exercise duration** should be instituted **as adaptation occurs** without signs of intolerance.

D.   FREQUENCY REFERS TO THE NUMBER OF EXERCISE SESSIONS PER DAY AND PER WEEK.

1. Frequency interacts with both intensity and duration.

2. **Deconditioned persons** with low functional capacity benefit from multiple daily bouts of short-duration/low-intensity exercise.

3. Individual goals, preferences, limitations, and time constraints may affect frequency.

E.   PROGRESSION (OVERLOAD) IS THE INCREASE IN ACTIVITY DURING EXERCISE TRAINING WHICH, OVER TIME, STIMULATES ADAPTATION.

1. The **rate of progression** depends on the participant's health/fitness status, age, goals, and compliance.

2. **Improvement depends upon systematic progression of frequency, intensity, and/or duration.** Increasing the frequency and duration of an activity before increasing the intensity is preferred.

3. **Adaptation** occurs when an individual physiology can adequately respond to the demands of a particular exercise stress.

   –depends on health/fitness status and the relative mix of frequency, intensity, duration, and the mode of exercise.

   a. Most participants adapt more easily and comfortably to **smaller increases** in the volume or intensity of exercise.

   b. There are few **objective markers for short-term adaptation** (1–3 weeks); some indications may be:

      –improvements in motor patterns.

      –lower RPE.

      –subjective evaluation by communication between the exercise professional and the individual.

   c. The **rate of adaptation** is affected by the participant's compliance with the exercise program.

III.   PRINCIPLES OF CARDIORESPIRATORY ENDURANCE EXERCISE

–The **ability to take in, deliver, and utilize oxygen** is dependent on the **function of the circulatory systems** and **cellular metabolic capacities.**

–The **degree of improvement** that may be expected in cardiorespiratory fitness is **directly related to the frequency, intensity, duration,** and **mode.**

–Maximal oxygen uptake ($\dot{V}O_{2\,max}$) **may increase between 5% and 30%** with training.

A.   MODE

–The best improvements in cardiorespiratory endurance occur when **large muscle groups** are engaged in **rhythmic, aerobic activity.**

–**Various activities** may be incorporated into an exercise plan **to increase enjoyment and improve compliance.** Appropriate activities include walking, jogging, cycling, rowing, stair climbing, aerobic dance ("aerobics"), water exercise, and cross-country skiing.

–The **potential for musculoskeletal injury,** such as shin splints and stress fractures, **increases when weight-bearing activity is performed excessively.** Comfortable, supportive walking or running shoes are important.

1. **Cycling**

   –This **non-weight-bearing** activity has a **low potential for musculoskeletal injury.**

   –An **ergometer** is recommended for accurate exercise testing and training so that workload can be quantified.

   –The major limiting factor to cycling is **local muscle fatigue of the upper leg.**

2. **Stair climbing**

   –Stair-climbing machines, including chain-driven machines, step-treadmills, and "steppers," are commonly found in fitness centers.

   –An **upright posture** is important **to avoid low back trauma.**

   –Weak **quadriceps and gluteals may cause dependence on handrails for support,** reducing the intensity of the exercise.

3. **Aerobics** is typically offered as a group activity.

   a. **Intensity** is usually controlled by music and choreographed movement patterns.

      –**HR is not a valid indicator of exercise intensity when excessive arm movements are used.

      –The use of **RPE** should be considered an **adjunct form of intensity monitoring.**

   b. **High-impact aerobics**

      –refers to **movements where both feet leave the ground simultaneously.**

      –may require **significant energy expenditure.**

      –increase the potential for **musculoskeletal injury.**

   c. **Low-impact aerobics**

      –refers to movement patterns where **one foot remains in contact with the floor at all times.**

      –produce **low impact forces** and **low injury potential**

      –are appropriate for even highly fit individuals.

      –**Exercise intensity** can be **increased** by using **greater horizontal displacement** during movement.

   d. **Step aerobics** involves the use of **choreographed movement patterns**

performed on and off bench steps varying in heights from 4 to 12 inches.

      –Energy cost ranges from **6–11** metabolic equivalents (**METs**).

      –**Cadence must be reduced for less fit individuals** (< 8 METs functional capacity).

   e. Organizations such as **the American College of Sports Medicine,** the **American Council on Exercise (ACE),** and the **Aerobics and Fitness Association of America (AFAA)** are excellent resources for more detailed aerobics information and continuing education.

4. **Water exercise** allows the **buoyancy** properties of water **to help reduce the potential for musculoskeletal injury** and **may even allow an injured person an opportunity to exercise** without further injury.

   a. **Activities**

      –include walking, jogging, and dance activity.

      –typically combine the benefits of the **buoyancy and resistive properties of water,** providing an **aerobic stimulus** as well as enhancing **muscular strength** and **endurance.**

   b. **Special population groups** such as the obese, pregnant, arthritic, and elderly may benefit from water exercise.

   c. **Intensity may be altered** by changing the speed of movement or the depth of the water, or by using resistive devices such as fins and hand paddles.

B.   INTENSITY

1. The ACSM recommends that exercise intensity be prescribed within a range of **70%–85% of maximum HR, 50%–85% of** $\dot{V}o_{2\,max}$, or 60%–80% of max METs, or HR reserve (HRR) (**Figure 8-1**).

   a. Lower intensities (40%–50% of $Vo_{2\,max}$) elicit a favorable response in individuals with **very low fitness levels.**

   b. Due to the variability in estimating maximal HR from age, whenever possible **use an actual maximal HR from a graded exercise test.**

2. **RPE may be used with HR** for regulating intensity.

   a. ACSM recommends an intensity that will elicit an **RPE within a range of 12–16** on the original 6–20 Borg scale.

Age		200	200
		-25	-25
Max Heart Rate		195	195
Resting Heart Rate		-75	-75
Heart Rate Reserve		120	120
50-85%		x .5	x .85
		60	102
Resting Heart Rate		+75	+75
Target Heart Rate	50% HRR=135		85% HRR=177

FIGURE 8-1 Calculation of 50%–85% heart rate reserve (HRR) based on a 25-year-old person with a resting heart rate of 75 beats per minute. (From Karvonen M, Keutala K, Mustala O: The effects of training on heart rate: A longitudinal study. *Annales Medicinae Experimentalis et Biological Fennial* 35:307–315, 1957.)

   b. RPE is considered a **reliable indicator of exercise intensity,** though some learning is required on the part of the participant.

   c. RPE is **particularly useful** when a participant (particularly the elderly) is **unable to monitor his/her pulse accurately** or when **HR response to exercise is altered by medications.**

3. The HR-VO$_2$ relationship can be plotted to determine exercise intensity **(Figure 8-2)**.

4. An **abnormal response** to a graded exercise test or individual exercise limitations must be considered when prescribing intensity.

   a. **Exercise at intensities where the following problems occur should be avoided:**

     –exercise-induced anginal pain.

     –inappropriate BP changes.

     –musculoskeletal discomfort.

     –leg pain.

     –any sign or symptom that caused premature termination of the exercise test.

   b. For any of the problems mentioned above, the **training HR may be 10 bpm lower than the HR** where a problem was evidenced.

C. DURATION

1. The ACSM recommends **20–60 minutes of continuous aerobic activity.**

   –Caloric expenditure and cardiorespiratory conditioning goals may be met with exercise sessions of moderate duration (20–30 min).

2. **Deconditioned individuals** may benefit from multiple, **short-duration exercise sessions** (< 10 minutes) with frequent interspersed rest periods.

3. An **inverse relationship** exists between the intensity and duration of training.

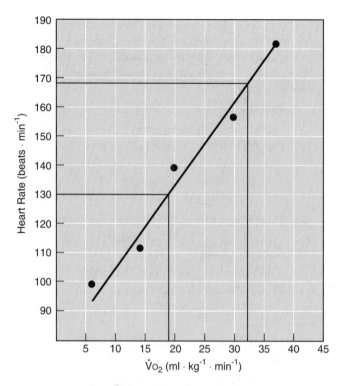

FIGURE 8-2 A line of best fit has been drawn through the data points on this plot of heart rate and oxygen consumption data observed during a hypothetical maximal exercise test in which $\dot{V}o_{2max}$ was observed to be 38 ml•kg^{-1}•min^{-1} and maximal heart rate was 184 beats•min^{-1}. A target heart rate range was determined by finding the heart rates that correspond to 50% and 85% of $\dot{V}o_{2max}$. For this individual, 50% of $\dot{V}o_{2max}$ was approximately 19 ml•kg^{-1}•min^{-1}, and 85% of $\dot{V}o_{2max}$ was approximately 32 ml•kg^{-1}•min^{-1}. The corresponding target heart rates are approximately 130 and 168 beats•min^{-1}. (From American College of Sports Medicine: *ACSM's Guidelines for Exercise Testing and Prescription,* 6th ed. Baltimore, Lippincott Williams & Wilkins, 2000, p. 148.)

4. There may be greater **musculoskeletal and cardiovascular risk with exercise performed at high intensities for short durations** as compared with lower intensity exercise for a longer duration.

5. **Interval training programs** that use bouts of higher intensity exercise with bouts of lower intensity exercise can be effective **for improving cardiorespiratory fitness.**

   a. Intermittent exercise may allow **increased caloric expenditure and interest level** compared with continuous aerobic activity and may be particularly **useful for beginning or deconditioned exercisers.**

   b. Intervals programmed for health/fitness purposes should be aerobic in nature and not exceed an intensity of 85% HRR.

D. FREQUENCY

1. The ACSM recommends that aerobic exercise be performed **3–5 days per week** for most individuals.

2. Although frequency, intensity, and duration of exercise are interrelated, frequency is also **influenced by lifestyle and convenience.**

3. **Less conditioned people** may benefit from lower intensity, shorter duration exercise performed at higher frequencies per day and/or per week.

E. PROGRESSION (OVERLOAD)

1. The **rate of progression** depends on health/fitness status, individual goals, and compliance rate.

2. The combination of frequency, intensity, and duration of activity dictates the **volume of work** that is done and may be expressed as **caloric expenditure.**

3. Frequency, intensity, and/or duration can be increased to provide overload.

4. It is reasonable to increase duration of activity initially. When the desired final goal of the exercise program is achieved, maintenance of functional capacity becomes the new goal.

5. The goal for most healthy individuals is 30 minutes, 3–4 days per week at 85% HRR.

F. WARM-UP

–consists of large muscle group activity performed rhythmically at a relatively low intensity.

1. **Physiological changes induced by appropriate warm-up exercises** include:

   –increase in muscle temperature.

   –increase in muscle blood flow.

   –increased dissociation of oxygen from hemoglobin.

   –enhancement of enzyme activity.

   –increase in nerve conduction velocity.

   –increases in elasticity of muscle and connective tissue.

   –decrease in muscle viscosity.

2. Benefits include possible **prevention of musculoskeletal and cardiovascular injury.**

3. **Five to ten minutes** should be allotted for the warm-up.

G. COOL-DOWN

–consists of large muscle activity performed at a low to moderate intensity for approximately 5–10 minutes.

–facilitates venous return.

–facilitates removal of metabolic by-products.

–promotes a gradual return of HR and BP to pre-exercise values.

Table 8-1. Contraindications to Exercise Testing*

Absolute

• A recent significant change in the resting ECG suggesting significant ischemia, recent myocardial infarction (within 2 days) or other acute cardiac event

• Unstable angina

• Uncontrolled cardiac arrhythmias causing symptoms or hemodynamic compromise

• Severe symptomatic aortic stenosis

• Uncontrolled symptomatic heart failure

• Acute pulmonary embolus or pulmonary infarction

• Acute myocarditis or pericarditis

• Suspected or known dissecting aneurysm

• Acute infections

Relative†

• Left main coronary stenosis

• Moderate stenotic valvular heart disease

• Electrolyte abnormalities (e.g., hypokalemia, hypomagnesemia)

• Severe arterial hypertension (i.e., systolic BP of > 200 mm Hg and/or a diastolic BP of > 110 mm Hg) at rest

• Tachyarrhythmias or bradyarrhythmias

• Hypertrophic cardiomyopathy and other forms of outflow tract obstruction

• Neuromuscular, musculoskeletal, or rheumatoid disorders that are exacerbated by exercise

• High-degree atrioventricular block

• Ventricular aneurysm

• Uncontrolled metabolic disease (e.g., diabetes, thyrotoxicosis, or myxedema)

• Chronic infectious disease (e.g., mononucleosis, hepatitis, AIDS)

*Modified from Gibbons RA, Balady GJ, Beasely JW, et al. ACC/AHA guidelines for exercise testing. J Am Coll Cardiol 1997;30:260–315.

†Relative contraindications can be superseded if benefits outweigh risks of exercise. In some instances, these individuals can be exercised with caution and/or using low-level end points, especially if they are asymptomatic at rest.

–Because the musculature and connective tissue are less viscous and more pliable after the exercise stimulus, the cool-down period is an **appropriate time to enhance flexibility through stretching.**

H. EXERCISE CONTRAINDICATIONS

–The ACSM specifies medical conditions that preclude safe participation in exercise testing and exercise programs. **Table 8-1** provides a complete listing of these conditions.

Table 8-2. Indications for Terminating Exercise Testing*	
Absolute Indications	**Relative Indications**
• Drop in systolic blood pressure of ≥ 10 mm Hg from baseline blood pressure despite an increase in workload, when accompanied by other evidence of ischemia	• Drop in systolic blood pressure of ≥ 10 mm Hg from baseline blood pressure despite an increase in workload, in the absence of other evidence of ischemia
• Moderate to severe angina	• ST or QRS changes such as excessive ST depression (> 2 mm horizontal or downsloping ST-segment depression) or marked axis shift
• Increasing nervous system symptoms (e.g., ataxia, dizziness, or near syncope)	• Arrhythmias other than sustained ventricular tachycardia, including multifocal PVCs, triplets of PVCs, supraventricular tachycardia, heart block, or bradyarrhythmias
• Signs of poor perfusion (cyanosis or pallor)	• Fatigue, shortness of breath, wheezing, leg cramps, or claudication
• Technical difficulties monitoring the ECG or systolic blood pressure	• Development of bundle-branch block or intraventricular conduction delay that cannot be distinguished from ventricular tachycardia
• Subject's desire to stop	• Increasing chest pain
• Sustained ventricular tachycardia	• Hypertensive response†
• ST elevation (≥ 1.0 mm) in leads without diagnostic Q-waves (other than V_1 or aVR)	

*Reprinted with permission from Gibbons RA, Balady GJ, Beasely JW, et al. ACC/AHA guidelines for exercise testing. J Am Coll Cardiol 1997;30:260–315.

†Systolic blood pressure of more than 250 mm Hg and/or a diastolic blood pressure of more than 115 mm Hg.

I. TERMINATION OF AN EXERCISE SESSION

–The ACSM specifies the conditions that require termination of a test or an exercise session.

Table 8-2 provides a complete listing of these conditions.

IV. FLEXIBILITY

–An appropriate range of motion (**joint mobility**) is necessary for optimal musculoskeletal health and physical activity.

–Activities that enhance or maintain musculoskeletal flexibility should be included in comprehensive preventive or rehabilitative exercise programs.

A. THREE STRETCHING TECHNIQUES

–Each technique has associated risk/benefit considerations.

1. **Static stretching**

   –involves **slow stretching to the point of discomfort** and holding that position for a period of 10–30 seconds.

   –involves **minimal risk of injury.**

   –has been shown to be **effective.**

2. **Ballistic stretching**

   –uses **repetitive bouncing movements** to produce muscle stretch.

   –**may produce residual muscle soreness** or **acute injury.**

   –may play a role in athletic training, but the **ACSM discourages prescribing ballistic stretching for the non-athlete.**

3. **Proprioceptive neuromuscular facilitation (PNF)**

   –**alternates contraction and relaxation** of both agonist and antagonist muscle groups.

   –is effective, but **may cause residual muscle soreness.**

   –is **time consuming.**

   –**requires a partner** to assist with stretching.

   –has the **potential for injury** if partner-assisted stretching is applied too vigorously.

B. RISKS OF STRETCHING

–Careful attention should be paid to body alignment and joint position to minimize risk of musculoskeletal injury.

–Some common stretching exercises may be potentially harmful to the musculoskeletal system and should be avoided or modified for the general population (**Figure 8-3**).

CONTRAINDICTATED/HIGH-RISK EXERCISE	ALTERNATIVE EXERCISE
Straight Leg Full Sit-ups Risk: Stress on lower back due to utilization of hip flexors with origin in the lumbar spine; exercise primarily targets hip flexors	Crunches
Double Leg Raises Risk: Hyperextends low back due to utilization of hip flexors with origin in the lumbar spine	Single Leg Raises-Opposite Knee Flexed
7.6t BW Tendon *Pateller Tendon* *on Full Squat* Full Squats Risk: Patellar tendon forces during deep knee bending are 7.6 times body weight (7), increasing the risk of chondromalacia meniscal tears; individuals with previous injury to ligamental structures and menisci are at increased risk for injury	Squats to 90 Degrees of Knee Flexion-Knee Over Ankle 90°
Hurdler's Stretch Risk: Knee flexion at end range of motion with rotational forces on hinge joint may stress the medial collateral ligament and menisci	Seated Hamstring Stretch
Plough Risk: Loaded neck flexion can sprain cervical ligaments and increase pressure in cervical disks	Double Knee to Chest
Back Hyperextension Risk: Hyperextension of the back	Back Extension to Normal Standing Lumbar Lordosis
Full neck rolls Risk: Stretches cervical ligaments, increases cervical disc pressure and may impinge arterial flow, resulting in dizziness	Lateral Neck Stretches
Flexion with rotation Risk: Flexion with rotation increases pressure on spinal disks	Supine Curl-ups with Flexion followed by Rotation
Standing toe touch Risk: Increases pressure in lumbar disks and overstretches lumbar ligament	Standing Hamstring Stretch, Back Flat

FIGURE 8-3 Common high-risk exercises and recommendations for alternative exercises. (Adapted from American College of Sports Medicine: *ACSM's Resource Manual for Guidelines for Exercise Testing and Prescription,* 3rd ed. Baltimore, Williams & Wilkins, 1998, p 644.)

V. MUSCULAR STRENGTH AND ENDURANCE

A. INTRODUCTION

1. **Muscular strength**

   –is the **maximal force generated by a muscle or muscle group.**

   –One repetition maximum (1-RM) is commonly used to assess muscular strength.

   –1-RM is the most weight that can be lifted at one time.

2. **Muscular endurance**

   –is the a**bility of a muscle** or group of muscles **to contract repeatedly against submaximal loads.**

3. **Maintenance or improvement of muscular strength and endurance**

   –is **critical to the performance of the activities of daily living.** Increased strength enables performance of normal physical activity with less physiologic strain and at reduced risk for musculoskeletal injury.

   –**Improvements** in muscular strength and endurance generally occur as a result of **enhanced neuromuscular function** and **increases in the size of individual muscle fibers.**

   –The ability to realize substantial **increases in muscle size** is **hormonally mediated** and probably **genetically limited.**

   –Resistance training should be included as an integral part of comprehensive preventive and rehabilitative exercise programs.

B. PROGRESSIVE RESISTANCE EXERCISE

–involves the **systematic increase of the resistance, repetitions, sets, and/or the frequency of exercise** in an effort to improve muscular strength and endurance.

–Contracting muscle can produce force as it shortens (**concentric**), lengthens (**eccentric**), or when it stays at the same length (**isometric**).

1. **Isometric contraction** occurs when **the length of the muscle does not change** during force production.

   a. Isometric activities have been shown to elicit **improvements in muscular strength.** However, these improvements seem to be **limited to the joint angle(s) at which the training is performed.**

   b. **Exaggerated BP response** may accompany isometric muscle contraction.

   c. Isometric activities have some application in the **management of select musculoskeletal injury.**

2. **Isotonic muscle contraction** occurs when the **length of the muscle changes during muscular action (contraction).**

   –**Concentric** as it shortens

   –**Eccentric** as it lengthens

   –**Isokinetic** as the speed of movement is held constant

   a. **Eccentric contractions** have been implicated as a cause for **delayed onset of muscle soreness (DOMS).**

   b. **Isokinetic exercise** is usually performed with a **dynamometer** to provide a speed-controlled movement.

C. EXERCISE PRESCRIPTION

–**Exercises that address major muscle groups** should be included in the exercise prescription.

–The order of the exercises may be left to individual preference; however, **arms should be exercised after the torso,** if possible. Fatigue of the smaller arm muscles may limit the ability to adequately stress the larger torso muscles (i.e., the triceps). Fatigue may limit bench press activity or the stimulus for chest musculature.

1. **ACSM recommendations**

   a. One set of **8–12 repetitions of each exercise** should be performed to volitional fatigue. **Volitional fatigue refers to the inability to move a resistance through the concentric range of motion with proper mechanical form.**

   b. A **5- to 10-minute warm-up,** consisting of aerobic activity or a light set (50%–75% of the training weight) of the specific resistance exercise, should precede the resistance exercise program.

   c. These exercises should be performed **at least 2 days per week.**

   d. If time permits, **different exercises for a given muscle group should be performed** in an effort to recruit different motor units.

2. **Intensity** is prescribed as the **percent of the maximal voluntary contraction (MVC).**

   a. The **number of repetitions** to volitional fatigue **varies inversely** with **resistance.**

b. Exercise to volitional fatigue is **safe, provided good technique is maintained.**

c. **Caution** should be used when prescribing exercise intensity **for individuals with cardiovascular disease, hypertension,** or those with **complications associated with diabetes.**

d. Relative exercise intensity should be **similar for men and women.**

e. A particular set of resistance exercise **should be terminated when the resistance cannot be moved through the full range of motion during successive repetitions,** with good technique, including proper breathing (volitional fatigue).

f. **Resistance may be increased** when 12 repetitions can be completed with good technique.

g. **One exercise session per week** has been shown **to maintain strength for up to 3 months** provided intensity remains constant.

D. SYSTEMS OF RESISTANCE TRAINING

–differ in the combinations of **sets, repetitions, and resistance** applied to overload the muscle.

1. **Pyramiding** is a training method where the resistance is increased (ascending pyramid) or decreased (descending pyramid) with each consecutive set.

2. **Circuit weight training** employs a series of exercises performed in succession with minimal rest between exercises.

3. **Super-sets** refer to consecutive sets for antagonistic muscle groups with no rest between sets or multiple exercises for a specific muscle group with little or no rest.

4. **Split routines** require exercising different body parts on different days or during different sessions.

5. **Plyometrics** is a method of strength and power training that involves an eccentric loading of muscles and tendons followed immediately by an explosive concentric contraction.

   a. The **eccentric phase** of the stretch-shortening cycle may allow for enhanced force generation during the concentric phase.

   b. The **explosive nature** of this type of activity may increase the **risk of musculoskeletal injury.**

   c. Plyometrics is **not considered a practical resistance exercise for health/fitness applications.** It may be appropriate for select athletic/performance needs.

6. **Periodization** is the gradual cycling of specificity, intensity, and volume of training in an effort to achieve peak performance at a desired time.

E. MODES OF EXERCISE FOR RESISTANCE TRAINING

–**Free weights** require that the participant have some skill to perform exercise properly and safely.

–**Machines** (such as Nautilus, Universal, Keiser) **may be safer** than free-weight exercise, particularly **for the novice participant.**

–**Springs, surgical tubing,** and **electronic devices** are also used for resistance training.

F. SAFETY OF RESISTANCE EXERCISE

1. **Breathing**

   –**Proper breathing instruction** for individuals unfamiliar with resistive training is necessary. Individuals should practice **exhaling as the exercised muscle contracts concentrically,** and **inhaling during the eccentric phase** of each repetition.

   –The **Valsalva maneuver** (a forced expiration against a closed airway) **should be discouraged** during resistance exercise because it **may be accompanied by a significant increase in arterial BP.**

2. **Spotting**

   –is assistance rendered by another person to allow safe completion of a repetition or set of an exercise.

   –is especially important for **exercises where the weight is lifted overhead, for bench press exercises, and for squats.**

3. **Speed of movement**

   –The ACSM recommends that resistance exercise training be performed at **moderate to slow speeds,** in a controlled manner, over the full range of motion.

4. **Proper mechanics**

   –Heavy resistance should never be performed at the expense of proper technique.

VI. EXERCISE LEADERSHIP

A. QUALIFICATIONS FOR SAFE AND EFFECTIVE EXERCISE LEADERSHIP

–An **understanding** of the **scientific concepts** of exercise

–The ability to **interpret and effectively teach** these concepts

–The ability to **motivate individuals**

–The ability to **identify the level of supervision required** for individuals based on their health/fitness status

B. THE EFFECTIVE EXERCISE LEADER:

1. Is a **resource for up-to-date, accurate information** regarding health/fitness
2. Serves as a **role model** for the participants
3. Creates the **atmosphere and opportunity for learning**
4. Establishes a **clear set of goals** for each individual
5. **Communicates effectively** by:
   –**giving direct and specific messages**
   –**presenting consistent, not contradictory, information**
   –**soliciting feedback** from participants to ensure understanding
   –**providing written material** to reinforce verbal instruction
6. Is **able to observe all participants** in a group exercise session

7. Is aware of **individual differences** in fitness level and **adapts the exercise prescription** accordingly

8. **Recognizes that motivation is individual** and that not all participants are driven by the same rewards

   a. Reasons cited for **noncompliance** include lack of time, boredom with the exercise program, inaccessibility of the exercise facility, lack of results, and degree of difficulty.

   b. **Periodic fitness assessments** may provide objective evidence of improvement for some participants.

   c. The exercise prescription should be within the individual's **physical and psychological capabilities.**

   d. **Continuous verbal encouragement** and reinforcement are important.

   e. Setting **attainable short-term goals,** especially when weight loss is an objective, is crucial.

   f. **Incentive programs** may be useful to enhance compliance.

   g. Establishing **instructor-client relationships and/or client-client relationships** gives a sense of belonging and may enhance compliance.

   h. Accurate and complete **records of exercise performance and attendance** may help motivational efforts and guide feedback.

VII. CONDITIONS REQUIRING MODIFICATION OF EXERCISE PROGRAMS

A. AGE

–An individual's **health and fitness is largely independent of chronological age,** differing greatly amongst individuals of the same chronological age. Hence, age should not be the primary consideration when developing or modifying an exercise prescription.

–It is **difficult to differentiate the effects of aging from those of deconditioning.**

–Research suggests that **regular exercise may slow changes that occur with aging.** Exercise **helps maintain the functional capacity** necessary for independence and a higher quality of life.

1. **Changes associated with aging**

   a. **Decreased function of cardiorespiratory, musculoskeletal, and neuromuscular systems**

   –There seems to be a gradual loss of aerobic capacity after the age of 20.

   –Decreased maximal HR and reductions in fat-free mass may be responsible for declining maximal oxygen uptake.

   –A decrease in fat-free mass is responsible for a decline in muscular strength.

   b. **Osteoporosis**

   –increases the **risk of fractures** of the wrists, hips, and lumbosacral regions.

   –Reductions in bone mass are **most prevalent in sedentary individuals** and **progress at a more rapid rate following menopause.**

   –**Weight-bearing exercise** is most effective in maintaining or increasing bone density.

c. **Joint inflammation, or arthritis**

–Exercise is not recommended during periods of active pain or inflammation.

d. **Connective tissue alterations**

–manifest in **reduced flexibility.**

–may contribute to a **loss of ability to perform activities of daily living.**

e. **Loss of balance and coordination**

–A decreased state of balance and coordination **may increase the risk of physical harm.**

–When prescribing exercise, particularly weight-bearing activities, ensure maximal safety by **utilizing proper spotting techniques and creating a safe exercise environment.**

2. **Exercise modifications for aging clients**

a. **Recommended exercise intensity** is 50%–70% of HR reserve (HRR).

b. **Duration**

–A **continuous duration of 20 minutes** during the initial stages of an exercise program may be difficult but should be the goal.

–**Intermittent 10-minute bouts of activity** interspersed within the exercise session or throughout the day **may be appropriate** for those who find a continuous 20-minute session difficult.

c. **Frequency**

–Recommended frequency is 3–5 days per week, with a day of recovery allowed between sessions.

d. **Appropriate exercise modalities**

–include walking, stationary cycling, water exercise, and machine-based stair climbing.

e. **Weight-bearing activity** is recommended for enhancing bone density.

f. **Resistance exercise training**

–**may counter the loss of muscle and bone** that accompanies aging.

–Maintenance of muscular strength is critical for activities of daily living and may assist independence and improve quality of life.

g. **Flexibility** should be part of a comprehensive health/fitness program for the older adult (ACSM).

B. EXERCISE-INDUCED ASTHMA (EIA)

1. **Definition and manifestations**

–EIA is a reversible airway obstruction that is a direct result of the ventilatory response to exercise. It is thought to occur as a consequence of fluid loss in the airways as the inspired air is **conditioned** (warmed, humidified, and filtered) during exercise. The **deconditioned** air is thought to trigger an immune or allergic response, which may manifest in bronchospasm. The nose warms, cleans, and humidifies.

–EIA is characterized by **coughing, wheezing, mucus production,** and general **shortness of breath.**

–**EIA attacks usually occur within 10 minutes after exercise,** but can occur at any time during exercise. They **usually subside spontaneously** with complete resolution within 1 hour.

2. **Medications that may prevent or reverse asthma attacks**

a. Beta$_2$-agonists

–most effective in preventing EIA

b. Glucocorticosteroids

–may be effective due to anti-inflammatory properties.

c. Cromolyn sodium

–free of side effects; is generally effective

d. Theophylline

–slow onset of action; associated side effects

3. **Exercise modifications for the client with EIA**

–Modifications in exercise programming coupled with the appropriate pharmacological regimen can minimize frequency and severity of episodes.

a. Use a prolonged, gradual warm-up.

b. Exercise in warm, humid environments when possible.

c. Intermittent exercise may be effective.

d. Use a mask or scarf over the nose and mouth in cold environments.

e. Avoid outdoor activity during periods of peak pollen count or air pollution.

C. HYPERTENSION

1. **Definition and manifestations**

–Hypertension is clinically defined as a **systolic BP > 140 mm Hg and/or a diastolic BP > 90 mm Hg.**

–The majority of hypertensive cases may be classified as **primary** (of unknown origin) and typically warrant **multidimensional management strategies,** which may include pharmacological management, dietary management, weight loss, and relaxation therapies.

2. **Exercise modifications for the client with hypertension**

–Exercise is an **effective** tool in managing hypertension, with an expected **reduction of 5–10 mm Hg in both systolic and diastolic pressure** after exercise training.

–**Cardiovascular endurance activities** such as walking, cycling, and swimming are appropriate. Guidelines for frequency, duration, intensity, and mode are similar to those for healthy adults. Intensity ≤ 70% HRR is recommended.

–**Activities that should be specifically avoided** include isometric exercise, Valsalva maneuvers, and maximal effort.

3. **Antihypertensive medications**

a. **Primary classifications**
–Beta-blockers
–Calcium channel blockers
–Diuretics
–Vasodilators
–Angiotensin-converting enzyme inhibitors

b. **Side effects**
–**Hypotension** is the most prevalent **side effect** of these medications, **particularly in conjunction with exercise.**

(1) A **prolonged cool-down** after exercise enhances venous return and reduces the risk of a hypotensive response.

(2) **Abrupt postural changes should be avoided.**

D. **DIABETES MELLITUS**

–is a metabolic disorder characterized by **hyperglycemia.**

–is associated with increased risk for cardiovascular disease, renal failure, neuropathic disorders, and blindness.

1. **Classification**
–The two major classifications of diabetes are:

a. **Type 1** or **insulin-dependent diabetes mellitus (IDDM),** which is caused by **insulin deficiency.**

b. **Type 2** or **non–insulin-dependent diabetes mellitus (NIDDM),** which is caused by **insulin resistance.**

2. **Complications**
–often necessitate modification of the exercise program.

–can include autonomic neuropathy, peripheral neuropathy, claudication, hypertension, retinopathy, and nephropathy.

3. **Exercise modifications for the client with diabetes mellitus**

–Exercise has an "insulin-like" effect. Therefore, avoidance of hypoglycemia during or after exercise is important.

a. **ACSM guidelines for pre-exercise blood glucose**

(1) **> 300 mg/dl:** Exercise may be contraindicated.

(2) **> 240 with ketones present:** Exercise may be contraindicated.

(3) **< 100:** Supplement with 20–30 g carbohydrate.

b. **Aerobic exercise** is a useful adjunct in a diabetes therapy regimen in which the goal is control of blood glucose.

(1) **Intensity, duration, and mode** guidelines are similar to those for healthy adults.

(2) **Recommended frequency**
–Type 1 diabetics: daily
–Type 2 diabetics: 3–5 times/wk

c. **Resistance exercise training** following ACSM guidelines may also be included as part of a comprehensive exercise program.

E. **OBESITY**

1. **Definition**
–A **body mass index (BMI) > 30.0** defines **obesity.**

2. **Exercise modifications for the obese client**

a. **Aerobic exercise**

(1) **Maximize caloric expenditure.**
–The ACSM recommends **300–500 kcal/day** as a **goal for caloric expenditure.**

–**Large muscle group, aerobic activity** is recommended for caloric expenditure and can result in significant fat loss over a period of time.

–**Frequency, intensity, and duration of exercise** must be manipulated in conjunction with a dietary regimen in an attempt to create a sensible caloric deficit. Exercise intensity should be reduced to allow for longer duration and/or increased frequency.

(2) Screen obese exercise participants carefully before allowing participation in an exercise program.

(3) Walking is a generally accessible activity and should be within the tolerance limits of most obese clients.

(4) Non-weight-bearing activities such as cycling or water exercise may be considered **for the client who has lower body orthopedic problems.**

b. **Resistance training** is recommended as an **adjunct** to an aerobic exercise program and not as the primary means for caloric expenditure.

c. **Cross-training** with combinations of weight-bearing and non-weight-bearing activities **may be effective.**

d. **Thermoregulation** may be a problem for the obese exerciser. Precautions should be followed in warm weather.

–Maintain hydration.

–Wear loose-fitting cotton clothing.

–Exercise during cooler parts of the day.

F. PREGNANCY

–**Exercise is contraindicated during any acute complications** of pregnancy.

–Although there is no published evidence that either labor or delivery is affected by exercise training, it is generally agreed that "reasonable" amounts of exercise are beneficial.

–The **American College of Obstetricians and Gynecologists (ACOG)** has published recommendations for exercise in pregnancy and postpartum (**Table 8-3**).

G. HEART DISEASE

1. Definition

–The following clients may fall within the category of those with heart disease:

a. Clients with angina pectoris, myocardial infarction (MI), valvular heart disease, congestive heart failure (CHF), left ventricular dysfunction (LVD)

b. Those who have recently undergone coronary artery bypass graft (CABG) surgery, heart transplant, or percutaneous transluminal coronary angioplasty (PTCA)

Table 8-3. American College of Obstetricians and Gynecologists (ACOG) Recommendations for Exercise in Pregnancy and Postpartum

- During pregnancy, women can continue to exercise and derive health benefits even from mild to moderate exercise routines. Regular exercise (at least 3 times per week) is preferable to intermittent activity.

- Women should avoid exercise in the supine position after the first trimester. Such a position is associated with decreased cardiac output in most pregnant women. Because the remaining cardiac output will be preferentially distributed away from splanchnic beds (including the uterus) during vigorous exercise, such regimens are best avoided during pregnancy. Prolonged periods of motionless standing should also be avoided.

- Women should be aware of the decreased oxygen available for aerobic exercise during pregnancy. They should be encouraged to modify the intensity of their exercise according to maternal symptoms. Pregnant women should stop exercising when fatigued and not exercise to exhaustion. Weight-bearing exercises may under some circumstances be continued at intensities similar to those prior to pregnancy throughout pregnancy. Non-weight-bearing exercises, such as cycling or swimming, will minimize the risk of injury and facilitate the continuation of exercise during pregnancy.

- Morphologic changes in pregnancy should serve as a relative contraindication to types of exercise in which loss of balance could be detrimental to maternal or fetal well-being, especially in the third trimester. Further, any type of exercise involving the potential for even mild abdominal trauma should be avoided.

- Pregnancy requires an additional 300 kcal/day to maintain metabolic homeostasis. Thus, women who exercise during pregnancy should be particularly careful to ensure an adequate diet.

- Pregnant women who exercise in the first trimester should augment heat dissipation by ensuring adequate hydration, appropriate clothing, and optimal environmental surroundings during exercise.

- Many of the physiologic and morphologic changes of pregnancy persist 4 to 6 weeks postpartum. Thus, prepregnancy exercise routines should be resumed gradually based on a woman's physical capability.

Reprinted with permission from American College of Obstetricians and Gynecologists. *Exercise During Pregnancy and the Postpartum Period (Technical Bulletin #189).* Washington, D.C., American College of Obstetricians and Gynecologists, 1994.

2. Exercise modifications for clients with heart disease

a. A **hospital-based program** is recommended initially.

b. **Cardiovascular endurance exercise** is a primary component of the exercise program. **Frequency, duration, and intensity guidelines are similar to those for healthy adults, unless:**

–restrictions have been imposed by the physician.

–restrictions are inherent because of the disease process (signs/symptoms).

c. The information necessary for exercise programming in cardiac patients should be derived from a **physician-supervised clinical exercise tolerance test.**

d. Patients with MI, angina, or severe left ventricular dysfunction progress more slowly and may not attain a functional capacity comparable to that of patients who have had a CABG or other revascularization surgery (e.g., PTCA) without MI.

e. **Resistance exercise training** is safe and effective for select groups of cardiac patients. It is indicated as a component of a comprehensive exercise program under the following conditions:

  –Low level resistance training as early as 2–3 weeks post MI

  –Free weight and machines 4–6 weeks after an MI

  –Range of motion and very light hand weights in CABG patients during convalescence and recovery

  –Traditional resistance exercise after 3 months post-CABG

  –The resistance exercise program is **preceded by 2 weeks of supervised and monitored aerobic exercise.**

  –The patient has a **resting diastolic BP < 105 mm Hg.**

  –The patient's **peak exercise capacity is > 5 METs.**

  –The patient is **clinically stable.**

f. The **side-effects of cardiovascular medications** must be considered when programming exercise for cardiac patients.

H. LOW BACK PAIN (LBP)

1. **Causes**

  –In most patients, LBP is **mechanical in origin,** implying that there is no systemic or visceral involvement.

  –**Obesity, poor abdominal strength,** and **lack of flexibility** in the low back and hamstring regions are associated with LBP.

  –Injuries to lumbar/sacral areas typically result from **cumulative microtrauma** that occurs over time, not a single episode of poor mechanical application.

  –Many episodes of low back pain will resolve over time and without treatment.

2. **Exercise modifications for the client with LBP**

  a. Exercise should be used as an intervention for **uncomplicated mechanical pain** when there is **no evidence of neurological deficit.**

b. Exercise programs for LBP management should be **administered in conjunction with the appropriate medical or allied health personnel.**

c. Exercise regimens for LBP patients should emphasize:

  –increasing muscular strength and endurance of abdominal and back extensor muscles.

  –improving the flexibility of the pelvic, lumbar, and posterior thigh regions.

d. **Aerobic exercise** improves overall muscular endurance in individuals with LBP, allowing performance of daily activities with less fatigue and lower risk of low back trauma. Aerobic activity should be performed consistent with **ACSM guidelines.**

e. **Lumbar flexion, extension, and flexibility exercises** may be performed daily. Flexibility exercises should **target the low back region and the hamstring muscle groups** following general flexibility exercise principles.

f. All exercise should be implemented **without exacerbating the existing condition.**

g. **Lumbar disc pressure** is generally **greatest in the seated position.** Clients may be more comfortable in a standing position.

h. **Swimming** is usually well tolerated.

i. Because not all back pain is secondary to excessive intravertebral disc loading, **weight-bearing activities such as walking and jogging may be appropriate** and should be considered on an individual basis.

j. **Spinal exercises** that are often used as part of a comprehensive back pain management program include:

  –**spinal flexion,** specifically the Williams flexion exercises.

  –**spinal extension,** namely McKenzie spinal extension exercises.

3. **Additional management modalities**

  –**Rest** is generally indicated for a short period but does little to resolve the underlying mechanical or musculoskeletal problems.

  –Back pain may also be managed with **physical therapy modalities, behavioral therapy,** and **medications** such as anti-inflammatory drugs and muscle relaxants.

VIII. ENVIRONMENTAL CONSIDERATIONS

–Excessive heat, humidity, cold, and air pollution change resting physiological state and its responses to exercise. **Heat and humidity impose the greatest environmental stress.**

A. HEAT AND HUMIDITY

–Exercise in thermally hostile conditions can **imperil the ability to properly thermoregulate.** Prolonged exposure results in a **gradual increase in core body temperature**, which inevitably results in **heat illness**, sometimes with devastating consequences.

–**Recommendations for exercise in the heat** focus on avoidance of the adverse environmental conditions and adequate hydration.

1. **Wet bulb globe temperature (WBGT)**

   –is **an index of environmental conditions.**

   –is dependent on air temperature, humidity, radiant heat from the sun, and wind speed.

   –**provides an index of relative risk for heat injury.**

2. **Heat illness**

   –can take several progressive forms, from **benign to life-threatening.**

   a. **Heat cramps** are not life threatening; they may result from dehydration.

   b. **Dehydration** is a result of excessive sweating and may be a precursor to heat injury. Water loss of as little as 1.5% of total body weight can decrease exercise performance.

   c. **Heat exhaustion** and **heat stroke** are **health- and life-threatening conditions** that result from a combination of metabolic heat generated during exercise accompanied by dehydration and electrolyte loss from sweating.

      (1) **Signs and symptoms** include uncoordinated gait, headache, dizziness, vomiting, and elevated body temperature.

      (2) **First aid**

      –If signs and symptoms of heat exhaustion or heat stroke are present:

      (a) **Discontinue exercise.**

      (b) **Place the person in the supine position with feet elevated.**

      (c) **Rehydrate the person immediately.**

      (d) **Cool the body** by any means possible.

   (3) **Prevent heat problems by:**

      (a) **acclimatizing properly (10–14 days).**

      (b) **exercising during cooler parts of the day.**

      (c) **reducing the duration and intensity or discontinuing exercise of WBGT > 88°F.**

      (d) **hydrating liberally before, during, and after exercise.**

B. ACUTE COLD EXPOSURE

–normally does not pose a significant health risk.

1. **Exercise generates metabolic heat** that warms the body.

2. **Clothing** can be used to help retain heat.

3. **Exercise performance** is not significantly reduced in a cold environment.

4. **Cold injury**

   –can occur during exercise in a cold and windy environment. **Types of cold injury** include:

   a. **Hypothermia**, a **potentially life-threatening** condition, occurs when metabolic heat production cannot compensate for heat loss to the environment, resulting in a gradual decrease in core temperature.

   b. **Frostbite** results from water crystallizing within tissues, with subsequent destruction of that tissue, which generally occurs when skin is exposed or insufficiently insulated.

   c. **Cold air does not usually damage lung tissue,** because inspired air is warmed adequately in the upper airways before reaching the lungs. **Inhalation of cold air may provoke anginal pain** in symptomatic cardiac patients or others with coronary artery disease.

5. **Prevention of cold injuries** requires a balance between exercise intensity and the insulating effect of protective clothing.

C. ALTITUDE

–Altitudes as low as 3000 feet can impose physiologic limitations on the human body.

1. **Physiology of high altitude exposure**

   –With increasing altitude, **barometric pressure decreases** along with **decrease in the partial pressure of oxygen** (PO_2).

–**A lower** P_{O_2} makes it more difficult for oxygen to move from the air (alveoli) into the blood (hemoglobin molecule), resulting in **reduced oxygen saturation** (Sa_{O_2}) of the blood. Consequently, **less oxygen is available for delivery to working tissue** resulting in a **reduced physical work capacity.**

–Physiological consequences include **an elevated HR** at rest and during exercise.

–Because $\dot{V}_{O_{2\,max}}$ decreases at altitudes above 3000 feet, all **submaximal tasks become relatively more difficult.**

–**Acclimatization** occurs gradually and is usually complete within 2 weeks.

2. **Medical problems associated with high altitude exposure**

   a. **Acute mountain sickness (AMS)**

   –**Common signs** include dehydration, severe headache, nausea and other gastrointestinal symptoms, decreased appetite, and insomnia.

   –If AMS is not partially resolved within 2–3 days, descent is recommended.

   b. **High-altitude pulmonary edema (HAPE)**

   –Although rare, it **can be life-threatening** if not attended to immediately.

   –Onset may be subtle, with signs including dyspnea, fatigue, chest pain, tachycardia, coughing, and cyanosis.

   –Immediate descent to lower altitude is essential.

   c. **Hypothermia** frequently compounds altitude problems.

3. **Prevention of high-altitude sickness**

   –**Avoidance of alcohol and caffeine-containing beverages** helps protect against dehydration.

–**Liberal fluid intake** should be encouraged to offset the fluid loss that occurs through hyperventilation, urination, and sweating.

–A **high-carbohydrate diet** helps maintain hydration and provides necessary energy for muscular work.

–**Unacclimatized persons should avoid vigorous exercise during early exposure to high altitude.**

–**Training HRs** prescribed at sea level apply to high altitude. However, exercise pace (i.e., running speed) will be reduced.

D. AIR POLLUTION

–is a health risk and can reduce exercise tolerance.

–may cause **bronchoconstriction** and **increased airway resistance.**

–**Reduced oxygen-carrying capacity** may occur due to competition for hemoglobin binding sites between oxygen and pollutants, particularly **when concentrations of carbon monoxide are high.**

1. **Persons at risk**

   –Persons with **reactive airways** are usually most affected by atmospheric pollutants.

2. **Exercise modifications**

   –**Avoid high pollution levels** by both timing and place of exercise.

   a. **Carbon monoxide levels** in cities are usually highest during rush hours.

   b. **Ozone levels** are usually lowest in winter and peak during afternoon hours in the late summer and early fall.

E. COMBINED ENVIRONMENTAL FACTORS

–Combinations of cold air, altitude, and air pollution may present significant limitations for exercise, particularly in those with EIA.

REVIEW TEST

DIRECTIONS: Carefully read all questions and select the BEST single answer.

1. All of the following statements are true regarding warm-up EXCEPT
   (A) muscle blood flow is increased as a result of warm-up.
   (B) peripheral vasodilation occurs as a result of warm-up.
   (C) peripheral vasoconstriction occurs as a result of warm-up.
   (D) 5–10 minutes should be allotted for a warm-up period.

2. All of the following statements are true regarding cool-down EXCEPT
   (A) the emphasis should be large muscle activity, performed at a low to moderate intensity.
   (B) increasing venous return should be a priority during cool-down.
   (C) the potential for improving flexibility may be improved during cool-down as compared with warm-up.
   (D) 1–2 minutes are recommended for an adequate cool-down.

3. All of the following are examples of aerobic exercise modalities EXCEPT
   (A) weight training.
   (B) walking.
   (C) bicycling.
   (D) stair climbing.

4. A target heart rate equivalent to 85% heart rate reserve (HRR) for a 25-year old male with a resting heart rate of 75 beats per minute would be equal to
   (A) 195 beats per minute.
   (B) 166 beats per minute.
   (C) 177 beats per minute.
   (D) 102 beats per minute.

5. The appropriate exercise heart rate for an individual on beta-blocking medication would generally be
   (A) 75% heart rate reserve.
   (B) 30 beats per minute above the standing resting heart rate.
   (C) 40% heart rate reserve.
   (D) (220 – age) × 0.85.

6. The recommended cardiorespiratory exercise training goal for apparently healthy individuals should be
   (A) 15 minutes, six times per week, at 90% HRR.
   (B) 30 minutes, three times per week, at 85% HRR.
   (C) 60 minutes, three times per week, at 85% HRR.
   (D) 30 minutes of weight training, three times per week, at 60% HRR.

7. In an effort to improve flexibility, ACSM recommends
   (A) proprioceptive neuromuscular facilitation (PNF).
   (B) ballistic stretching.
   (C) the plough and hurdler's stretches.
   (D) static stretches held for 10–30 seconds per repetition.

8. An appropriate exercise for improving the strength of the lower back muscles are
   (A) straight leg lifts.
   (B) parallel squats.
   (C) spinal extension exercises.
   (D) sit-ups with feet anchored.

9. Which of the following statements is NOT true regarding exercise leadership?
   (A) The exercise leader should be fit enough to exercise with any of his or her participants.
   (B) Most people are not bored by exercise and can easily find time to participate in an exercise program.
   (C) The exercise leader should adjust exercise intensity based on individual differences in fitness.
   (D) Periodic fitness assessment may provide evidence of improvement in fitness for some participants.

10. Which of the following statements is NOT true regarding exercise for the elderly?
    (A) A decrease in maximal heart rate is responsible for reductions in the maximal oxygen consumption as we age.
    (B) A loss of fat-free mass is responsible for a decrease in muscular strength as we age.
    (C) ACSM recommends a cardiorespiratory training intensity of 50–70% HRR for older adults.
    (D) Resistance exercise training is not recommended for older adults.

11.   Which of the following medications have been shown to be the most effective in preventing or reversing exercise-induced asthma?
(A)   Beta$_2$-agonists
(B)   Beta-blockers
(C)   Diuretics
(D)   Aspirin

12.   The exercise leader or health/fitness instructor should modify exercise sessions for hypertensive participants by
(A)   shortening the cool-down to less than 5 minutes.
(B)   eliminating resistance training completely.
(C)   prolonging the cool-down.
(D)   implementing high-intensity (> 85% HRR) short duration intervals.

13.   Normal values for fasting blood sugar are
(A)   > 140 mg/dl.
(B)   60–140 mg/dl.
(C)   < 60 mg/dl.
(D)   200–400 mg/dl.

14.   The goal for the obese exercise participant should be to
(A)   sweat as much as possible.
(B)   exercise at 85% HRR.
(C)   perform resistance exercise three to five times per week.
(D)   expend 300–500 calories per exercise session.

15.   Which of the following statements is true regarding exercise for persons with controlled cardiovascular disease?
(A)   Resistance exercise training is dangerous and should be avoided.
(B)   A physician-supervised exercise test is not necessary to establish exercise intensity.
(C)   Anginal pain is normal during exercise and participants should be pushed through the pain.
(D)   Exercise intensity should be set at a heart rate of 10 bpm less than the level where signs/symptoms were evidenced during an exercise test.

16.   All of the following factors are important to consider when determining exercise intensity EXCEPT
(A)   individual's level of fitness.
(B)   risk of cardiovascular or orthopedic injury.
(C)   previous history participating in organized sports.
(D)   individual preference and exercise objectives.

17.   When determining the intensity level, rating of perceived exertion (RPE) is a better indicator than percent of maximal heart rate for all of the following groups EXCEPT
(A)   individuals on beta-blockers.
(B)   aerobic classes that involve excessive arm movement.
(C)   individuals over 65.
(D)   individuals involved in high-intensity exercise.

18.   Using the original Borg scale, it is recommended that the exercise intensity elicit a rating of perceived exertion (RPE) within the range of
(A)   8–12.
(B)   12–16.
(C)   14–18.
(D)   6–10.

19.   The MINIMAL duration of exercise necessary to achieve improvements in health for deconditioned individuals is:
(A)   20 minutes continuously.
(B)   30 minutes continuously.
(C)   multiple sessions of < 10 minutes duration throughout the day.
(D)   two sessions of 20 minutes throughout the day.

20.   _____ is a method of strength and power training that involves an eccentric loading of muscles and tendons followed immediately by an explosive concentric contraction.
(A)   Super sets
(B)   Split routines
(C)   Plyometrics
(D)   Periodization

21.   The safety of resistance exercise is dependent on all of the following EXCEPT
(A)   having a personal trainer.
(B)   proper breathing.
(C)   speed of movement.
(D)   body mechanics.

22.   The recommended muscular strength and endurance training program for apparently healthy individuals should be
(A)   1 set of 8–12 reps, 8–10 separate exercises, 2 days/week.
(B)   2 sets of 6–8 reps, 8–10 separate exercises, 2 days/week.
(C)   1 set of 8–12 reps, 8–10 separate exercises, 4–5 days/week.
(D)   2 sets of 6–8 reps, 8–10 separate exercises, 4 days/week alternating days for legs and upper body.

23. All of the following statements are true with regard to intensity of resistance training EXCEPT
    (A) the number of repetitions to volitional fatigue will vary inversely with resistance.
    (B) it is necessary to determine the 1 RM to establish training intensity.
    (C) exercise to volitional fatigue is not dangerous from a musculoskeletal standpoint, provided good exercise form is maintained.
    (D) exercise intensity should be similar for males and females.

24. The recommended cardiorespiratory endurance exercise training program for older individuals should be
    (A) 40%–60% of HR_{max}, 20–30 minutes continuously, 3 days/week.
    (B) 50%–70% of HRR, 20–30 minutes (multiple sessions of 5–10 minutes), 3 days/week.
    (C) 40%–60% of HR_{max}, 20–30 minutes (multiple sessions of 5–10 minutes), 3 days/week.
    (D) 50%–70% of HRR, 20–30 minutes continuously, 3 days/week.

25. Osteoporosis is more prevalent in
    (A) women who have never been pregnant.
    (B) African-American women.
    (C) women involved in activities that place stress on the wrists, hips, or lumbosacral region.
    (D) postmenopausal women.

ANSWERS AND EXPLANATIONS

1–C. Peripheral vasoconstriction would be a negative consequence of warm-up if it did occur. Appropriate warm-up activities promote an increase in muscle blood flow and an increased oxygen delivery. This is accomplished through peripheral vasodilation. Typically a 5- to 10-minute time frame will allow for a gradual increase in heart rate, an increase in body temperature, and a slight reduction in pH. These changes will facilitate increased oxygen consumption. Although more research is needed to determine the effects of warm-up on musculoskeletal injury rates, it seems, that even from a psychological perspective, warm-up may prevent injury during exercise.

2–D. The primary purpose for cool-down is to increase venous return and is accomplished by low-intensity, large-muscle activity. This type of activity will also aid in the removal of lactic acid. Evidence of an effective cool-down is a heart rate less than 100 beats per minute and a systolic blood pressure within 10 mm Hg of pre-

exercise levels. Five to ten minutes will allow for these changes to occur and for some attention to flexibility exercises. The potential for improving flexibility is increased when the body is warm and muscles and connective tissue are more pliable, as is the case after exercise versus before.

3–A. Weight training is not considered an aerobic exercise. Although some increases in maximal oxygen consumption have been shown from circuit weight training, this is not considered to be the most effective means for improving cardiorespiratory fitness. Large-muscle group activity, performed in rhythmic fashion for a prolonged period, is the most efficient means for taxing the aerobic energy system.

4–C. Using 220 minus age (25) yields 195. Subtract 75 (resting heart rate) to yield heart rate reserve (120). Multiply 120 by .85 (85%) to yield 102, then add the resting heart rate (75) back in, to yield 177 as target heart rate.

5–A. Beta-blocking medications blunt the heart rate response at rest and during exercise, but the linear relationship between heart rate and oxygen consumption remains consistent with beta-blocking medication. It is appropriate to program exercise at a percentage of HRR; 75% is well within the correct range, but 40% HRR is not within Guidelines Standards.

6–B. Although additional improvements in maximal oxygen consumption may be seen when exercise is performed at greater than 85% HRR, or when duration exceeds 30 minutes, and at frequencies greater than three times per week, these improvements are minimal and are accompanied by increased musculoskeletal injury risk.

7–D. PNF is impractical because it requires a partner and potential for injury exists if the stretch is applied too vigorously. Ballistic stretching may induce soreness and actually impede the ability to stretch. The plough and hurdler's stretches are potentially harmful exercises that compromise the neck and knee, respectively. Isometric activity involves exerting force against an immovable object and is considered an inefficient form of muscle strengthening exercise. Static stretches held for 10–30 seconds per repetition have been shown to be effective, with low risk of injury.

8–C. Straight leg lifts are potentially harmful to the lower back and actually tax the hip flexors and the abdominals. Squats primarily involve the gluteals and the quadriceps. The erector spinae are the prime movers for spinal extension. Spinal flexion requires the abdominals to contract, while placing the low back muscles on a slight stretch. Sit-ups exercise the abdominal musculature and if performed with the feet anchored or to a full range of motion will involve the hip flexors.

9–B. Unless creative program strategies are employed, most people become bored with exercise. The exercise leader may be able to increase exercise program compliance by offering variety in programming; providing adequate instruction and encouragement; keeping participants injury free; and demonstrating progress through exercise testing. A comprehensive exercise program that can be completed in no more than 1 hour, three times per week should be developed for all participants who are interested in health/fitness. The idea is to minimize the time commitment and at the same time provide for maximal response.

10–D. Resistance exercise training for older adults is highly recommended to slow the typical age-related loss of lean tissue. Additional benefits include increases in bone density and improved functional capacity. Attention should be given to the overall health status of the individual and appropriate modifications made if there is presence of cardiovascular, metabolic, or musculoskeletal problems.

11–A. Beta$_2$ agonists provide effective bronchodilation with relatively minimal side effect. Beta-blockers are prescribed for cardiovascular concerns, including hypertension. Diuretics are also used to treat hypertension and congestive heart failure. Aspirin is used to reduce pain and fever, but provides no pulmonary effect. Theophylline has a slow onset of action and many associated side effects.

12–C. A prolonged cool-down of 5–10 minutes will enhance venous return and the hypotensive effects that are associated with many antihypertensive medications.

13–B. Blood sugar levels less than or equal to 60 mg/dl are considered to be hypoglycemic, whereas levels that are greater than or equal to 140 mg/dl are indicative of hyperglycemia.

14–D. The goal for weight loss would be to expend 300–500 kcal/exercise session in combination with a reduced caloric intake that would yield a total caloric deficit of no more than 1000 kcal/day or 7000 kcal/week. The recommended rate of weight loss should not exceed one to two pounds per week to ensure adequate nutrition and health. The emphasis for weight-loss exercise programs should be large muscle group aerobic type exercise at a level of intensity that will allow for the greatest caloric expenditure for the time spent exercising, with attention given to musculoskeletal and cardiovascular safety.

15–D. According to ACSM, individuals with known disease should have a clinical exercise test prior to exercise participation. A purpose of this test is to determine safe levels of exercise for the participant. Exercise intensity should be set at one MET below the level where signs/symptoms are evidenced. A heart rate 10 beats/minute less than the heart rate where signs/symptoms are evidenced may also be used. Whenever anginal pain is evidenced during exercise, the exercise should be terminated and appropriate medical attention sought.

16–C. The risk of orthopedic and perhaps cardiovascular complications may be increased with high-intensity activity. Factors to consider when determining intensity include the individual's level of fitness, presence of medications that may influence exercise performance, risk of cardiovascular or orthopedic injury, and the individual preference for exercise and individual program objectives.

17–D. The RPE is particularly useful when participants are incapable of monitoring their pulse or when medications such as beta-blockers alter the heart rate response to exercise. Excessive arm movements (such as in high-intensity exercise) makes it difficult to feel and accurately count the pulse rate.

18–B. The RPE is particularly useful when participants are incapable of monitoring their pulse or when medications such as beta-blockers alter the heart rate response to exercise. The ACSM recommends an exercise intensity that will elicit an RPE within a range of 12–16 on the original Borg scale.

19–C. The ACSM recommends 20 to 60 minutes of continuous aerobic activity. Typically, adequate caloric expenditure and cardiorespiratory conditioning goals may be met with exercise sessions of moderate duration (20 to 30 minutes). Individuals who are very deconditioned may benefit from multiple exercise sessions of short (< 10 minutes) duration. Increases in duration may be instituted as evidence of adaptation occurs without undue fatigue or injury.

20–C. Plyometrics is a method of strength and power training that involves an eccentric loading of muscles and tendons followed immediately by an explosive concentric contraction. This stretch-shortening cycle may allow for an enhanced force generation during the concentric (shortening) phase.

21–A. The safety of resistance exercise is dependent on the proper execution of a given exercise. Spotting, proper breathing, speed of movement, and body mechanics are all central to safe exercise performance.

22–A. The ACSM recommends that one set of 8–12 repetitions of exercise should be performed to volitional fatigue at least two days each week.

23–B. Intensity is defined as a percent of one's momentary ability to perform an activity; that is, how difficult the exercise is, or the amount of effort during the exercise. It is the percentage of the maximal voluntary contraction in resistance exercise. It is not the percent of 1 RM unless all other variables (i.e., the individual exercise, speed of movement, number of repetitions) are kept constant.

24–B. The health status of the individual should be carefully considered when establishing intensity. Generally, a conservative approach should be taken initially. The ACSM recommends an intensity of 50%–70% of heart rate reserve for older adults.

25–D. Osteoporosis is the reduction in bone mass per unit volume. Reduced bone mass is more prevalent in sedentary individuals and progresses at a more rapid rate in women following menopause. This condition increases the risk for fractures of the wrists, hips, and lumbosacral regions and is considered a significant source of debilitation in older adults.

CHAPTER 9

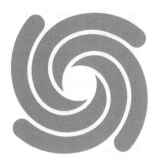

Nutrition and Weight Management
MAUREEN SMITH PLOMBON AND JANET R. WOJCIK

I. ESSENTIAL NUTRIENTS

–There are **six major categories of nutrients,** representing over 50 known nutrients used by the body for daily functioning. These categories are **carbohydrates, proteins, fats, vitamins, minerals, and water.**

A. MACRONUTRIENTS CONSIST OF CARBOHYDRATES, PROTEIN, AND FAT.

1. **Carbohydrates (CHO)**

   –are compounds made up of **carbon, hydrogen, and oxygen** whose primary function is to provide a **continuous energy source** to all cells.

   –are easily metabolized to produce energy in the form of **adenosine triphosphate (ATP).**

   a. There are **two types of carbohydrates:**

      (1) Simple carbohydrates are the **sugars:** glucose, fructose, galactose not found free in nature, a breakdown of lactose (disaccharide), sucrose, and lactose.

      (2) Complex carbohydrates (starches)

      –are composed of **chains of single sugars.**

      –are found in such foods as pasta, bread, cereal, rice, fruits, and vegetables.

   b. **Blood glucose** is the most immediate energy source.

      (1) Regardless of type or food source, all carbohydrates (simple and complex) are broken down to glucose for metabolic purposes.

      (2) Glucose is **stored as glycogen** in liver, muscle, and other tissues.

   c. **Fiber (roughage)** is a type of carbohydrate that **passes through the alimentary canal without being broken down** by the enzymes of the digestive system.

      –Intakes of fiber at the recommended level of 20–35 g/day have been linked to the prevention of certain diseases, including heart disease, diabetes, and some types of cancer.

      (1) Insoluble fiber

      –absorbs water in the large intestine; softens stool.

      –is theorized to reduce colon cancer risk.

      –includes cellulose, hemicellulose, or lignin.

      –is found in whole-grain products such as high-fiber cereals and breads, and in vegetables.

      (2) Soluble fiber

      –dissolves in water.

      –reduces blood cholesterol levels; offers protection against CAD.

      –is found in fruits (especially apples, oranges, pears, peaches, and grapes), vegetables, legumes, and brans.

      –includes pectin and gums.

2. **Protein**

   –is made up primarily of **carbon, hydrogen, and oxygen,** but also includes **nitrogen.**

   –All proteins in the body are **synthesized from 20 amino acids.** These amino acids are combined and modified to make specific long-sequenced chains of proteins that can be used to synthesize many structures such as **muscle, hormones, enzymes, and hemoglobin.**

  a. The **eight essential amino acids** cannot be manufactured from other sources; they **must be obtained by dietary intake.**

  b. **Complete proteins**

   –are foods that **provide all the essential amino acids.**

   –include **animal products** such as eggs, milk, cheese, meat, poultry, and fish.

  c. **Incomplete proteins**

   –are a narrow selection of amino acids, as found in **plant sources.**

   –**Combining a wide variety of incomplete proteins** within the meal or throughout the day **helps to provide a complete intake of essential amino acids.**

3. **Fat**

 –Dietary fat includes triglycerides, cholesterol, and phospholipids.

  a. **Triglycerides**

   –are **glycerol molecules** connected to **three fatty acid molecules.**

   –represent **> 90% of the fat** stored in the body.

   –Fats stored as triglycerides in adipose tissue and surrounding muscle tissue provide the body with a **large energy reserve.**

   –Fat also **surrounds and protects vital organs and the spinal cord, preserves body heat,** and acts as a **store for the fat-soluble vitamins A, D, E, and K.**

   –**Fatty acids** are classified by the number of chemical bonds that link the carbon atoms.

   (1) Saturated fatty acids

   –have only **single bonds.**

   –typically come from **animal sources.**

   –also include **palm oil, palm kernel oil, coconut oil, and cocoa butter.**

   –Foods that contain a large number of saturated fats are **solid at room temperature.**

   (2) Monounsaturated fatty acids

   –have **one double bond.**

   –are **liquid at room temperature.**

   –include **olive, rapeseed (canola), and peanut oils.**

   (3) Polyunsaturated fatty acids

   –have **two or more double bonds.**

   –are **liquid at room temperature.**

   –include **corn, safflower, soybean, and cottonseed oils.**

  b. **Cholesterol**

   –is a waxy, fat-like compound present in membranes of all **animal cells.**

   –is **not found in plants** or plant products.

   –is **synthesized in the liver.**

   –is used in the **digestion and absorption of fat.**

   –is used in **the production of all steroid hormones,** i.e., cortisol, estrogen, progesterone, and adrenal androgens.

  c. **Phospholipids**

   –All cells contain phospholipids, which are essential for absorption and digestion of fats.

   –Phospholipids facilitate uptake of fatty acids by cells.

   –Phospholipids comprise a significant proportion of blood lipoproteins.

B. MICRONUTRIENTS CONSIST OF VITAMINS AND MINERALS.

1. **Vitamins**

 –are **organic compounds** derived from living substances.

 –are **required in small amounts** to maintain life.

 –provide no energy.

 –are essential for a variety of roles in the body, from **nutrient processing** to **formation of red blood cells.**

 –Most act as **co-factors** that **help enzymes** function.

 –The **13 vitamins** are categorized as **fat-soluble or water-soluble.**

  a. **Fat-soluble vitamins (A, D, E, K)**

   –are **absorbed through intestinal membranes** and **stored in body fat.**

   –Excessive intake of fat-soluble vitamins, especially A and D, may lead to **toxicity** manifesting in physical symptoms and **may** adversely affect the balance of other vitamins.

Table 9-1. Function, Source and Recommended Dietary Allowances (RDA) for Vitamins*

Vitamin	Main Function	Good Sources	RDA (adult)
A	Maintenance of skin, bone, growth, vision, and teeth	Eggs, cheese, margarine, milk, carrots, broccoli, squash, and spinach	m: 1000 μg f: 800 μg
D	Bone growth and maintenance of bones	Milk, egg yolk, tuna, and salmon (sunlight)	m: 5 μg f: 5 μg
E	Antioxidant	Vegetable oils, whole-grain cereal, bread, dried beans, & green leafy vegetables	m: 10 mg f: 8 mg
K	Blood clotting	Cabbage, green leafy vegetables, milk	m: 80 μg f: 65 μg
Thiamine (B_1)	Energy-releasing reactions	Pork, ham, oysters, breads, cereals, pasta, green peas	m: 1.5 mg f: 1.1 mg
Riboflavin (B_2)	Energy-releasing reactions	Milk, meat, cereals, pasta, mushrooms, dark green vegetables	m: 1.7 mg f: 1.3 mg
Niacin	Energy-releasing reactions	Poultry, meat, tuna, cereal, pasta, bread, nuts, legumes	m: 19 mg f: 15 mg
Pyridoxine (B_6)	Metabolism of fats & proteins & formation of red blood cells	Cereals, bread, spinach, avocados, green beans, bananas	m: 2.0 mg f: 1.6 mg
Cobalamin (B_{12})	Formation of red blood cells & functioning of nervous system	Meat, fish, eggs, milk	m: 2.0 μg f: 2.0 μg
Folacin	Assists in forming proteins & in formation of red blood cells	Dark green leafy vegetables, wheat germ, oranges, bananas	m: 200 μg f: 180 μg
Pantothenic acid	Metabolism of proteins, CHO, & fats, formation of hormones	Bread, cereals, nuts, eggs, & dark green vegetables	ESADDI = 7–9 mg
Biotin	Formation of fatty acids & energy-releasing reactions	Egg yolk, leafy green vegetables	ESADDI = 30–100 μg
C	Maintenance of bones, teeth, blood vessels, & collagen: antioxidant	Citrus fruits, tomatoes, strawberries, melons, green peppers, potatoes	m: 60 mg f: 60 mg

m = male; f = female; ESADDI = Estimated Safe and Adequate Daily Dietary Intake.

*With permission from the National Resource Council. *Recommended Dietary Allowances,* 10th ed. Washington, DC: National Academy of Sciences, 1989.

b. **Water-soluble vitamins (C and the eight B vitamins)**

–are not typically stored in the same manner as fat-soluble vitamins; they require **regular intake.**

–Toxic levels may occur with oversupplementation of C, B_6, and niacin.

2. **Minerals**

–are inorganic substances.

–**provide structure** for teeth and bones.

–serve as **important parts of enzymes (co-enzymes) and hormones.**

–are responsible for **acid-base balance.**

–aid in the **conduction of electrical impulses** throughout the body.

a. **Macrominerals** (needed in relatively large doses)

–Calcium

–Phosphorus

–Magnesium

–Potassium

–Sulfur

–Sodium

–Chloride

b. **Microminerals** (needed in small amounts)

–Iron

–Zinc

–Selenium

–Manganese

–Molybdenum

–Iodine

–Copper

–Chromium

–Fluoride

Table 9-2. Function, Source and Recommended Dietary Allowances (RDA) for Minerals*

Mineral	Main Function	Good Sources	RDA (Adult)
Calcium	Formation of bones, teeth, maintenance of nerve impulses, blood clotting	Cheese, sardines, dark green vegetables, vegetables, clams, milk	m: 800 mg f: 800 mg
Phosphorus	Formation of bones & teeth, acid-base balance	Milk, cheese, meat, fish, poultry, nuts, grains	m: 800 mg f: 800 mg
Magnesium	Activation of enzymes and protein synthesis	Nuts, meat, milk, whole-grain cereal, green leafy vegetables	m: 350 mg f: 280 mg
Sodium	Acid-base balance, body water balance, nerve function	Most foods	min. = 500 mg
Potassium	Acid-base balance, body water balance, nerve function	Meat, milk, many fruits, cereals, vegetables, legumes	min. = 2000 mg
Chloride	Gastric juice formation & acid-base balance	Table salt, seafood, milk, meat, eggs	
Iron	Component of hemoglobin & enzymes	Meats, legumes, eggs, grains, dark green vegetables	m: 10 mg f: 15 mg
Zinc	Component of many enzymes	Milk, shellfish, & wheat bran	m: 15 mg f: 12 mg
Iodine	Component of thyroid hormone	Fish, dairy products, vegetables, iodized salt	m: 150 mg f: 150 mg
Copper	Component of enzymes, delivers iron from storage	Shellfish, grains, cherries, legumes, poultry, oysters, nuts	ESADDI = 1.5–3 mg
Manganese	Component of enzymes, fat synthesis	Greens, blueberries, grains, legumes, fruit	ESADDI = 2–5 mg
Fluoride	Maintenance of bones and teeth	Water, seafood, rice, soybeans, spinach, onions, and lettuce	ESADDI = 1.5–4 mg
Chromium	Glucose and energy metabolism	Fats, meats, clams, cereals	ESADDI = 50–200 μg
Selenium	Functions with vitamin E antioxidant	Fish, poultry, meats, grains, milk, vegetables	m: 70 μg f: 55 μg
Molybdenum	Component of enzymes	Legumes, cereals, dark green leafy vegetables	ESADDI = 70–250 μg

m = male; f = female; ESADDI = Estimated Safe and Adequate Daily Dietary Intake.

*With permission from the National Resource Council. *Recommended Dietary Allowances,* 10th ed. Washington, DC: National Academy of Sciences, 1989.

3. Recommended Dietary Allowances (RDAs) for Vitamins and Minerals (**Tables 9-1 and 9-2**)

–RDAs are **dietary standards established by the Food and Nutrition Board of the National Academy of Sciences.** They are intended to be **recommendations for the dietary intake of a population group** (i.e., children, pregnant women) over a period of time.

–RDAs are defined as "levels of intake of essential nutrients considered to be adequate to meet the known nutritional needs of practically all healthy persons." If no RDA level has been set, an "estimated safe and adequate intake" has been established.

–Although RDAs are commonly used to assess the adequacy of daily diet, their purpose is broader. They are specifically set to provide a

margin of safety to ensure that the needs of nearly all the population are met.

–Although intakes below the RDA are not necessarily inadequate, over a long period of time this may result in a deficiency of a nutrient.

–RDAs are **not intended to define the special nutritional needs of persons with certain medical conditions** that may alter the nutritional balance and needs.

C. **WATER**

–makes up approximately **60%–70% of total body weight.**

–is **an essential nutrient** because its absence limits survival. Essential body functions cannot occur without water.

–**Maintaining adequate hydration** is an important concern.

1. **It is recommended that the average adult consume 2–3 liters of water daily.** This is approximately the amount of water that is lost per day through sweat, breathing, and urination.

2. **Groups particularly at risk for dehydration** are:

   –the physically active.

   –infants and young children.

   –the elderly.

   –the ill.

3. **Sweating** is part of the heat-regulatory mechanism. Consumption of plain, cool water is usually sufficient for maintaining proper hydration during heat stress or activity. However, for exercise sessions longer than 90 minutes in duration, or for physical activities conducted in hot environments, **sport beverages** are often recommended because they also replenish electrolytes and supply energy.

4. **Exercise hydration recommendations**

   –**Pre-exercise:** Consume 8–16 oz 10–15 minutes prior.

   –**During exercise:** Consume 8–10 oz every 20 minutes.

   –**Post exercise:** Consume 16–32 oz for every pound of weight lost.

II. ENERGY

–**Food provides energy** for all biochemical reactions involved in physical work, movement, body temperature regulation, cell development, maintenance, and growth. The energy contained in ingested foods and body stores is turned into a usable form of chemical energy.

A. CALORIES

1. **Energy intake and expenditure** is often expressed in terms of **calories.**

   –**One calorie** represents the **amount of heat required to raise the temperature of one kilogram of water by one degree Celsius.**

   –Most scientific publications use the term *kilocalorie (kcal),* which can be used interchangeably with the term *calorie.*

2. **Energy requirements** are determined by a variety of factors such as age, size, metabolic rate, and level of physical activity.

3. **Carbohydrates and proteins** each provide approximately **4 kcal of energy per gram.**

4. **Fat provides 9 kcal of energy per gram.**

5. **One pound of body fat,** like all other triglycerides, contains energy in the amount of **3500 kcal.**

B. ENERGY BALANCE

–is achieved when **caloric intake is equivalent to total body energy needs,** leading to **maintenance of body weight.**

1. **Negative energy balance** occurs when more calories are expended than are consumed, resulting in **weight loss.**

2. **Positive energy balance** occurs when more calories are consumed than expended, resulting in **weight gain.** Excess kcal are stored in the body as triglycerides in fat cells (adipose tissue).

C. CALCULATION OF TOTAL ENERGY NEEDS

–A quick approximation of current energy needs—the amount of energy required for energy balance or to maintain weight—may be calculated using **Table 9-3**, which provides an estimate of daily energy allowances.

D. MACRONUTRIENT RECOMMENDATIONS

1. **Carbohydrates**

   –should compose at least **55% of total energy intake** (about 15% from simple sugars).

   –**Male athletes** may consume up to **70% total energy** from carbohydrates.

   –**Female athletes,** who typically consume less overall energy than male athletes, may consume at least **60% total energy** from carbohydrates.

2. **Protein**

   –Approximately **10%–15% of total energy intake** should come from protein.

   –Persons involved in **strength and power training may require more** than the RDA of **0.8 g/kg body weight.** Even for these particular athletes, there is likely **no benefit in exceeding protein intake of 1.5 g/kg body weight.**

Table 9-3. Estimation of Daily Energy Allowances at Various Levels of Physical Activity for Men and Women Aged 19–50*

Level of Activity (kcal/kg per day)	Energy Expenditure
Very Light	
Men	31
Women	30
Light	
Men	38
Women	33
Moderate	
Men	40
Women	47
Heavy	
Men	50
Women	44

- *Very light activity* is defined as mostly seated and standing activities such as driving, typing, ironing, cooking, or playing cards.
- *Light activity* is defined as walking on level surfact at 2.5 to 3.0 mph such as housecleaning, child care, golf, restaurant trades.
- *Moderate activity* is defined as walking 3.5 to 4 mph, weeding and hoeing, cycling, skiing, and dancing.
- *Heavy* is defined as walking with a load or uphill, heavy manual labor, basketball, climbing, football, or soccer.

*With permission from Food and Nutrition Board. *Recommended Dietary Allowances,* 10th ed. Washington, DC: National Academy Press, 1989.

Source: ACSM Resource Manual 3/e

3. **Fat**

   –A healthy diet **should not exceed 30%** of **total energy intake** from fat, with **saturated fat comprising no more than 10%** of total intake.

   –**Very low fat intake** usually results in high carbohydrate intake, which **may reduce the intake of fat-soluble vitamins.**

4. **Calculation of macronutrient intake**

   –Macronutrient intake is derived by **multiplying the total caloric daily requirement by the recommended macronutrient proportion,** and **dividing the product by the number of calories-per-gram of the macronutrient.** For example, an individual whose caloric needs are estimated at 2000 kcal per day should consume 275 g of CHO ([2000 × 0.55]/4), 75 g of protein ([2000 × 0.15]/4), and no more than 67 g of fat ([2000 × 0.30]/9).

E. **ENERGY AND WEIGHT LOSS**

1. **Weight loss of about 1–2 pounds (0.5–1.0 kg) per week is recommended** for overweight persons.

2. **Reducing 1 pound of body weight (0.45 kg) by achieving a negative energy balance of 3500 kcal per week** can be accomplished by several methods:

   a. Reducing energy intake by 500 kcal/day

   b. Increasing energy expenditure through physical activity by 500 kcal/day

   c. Reducing energy intake by 250 kcal/day plus increasing energy expenditure by 250 kcal/day for a total negative energy balance of 500 kcal/day

      –This may be the most practical method for the short term and the most successful for the long term.

      –Exercise can help promote more fat loss while maintaining lean body mass.

3. **Common recommendations of energy intakes for weight loss**

   –**Men: 1800–2000 kcal/day**

   –**Women: 1200–1500 kcal/day**

   –These ranges **should be adjusted upward if weight loss exceeds 2 pounds per week after the first 2 weeks** of reduced energy intake.

III. BODY COMPOSITION

–"Body composition" generally refers to **partitioning the body into fat and fat-free components.** The fat component is often expressed as **percent body fat;** the fat-free component is also known as **lean body mass.**

A. THE ROLE OF BODY COMPOSITION IN HEALTH IS SUPPORTED BY SUBSTANTIAL RESEARCH.

1. **Excess body fat** is associated with a higher risk of **diabetes, coronary artery disease, high blood pressure,** and some types of **cancers.**

2. **Very low body fat** is often associated with **disease states, malnourishment,** and **mortality.**

3. **Low fat-free mass** can signal **low functional capacity, low energy expenditure,** and **increased risk of osteoporosis.**

B. **BODY FAT DISTRIBUTION MAY BE AN INDICATOR OF RISK FOR CORONARY ARTERY DISEASE AND TYPE II DIABETES. FROM A HEALTH PERSPECTIVE, IT IS MORE IMPORTANT TO LOSE EXCESS BODY WEIGHT AT THE WAIST.**

1. **Male-type distribution**

   –is defined as excess weight around the waist **(android-type obesity).**

   –is very labile (can be gained or lost fairly quickly).

2. **Female-type distribution**

   –is defined as excess weight around the hips/buttocks **(gynoid-type obesity).**

   –is more resistant to weight loss.

   –confers no known health risk.

C. **WAIST/HIP RATIO**

   –is indicator of body weight distribution.

   –A waist-to-hip ratio **> 0.86 for women** and **> 0.95 for men** has been associated with an **increased risk of type II diabetes, heart disease, and hypertension.**

D. **OVERWEIGHT**

   –is defined as **body weight in excess of some standard.**

1. The **NIH Consensus Conference on the Health Risks of Obesity** in 1985 defined overweight as **20% greater than the ideal weight range for a given height.**

2. The most commonly used standards are the 1959 and 1983 **Metropolitan Life Insurance Company weight tables** (established in 1959 and updated in 1983).

3. Total body weight does not reflect body composition (fat/lean weight ratio). Excess body weight may not confer a health risk.

E. **OBESITY**

   –is often defined as the **accumulation and storage of excess body fat.**

–**Body mass index (BMI)** is commonly used **to assess obesity** both individually and in large population studies, and is used **to assign health risk.**

–BMI is calculated using the **Quetelet equation:**

   body weight (in kg)/height (in meters)²

–A healthy weight target representing a **BMI < 25 for everyone over age 20 is recommended.**

–A person with a **BMI > 25** is considered **mildly obese** and is at a **higher risk for diseases** such as cardiovascular disease and Type II diabetes.

–**Weight loss and other lifestyle changes** are especially encouraged for those with **BMI ≥ 27.**

F. **RECOMMENDATIONS ON WEIGHT-LOSS PROGRAMS**

   –The **ACSM Position Stand on Weight-Loss Programs** states that a **desirable weight-loss program:**

1. Provides **at least 1200 calories per day** for normal adults to meet nutritional requirements.

2. Includes **food acceptable to the individual** in terms of sociocultural background, usual habits, taste, cost, and ease in acquisition and preparation.

3. Provides a **negative caloric balance** (not to exceed 500–1000 calories per day lower than recommended intake), **resulting in gradual weight loss** without metabolic abnormalities; **maximal weight loss should not exceed 2.2 lb (1 kg) per week.**

4. Includes the use of **behavior modification** to identify and eliminate dieting habits that contribute to improper nutrition.

5. Includes an **endurance exercise** program of at least **3 days a week, 20–30 minutes** per exercise session, at a minimum intensity of **60% of maximum heart rate.**

6. Provides for **new eating and physical activity habits** that can be continued for life in order to maintain the achieved lower body weight.

IV. DIET, EXERCISE, AND CARDIOVASCULAR DISEASE RISK

A. **HEALTH RISKS OF A HIGH-FAT DIET**

   –A diet high in fat, especially saturated fatty acids and cholesterol, raises **blood cholesterol levels** in many people. Elevated blood cholesterol is a major risk factor for **coronary heart disease.**

–A high-fat diet is linked to other health problems such as **obesity** and some types of **cancer**

–A diet rich in fats, sugars, and excess calories can also raise **blood triglycerides,** which also increases the risk for **heart disease.**

B. LIPOPROTEINS AND RISK OF HEART DISEASE

–Cholesterol must combine with protein to be carried in the blood. These lipoprotein molecules are differentiated by their density.

1. **Very low-density lipoproteins (VLDL)** are **the primary carriers of triglycerides** in the blood.

2. **Low-density lipoproteins (LDL)**

   –are the **primary carriers of cholesterol.**

   –attach to the artery wall at sites of injury and deposit cholesterol.

3. **High-density lipoproteins (HDL)**

   –**may inhibit LDL from attaching to the walls of the artery.**

   –**play a protective role by removing the cholesterol** from the wall of the artery and returning it to the liver where it is metabolized and excreted.

C. DIETARY CHANGES AND THE BLOOD LIPID PROFILE

–A **1% reduction in blood cholesterol** results in a **2% reduction in the risk of a heart attack.**

–The **National Cholesterol Education Program (NCEP II)** provides guidelines for lowering blood cholesterol and/or altering LDL/HDL ratio:

1. The **Step I diet** is the first-line of treatment and includes:

   a. **Total fat no more than 30%** of total kcal

   b. **Saturated fat no more than 8%–10%** of total kcal

   c. **Cholesterol** intake **less than 300 mg/day**

2. Persons unresponsive to the Step I diet may go to a **Step II diet.**

   a. The Step II diet **further restricts saturated fat to 7%** of total kcal and **cholesterol to 200 mg/day.**

   b. **Other dietary recommendations** to help lower cholesterol include:

      –**folic acid** supplements to lower blood homocysteine levels.

      –**omega-3 fatty acid** supplements (or increasing dietary intake of fish in the form of salmon, tuna, halibut, sardines and whitefish, or increasing dietary intake of canola oil and soybean oil).

      –using **soy proteins** instead of animal proteins.

      –increasing dietary intake of soluble fiber.

D. EXERCISE AND THE BLOOD LIPID PROFILE

a. Accumulating a weekly energy expenditure of 1000–1200 kcal by performing **aerobic exercise** 45 min/day **may increase HDL cholesterol.**

b. Aerobic exercise **may also decrease serum triglyceride levels.**

c. **Combination of weight loss and fat loss** amplifies the increase in HDL from aerobic exercise training.

V. GENERAL DIETARY GUIDELINES FOR HEALTH

–The U.S. Department of Agriculture (USDA) provides the most current advice from health and nutrition experts.

A. U.S. DIETARY GUIDELINES FOR AMERICANS

—**emphasize variety, balance, and moderation** in the total diet.

–**apply to the total diet,** i.e., not just one meal or one day, but all food choices over time.

–include **seven general recommendations.**

> **Recommendations of the U.S. Dietary Guidelines for Americans (1995)**
> 1. Eat a variety of foods.
> 2. Balance the food you eat with physical activity–maintain or improve your weight.
> 3. Choose a diet with plenty of grain products, vegetables, and fruit.
> 4. Choose a diet low in fat, saturated fat, and cholesterol.
> 5. Choose a diet moderate in sugars.
> 6. Choose a diet moderate in salt and sodium.
> 7. If you drink alcoholic beverages, do so in moderation.

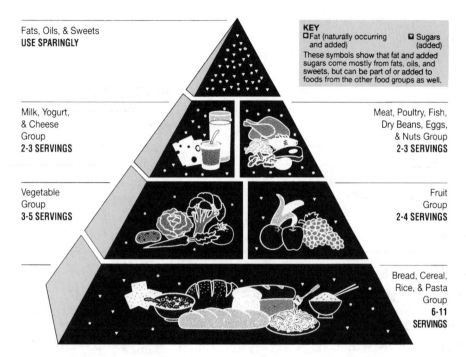

FIGURE 9-1 The USDA Food Guide Pyramid. (U.S. Department of Agriculture / U.S. Department of Health and Human Services.)

B. USDA FOOD GUIDE PYRAMID (Figure 9-1)

–is an educational tool designed to **simplify the U.S. Dietary Guidelines** by enabling people to visualize the recommended distribution among the basic 5 food groups.

–The **base of the pyramid** represents those foods (**carbohydrates**) that should make up the **largest portion of the diet.**

–Smaller intakes are recommended as one moves up the pyramid.

> **Basic 5 Food Groups**
> • Grain products (bread, cereal, rice, and pasta)
> • Vegetables
> • Fruits
> • Milk (milk, yogurt, cheese)
> • Meat and beans group (meat, poultry, fish, dry beans, eggs, and nuts)

–The **peak of the pyramid** represents **fats, oils, and sweets,** which **should be eaten least often.**

VI. MYTHS, FADS, AND MISCONCEPTIONS ABOUT WEIGHT LOSS

A. SPOT REDUCTION

–refers to **losing fat mass in specific body parts** by concentrating exercise on those selected areas.

–**does not work** because the body gains and loses fat in a genetically predetermined way.

–**may give the illusion of localized fat loss.** Repeated exercise on selected muscles may improve the local muscle strength, resulting in the appearance and "feel" of fat loss.

B. VERY LOW CALORIE DIETS (VLCDS) AND RAPID WEIGHT LOSS

–VLCDs are designed to maximize weight loss in a minimum of time. These diets are **usually not effective in the long term.**

–Total daily energy intake is in the range of **400–800 kcal/day.** With minimal energy intake (< 800 kcal), **the body is not able to maintain normal glucose levels** and is **in danger of receiving an inadequate supply of nutrients.**

–VLCDs **may be dangerous to individuals at risk for diabetes or heart disease.** The body enters a state of semistarvation, lowering metabolic rate, depleting glycogen stores from the muscle, and incompletely oxidizing fats for energy (which produces ketone bodies).

–**Most weight loss results from water that is released** when glycogen is broken down within the muscle. **Lean body mass may be lost as well, resulting in sustained lower metabolic rate and energy needs.** When normal eating is resumed, glycogen stores are replenished, but lean body mass is unchanged. As fat is regained, the result is a higher body fat percentage as a result of lowered lean body mass.

C. SAUNAS, BODY WRAPS, AND "SWEAT" SUITS

–Heat treatments such as these cause weight loss to occur as **water weight,** based on the premise that weight can be "sweated off." **Weight loss is only temporary;** weight is regained when fluids are consumed.

–The resulting **dehydration can be serious and potentially lethal** as a result of electrolyte imbalances and risk of heat-related illness.

–Dehydration reduces ability to perform work.

D. VIBRATING BELTS AND ELECTRIC STIMULATORS

–are not effective because mechanical, passive manipulation of muscles or skin results in **negligible energy expenditure,** and, therefore, **cannot impact fat loss.**

VII. ERGOGENIC AIDS

–Ergogenic aids are **substances believed to improve muscle size, strength, endurance, or athletic performance.** Some products may be benign, but others may have serious side effects. For additional information, refer to the American Dietetic Association Position Paper, "Nutrition for Physical Fitness and Athletic Performance for Adults," endorsed by the ACSM.

A. CARBOHYDRATE SUPPLEMENTS

1. Rationale for use
   a. A pre-event meal with adequate CHO is important for the **maintenance of blood glucose levels during exercise.**
   b. Maintenance of blood glucose during exercise **to prolong endurance** may be achieved by drinking a **6%–8% carbohydrate or carbohydrate/electrolyte solution.**

      –20 to 40 oz per hour should provide 60–70 g of CHO.

      –A drink containing more than 17 g CHO per 8 oz of fluid may lead to stomach irritation and cramps.
   c. **Replenishing muscle glycogen stores following exercise** is best achieved when an athlete consumes 1.0–1.5 g CHO per kg body weight within 30–60 minutes after exercise. (*Note:* This amount is difficult to consume within 30 minutes; some recommend consumption within the first 2 hours after exercise.)

2. Caveats

   –Too much carbohydrate in excess of energy needs will be converted to **body fat,** but otherwise there are no known health risks of oversupplementation.

–**Glucose or glucose polymer solutions** are recommended because fructose tends to irritate stomach.

3. Summary

   –Experimental research **supports efficacy and safety.**

B. PROTEIN AND AMINO ACID SUPPLEMENTS

1. Rationale for use

   –Advocates believe that more amino acids will be available for synthesis of new muscle protein **to increase muscle mass.**

2. Caveats

   –**Amino acids are very labile and not stored in the body** in a manner similar to glycogen.

   –**Research does not support benefit of consuming more than 1.5 g protein/kg body weight,** even in strength/power athletes.

   –Use may lead to **dehydration** and **excess protein in the urine,** and may unduly **stress the kidneys.**

   –Adequate protein can be easily obtained by food intake.

   –**Research does not support benefit** of supplementation with amino acids.

3. Summary

   –Experimental research **does not support** use.

C. VITAMINS AND MINERALS

1. Rationale for use

   –Advocates believe that vitamin and mineral supplements provide additional benefits to improve athletic performance.

2. Caveats

   –**Toxic levels** may build up.

–Athletes eating adequate diets rarely experience nutritional deficiencies.

–**Supplements cannot substitute for lack of adequate diet;** nutrient co-factors only found in whole foods are not present in supplements.

–Supplementation of a single vitamin or mineral may affect metabolism of other nutrients.

3. **Summary**

–Vitamin and mineral supplements are **generally not recommended** except under guidance of a physician or registered dietitian to correct nutritional deficiencies.

D. SODIUM BICARBONATE

1. **Rationale for use**

–Advocates believe that sodium bicarbonate will **enhance performance in short-term, high-intensity exercise** by inducing alkalosis (raise blood pH) to buffer hydrogen ion (H^+) and lactic acid.

2. **Caveats**

–Sodium bicarbonate often results in **abdominal cramps and diarrhea** approximately 1 hour after ingestion.

–**Safety is unknown.**

–**Research results are equivocal.**

3. **Summary**

–The use of sodium bicarbonate is **not recommended.**

E. BEE POLLEN

1. **Rationale for use**

–Advocates believe that bee pollen contains vitamins and minerals that act as **antioxidants to promote exercise endurance.**

2. **Caveats**

–Experimental studies **fail to support** an ergogenic effect.

–There is a potential to produce **serious allergic reaction** in sensitive persons.

3. **Summary**

–The use of bee pollen is **not recommended.**

F. CREATINE

1. **Rationale for use**

–Advocates believe that:

   a. Intake of creatine increases the muscle free creatine pool, thereby decreasing lag time in the synthesis of creatine phosphate, leading to **increased amount of work** during short-term,

high-intensity exercise, or bouts of short-term exercise.

   b. Creatine will buffer the hydrogen ion (H^+) to **increase the amount of work performed** during exercise.

   c. Creatine **may possibly increase lean body mass.**

2. **Caveats**

–Experimental studies suggest a **possible ergogenic benefit in short-term, high-intensity anaerobic exercise.**

–There are **no known benefits in endurance exercise.**

–The mechanism of action is unknown.

–Increased lean body mass may be a result of increased cell volume from water weight.

–**Long-term effects** of creatine supplementation are **unknown.**

3. **Summary**

–**Research on long-term safety is needed** before recommendations can be made.

G. SALT TABLETS

1. **Rationale for use**

–Advocates believe that salt tablets replace electrolytes lost from endurance exercise or exercise in the heat.

2. **Caveats**

–Salt tablets may irritate the stomach lining, cause **nausea,** and further **increase the need for water.**

3. **Summary**

–Salt tablets are **not recommended;** water is lost at a faster rate than electrolytes during exercise.

H. DIET PILLS

1. **Rationale for use**

–Diet pills may be used by athletes **to suppress appetite.**

–Some users believe that diet pills, because they mimic the actions of epinephrine and norepinephrine, will **increase alertness and exercise performance.**

2. **Caveats**

–Diet pills may become **addictive.**

–They can cause **headaches, dizziness,** or **agitation.**

–They may cause **increases in blood pressure, heart rate, cardiac output, respiration, and blood sugar.**

–They **may interfere with normal perception mechanisms for pain, fatigue, or heat stress.**

3. **Summary**

–Diet pills are **not recommended.**

I.   CHROMIUM PICOLINATE

1. **Rationale for use**

   a.   Advocates believe that chromium picolinate will **increase glucose tolerance, decrease body fat, and increase lean body mass,** because chromium **deficiency** results **in impaired glucose tolerance,** increased cholesterol and triglyceride levels, and **decreased HDL cholesterol.**

   b.   Some studies show that **exercising individuals may have lower levels of chromium** that may affect performance as a result of changes in carbohydrate and lipid metabolism.

2. **Caveats**

   –Experimental research is **inconclusive** about the benefits of chromium picolinate.

–The **toxicity** of chromium supplementation has recently been hypothesized.

3. **Summary**

–Chromium picolinate supplements are **not recommended** because their efficacy and safety are unknown.

J.   MEAL REPLACEMENTS AND ENERGY BARS

1. **Rationale for use**

   –Advocates believe that they provide energy or macronutrients as **alternatives to regular foods.**

2. **Caveats**

   –Even the best-designed products **cannot substitute for all the benefits and unknown components of whole foods.**

3. **Summary**

   –They may be safe to use on an **occasional basis.**

VIII.   DIET AND EXERCISE CONCERNS FOR WOMEN'S HEALTH

–Certain nutrition-related deficiencies and disorders are more common in women, although in some instances **men may also be at risk.**

A.   ANOREXIA NERVOSA

1. Signs and symptoms

   –Body weight 15% below expected

   –Distorted body image

   –Fear of weight gain

   –Preoccupation with food

   –Perfectionist behavior

2. **Treatment**

   –Exercise personnel may need to **refer client** for assistance from professionals specializing in eating disorders.

   –Exercise personnel may assist other professionals in treatment by **developing an exercise program to maintain basic health** in the patient and **focus less on weight.**

B.   BULIMIA

1. **Signs and symptoms**

   a.   Regular **binge eating** (consumption of large amounts of food in a short amount of time) 2 times a week for at least 3 months

   b.   **Feelings of guilt or lack of control** over binges

   c.   **Purging behaviors** to avoid weight gain:

      –**Vomiting**

      –Use of **laxatives**

      –**Excessive exercise**

   d.   **Strict dieting or fasting**

   e.   **Overpreoccupation** with weight and body shape

   f.   Body weight is **not** always an indicator of bulimia; the person may be of **normal weight, overweight, or underweight.**

2. **Treatment**

   –Exercise personnel may need to **refer client** for help from professionals specializing in eating disorders.

C.   MINERAL DEFICIENCIES COMMON IN WOMEN

1. **Causes of iron deficiency**

   –**Overall lower energy consumption compared with men**

   –**Low consumption of meat products** that are **iron-rich**

   –**Losses as a result of menstruation**

2. **Causes of calcium deficiency**

   –**Overall lower energy consumption** compared with men

   –**Lower consumption of dairy products,** resulting in less than RDA

3. **Treatment**

   –**Appropriate dietary counseling** may help correct these deficiencies.

   –**Supplementation** may be indicated under the guidance of a physician or registered dietitian.

D. **FEMALE ATHLETE TRIAD**

–This is the name given by the ACSM to **three distinct but often interrelated conditions** seen more commonly in exercising females than in the general population.

–The long-term health consequences are **serious and potentially life threatening.**

–These individuals usually need **medical and psychological (disordered eating) assistance.**

   1. **Disordered eating**

      –occurs on a **continuum** from preoccupation with food and body image to the syndromes of anorexia nervosa and bulimia.

   –Any degree of disordered eating may affect the eating pattern of the exercisers and place them at risk for nutritional deficiencies.

2. **Amenorrhea**

   –can be defined as the **cessation of menses,** missing 3–6 consecutive menstrual periods, or having < 3 cycles per year.

   –is associated with **high volumes of exercise** and **low levels of body fat.**

3. **Osteoporosis**

   –is the **loss of bone mineral density,** especially in the spine and hip, making bones brittle and susceptible to fracture.

   –Although more common in older, postmenopausal women, **young amenorrheic women are also at risk.**

   –**Chronic low dietary calcium intake** may contribute to low bone mineral density.

   –**Stress fractures** may be an indicator of reduced bone mineral density.

   –Women sometimes respond to **estrogen therapy or medications,** but bone losses are occasionally irreversible.

REVIEW TEST

DIRECTIONS: Carefully read all questions and select the BEST single answer.

1.   The eating habits of an athlete involved in long-distance running should differ from those of a sedentary individual of the same body weight as follows:
     (A)   The athlete should reduce fat intake to 10% of total calories.
     (B)   The athlete should increase protein intake to three times the RDA.
     (C)   The athlete should have a greater intake of grains, fruits, and vegetables.
     (D)   There should be no change in calories.

2.   Carbohydrates are compounds composed of carbon, hydrogen and oxygen. They are commonly known as sugars (simple carbohydrates) or starch (complex carbohydrates). Which of the following would contain complex carbohydrate?
     (A)   Milk
     (B)   Candy
     (C)   Pasta
     (D)   Butter

3.   Regardless of the sugar source, once ingested all sugars return to which state?
     (A)   Sucrose
     (B)   Glucose
     (C)   Fructose
     (D)   Galactose

4.   Fiber is a type of complex carbohydrate that is not digestible. This means that it will pass through the digestive system without being absorbed. There are water-soluble and water-insoluble fibers. Sources of water-soluble fibers include
     (A)   fruits.
     (B)   vegetables.
     (C)   brans.
     (D)   all of the above.

5.   Which of the following has the unique quality of having nitrogen as part of its atomic structure?
     (A)   Carbohydrates
     (B)   Proteins
     (C)   Fats
     (D)   Fibers

6.   Which of the following dietary fats represent more than 90% of the fat stored in the body?
     (A)   Cholesterol
     (B)   LDL-cholesterol
     (C)   HDL-cholesterol
     (D)   Triglycerides

7.   Vitamins are organic substances derived from living substances that are required in small amounts to maintain life. Vitamins do not provide any calories but are essential for a variety of roles, from the processing of nutrients to the formation of red blood cells. The 13 vitamins are categorized as either fat-soluble or water-soluble. Which of the following is fat-soluble?
     (A)   Vitamin C
     (B)   Vitamin A
     (C)   Vitamin B_6
     (D)   Vitamin B_{12}

8.   Minerals are considered either macrominerals (needed in large amounts) or microminerals (needed in very small amounts). Which of the following is an example of a macromineral?
     (A)   Calcium
     (B)   Iron
     (C)   Zinc
     (D)   All of the above

9.   Water makes up approximately what percentage of total body weight?
     (A)   40%
     (B)   60%
     (C)   80%
     (D)   99%

10. Groups particularly at risk for dehydration include the
     (A)   elderly.
     (B)   physically active.
     (C)   infants.
     (D)   all of the above.

11. Body mass index is calculated by using which of the following formulas?
     (A)   Weight/hip circumference
     (B)   Weight/height^2
     (C)   Height/weight^2
     (D)   Hip circumference/height

12. A common measure to assist in the evaluation of body fat distribution is
     (A)   height/weight charts.
     (B)   total body weight.
     (C)   waist/hip ratio.
     (D)   total body water.

13. According to the U.S. Senate Select Committee on Nutrition and Human Needs and professional nutrition organizations, which of the following percentages of carbohydrate, fat, and protein, respectively, are indicative of a healthy diet?
    (A) 55, 30, 15
    (B) 45, 35, 25
    (C) 65, 25, 10
    (D) 55, 15, 30

14. Carbohydrate, protein, and fat (respectively) provide which of the following amounts of energy (kcal/g)?
    (A) 2, 4, 6
    (B) 4, 6, 8
    (C) 6, 8, 9
    (D) 4, 4, 9

15. If total daily caloric consumption is 2400 kcal and the total fat in that diet is 30%, how many fat grams per day would be consumed?
    (A) 80 grams
    (B) 70 grams
    (C) 90 grams
    (D) 75 grams

16. When the body consumes more calories than it uses, the condition is called
    (A) ketogenesis
    (B) positive caloric balance
    (C) positive electrolyte balance
    (D) negative energy balance

17. Which of the following vitamins functions to maintain and/or improve vision, healthy skin, bone, and growth?
    (A) A
    (B) D
    (C) E
    (D) K

18. The most common dietary deficiency in young women is
    (A) fat and vitamin C deficiency.
    (B) protein and vitamin K deficiency.
    (C) iron and calcium deficiency.
    (D) magnesium and zinc deficiency.

19. Diets high in fat have been scientifically linked to which of the following health problems?
    (A) Heart disease
    (B) Cancer
    (C) Obesity
    (D) All of the above

20. Blood cholesterol is a modifiable risk factor for coronary heart disease. In fact,
    (A) a reduction of 1% in blood cholesterol can mean a 2% reduction in risk.
    (B) a reduction of 5% in blood cholesterol eliminates the risk of heart attack.
    (C) elevated blood cholesterol increases the proportion of triglycerides.
    (D) an increase of total cholesterol in foods also increases HDL-cholesterol.

21. Truly healthy weight-loss programs should set a goal of how many pounds per week?
    (A) 10 pounds
    (B) 3–5 pounds
    (C) 1–2 pounds
    (D) None of the above

22. The American College of Sports Medicine Position Stand on Weight Loss Programs states that a desirable weight loss program
    (A) provides at least 1200 calories per day for normal adults to meet their nutritional requirements.
    (B) provides a negative caloric balance resulting in gradual weight loss without metabolic abnormalities.
    (C) includes the use of behavior modification to identify and eliminate dieting habits that contribute to improper nutrition.
    (D) all of the above

23. At the start of an exercise program, a participant may actually experience a weight gain rather than a weight loss even though he or she was in negative caloric balance. This weight gain is caused by
    (A) an intense increase in bone density.
    (B) a gain of muscle mass.
    (C) a gain of fat weight.
    (D) all of the above.

24. The primary carriers of cholesterol in the bloodstream are
    (A) triglycerides.
    (B) low-density lipoproteins.
    (C) high-density lipoproteins.
    (D) free fatty acids.

25. Athletes who exercise in the heat and humidity have a special need for fluid replacement. Current guidelines suggest that athletes in these environments

    (A) drink 16–32 fluid ounces of water for every pound of weight lost.
    (B) drink nothing but alcoholic beverages after engaging in exercise.
    (C) avoid drinking water after exercise because of the danger of cramps.
    (D) eat salt tablets with every meal during the hot summer months.

ANSWERS AND EXPLANATIONS

1–C. Important to any physical activity program is a plan for healthy eating. The nutritional needs of physically active individuals do not differ significantly from those of healthy adults with the exception of energy or calorie intake. The primary source of additional calories will be from carbohydrates, that is, grains, fruits, and vegetables.

2–C. Pasta is a complex carbohydrate. Milk would contain lactose and candy would contain sucrose (both simple carbohydrates). Butter is a fat.

3–B. Sugar is found in foods under a variety of different names such as brown sugar, corn syrup, corn sugar, fructose, dextrose, honey, molasses, sorbitol, and sorghum. Despite the different names, the body does not differentiate between the sources and converts each of these sugar sources to glucose for metabolic purposes.

4–D. Insoluble fiber sources include fruits, vegetables, dried beans, wheat bran, brown rice, whole-grain breads, cereals, pasta, seeds, and popcorn. Soluble fiber is found in fruits (especially apples, oranges, pears, peaches, and grapes), vegetables, oat bran, oatmeal, rye, barley, and dried beans.

5–B. Protein is composed of hydrogen, carbon dioxide, oxygen, and nitrogen (which makes it unique). Fats, carbohydrates and fibers only have carbon dioxide, oxygen, and hydrogen.

6–D. Dietary fats include cholesterol, triglycerides, and phospholipids. Triglycerides represent more than 90% of the fat stored in the body. A triglyceride is a glycerol molecule base attached to three fatty acids. Although cholesterol is present in all cells, it is not stored in the same quantity as triglycerides. Fat stored as triglycerides in adipose tissue and surrounding muscle tissue provides the body with a tremendous energy reserve. Fat also serves to surround and protect vital organs and the spinal cord, preserves body heat, and manufactures and transports the fat-soluble vitamins A, D, E, and K.

7–B. The fat-soluble vitamins are absorbed through the intestinal membranes and are stored in body fat; they include A, D, E, and K. An abnormally high intake of fat-soluble vitamins can lead to toxic levels with symptoms and may also result in deficiency-like symptoms for other vitamins. The water-soluble vitamins are typically not stored in the body in the same manner, so they require a more regular intake. The water-soluble vitamins include C and the B vitamins.

8–A. Calcium, phosphorus, magnesium, potassium, sulfur, sodium, and chloride are considered to be the macrominerals because they are required in relatively large dosages. The microminerals include iron, zinc, selenium, manganese, molybdenum, iodine, copper, chromium, and fluoride.

9–B. Water makes up approximately 60% of the total body weight. Water is essential to human life. Every chemical reaction in the body relies on water and every cell depends on water for providing nourishment, elimination of waste, insulation, and cooling.

10–D. Individuals at risk for dehydration include those whose sweat mechanisms are immature or compromised for some reason (infants and the elderly), and those who may be physically active beyond their body's ability to keep up with the cooling process owing to physiological conditioning or environmental conditions.

11–B. Body mass index (BMI) is used more frequently than other measures to assess body fat. It eliminates the use of frame size and is calculated as weight (kg)/[height (m)]^2.

12–C. The waist/hip circumference ratio will help assess the distribution of body fat on the body. Men and women tend to have body fat distribution at different sites; men tend to exhibit extra weight around the waist, whereas women tend to have extra weight distributed around the hips and buttocks.

13–A. Dietary goals recommend that between 55% and 58% of total calories be derived from carbohydrate, less than 30% from fat, and between 12% and 15% from protein. The total carbohydrate intake may include approximately 15% refined and processed sugars. The fat component should be divided equally among saturated, monounsaturated, and polyunsaturated fats (approximately 10% each).

14–D. Each gram of carbohydrate and protein provides approximately 4 kcal of energy. Fat provides more than twice this energy at 9 kcal/g. The degree of fat saturation (saturated, monounsaturated, polyunsaturated) does not change the 9 kcal/g amount of energy.

15–A. Using the percentage distribution of 4 kcal of energy from carbohydrates and proteins and 9 kcal of energy from fat, a diet consisting of 2400 kcal with 30% fat would consist of 80 grams of fat (2400 kcal × 30% = 720 fat calories ÷ 9 kcal/gram = 80 grams).

16–B. When the body consumes more calories than it uses, the body is in a state of positive caloric, or energy, balance. A negative balance occurs when the body utilizes more energy than it consumes. Ketogenesis is a condition in which the body metabolizes ketone bodies for energy, typically during carbohydrate restriction. A positive electrolyte balance would reflect a greater supply of electrolytes than required by the body.

17–A. Many vitamins have multiple tasks and may assist other vitamins in their function. Vitamin A maintains and/or improves vision, healthy skin, and bone growth.

18–C. The most common dietary deficiency today is that of iron and calcium in young women. As a result of very low caloric intakes and an absence of or marginal intakes of meat and dairy products, these deficiencies can affect long-term health. If dietary changes including the use of fortified food products do not increase the intake of these nutrients, supplementation is recommended to decrease the risk of osteoporosis and anemia.

19–D. Diets high in fat have been linked to health problems such as heart disease, cancer, and obesity. Elevated blood cholesterol levels is one of the major risk factors for coronary artery disease. A diet high in fat, especially saturated fatty acids and cholesterol, raises blood

cholesterol levels in many people. A diet rich in fats, sugars, and excess calories can also raise blood triglycerides, which also increases the risk for heart disease.

20–A. For every 1% reduction in blood cholesterol, there is a 2% reduction in the risk of a heart attack.

21–C. Healthy weight loss programs should set a goal of 1–2 pounds per week. The most effective method for achieving and maintaining weight loss is a combined program of caloric management and regular physical activity.

22–D. All of these are true. In addition, sound weight loss programs include foods that are acceptable to the individual in terms of sociocultural background, usual habits, taste, cost and ease in acquisition and preparation. A regular exercise program should also be included.

23–B. At the start of an exercise program, a participant may actually experience no weight loss or a slight increase in body weight even though he or she was following a diet. This is typically due to a short-term gain in muscle mass, which may increase 3–5 pounds (1.5–2.5 kg) during the first 12 weeks of training. Any increase in bone density would not be detected on the scale.

24–B. Low-density lipoproteins (LDLs) are the primary source of cholesterol in the bloodstream. High-density lipoproteins (HDLs) do carry cholesterol, but in a smaller amount than LDLs. Triglycerides are made up of a glycerol molecule and three fatty acids; they do not carry any cholesterol.

25–A. Physically active individuals should drink plenty of cool, plain water before, during, and after activity even if they do not feel thirsty. Before exercise, hyperhydrate by drinking at least one to two cups (8 to 16 ounces) of water 10–15 minutes prior to activity. During hard exercise, drink 8–10 ounces every 20 minutes. After exercise, drink to quench thirst and then even more. It is recommended that every pound lost during activity be replaced with at least 16–32 ounces of water.

CHAPTER 10

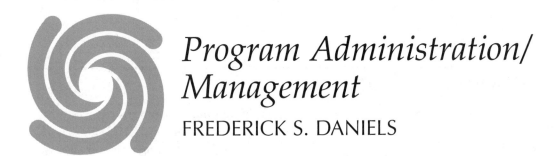

Program Administration/ Management

FREDERICK S. DANIELS

I. INTRODUCTION

–Effective program administration creates safe, successful programs and reduces the risk of problems and legal situations.

–Management skills are used at all levels of exercise program implementation, from fitness instructors to managers of programs, departments, or facilities.

II. CHARACTERISTICS OF A GOOD MANAGER

–A good manager:

A. DESIGNS AND MONITORS IMPLEMENTATION OF EXERCISE PROGRAMS BY:

–organizing the required resources.

–arranging the schedule.

–guiding the staff or clients through the program.

–purchasing equipment and supplies.

B. ASSESSES PROGRAM AND CLIENT NEEDS BY:

–establishing goals for the program.

–monitoring program and facility safety.

–ensuring program evaluation.

–implementing changes warranted by evaluation.

C. DEVELOPS AND MOTIVATES STAFF AND CLIENTS BY:

–demonstrating good communication skills with staff and clients.

–coordinating staff and program development.

–evaluating staff and programs.

D. PROVIDES EDUCATION AND TRAINING AS DEMONSTRATED BY:

–developing and implementing a staff training program.

–possessing strong teaching skills.

–soliciting feedback.

E. PROVIDES A ROLE MODEL AS AN EXERCISE LEADER BY:

–providing feedback.

–being motivated and a good motivator.

–controlling the situation and assuming a position of leadership.

F. MOTIVATES INDIVIDUALS BY:

–demonstrating strong communication skills.

–being persuasive and influential.

–demonstrating enthusiasm.

–inciting action and giving impetus to the program.

G. ACTS AS A COUNSELOR BY:

–advising staff and clients.

–possessing listening skills.

–expressing opinions, but being willing to listen to others.

–consulting with staff and clients.

–suggesting changes and recommending action.

III. MANAGING A PROGRAM OR FACILITY

A. RESPONSIBILITIES OF THE EXERCISE PROGRAM MANAGER

–The exercise program manager:

1. **Assesses client interest** with surveys, through client and staff feedback, and by observing programs.

2. **Describes the program and target audience** in detail, including:

   –the type of client expected.

   –the number of clients expected.

   –minimal and maximal enrollments.

   –procedures to be followed.

3. **Determines resource availability,** including equipment, supplies, space, and staff.

4. **Analyzes cost/benefits,** including:

   –budget of costs and expected revenues.

   –determination of profitability and break even point.

   –determining whether direct and indirect benefits outweigh costs.

5. **Promotes the program** through marketing efforts and designs promotions that attract participants.

6. **Schedules classes/programs** appropriately with target audience in mind and with consideration of other programs.

7. **Evaluates programs** using outcome evaluation tools, including:

   –assessment of financial outcomes (net income).

   –class size.

   –general feedback.

B. RESPONSIBILITIES OF THE MANAGER OF A FITNESS DEPARTMENT OR SHIFT

–The manager of a fitness department or shift is responsible for:

1. **Scheduling of staff**

H. POSSESSES THE ABILITY TO PROMOTE PROGRAMS, AS DEMONSTRATED BY:

–encouraging participation.

–understanding the benefits of the program.

–demonstrating the ability to communicate benefits to staff and clients.

2. **Implementing policies and procedures,** including:

   –assisting staff in understanding and enforcing all rules and policies.

   –communicating emergency procedures clearly.

   –confirming understanding in the day-to-day operations of the facility.

   –practicing emergency procedures and planning regularly.

3. **Evaluating and appraising performance,** including:

   –evaluating programs and staff through observation and through written feedback and appraisal.

   –reinforcing positive behaviors with praise and positive reinforcement.

   –establishing goals and/or standards for the next appraisal period.

   –correcting problem areas.

4. **Using client and staff feedback** about programs and management style

5. **Monitoring testing and evaluation** of clients using American College of Sports Medicine (ACSM) and other appropriate guidelines and standards

C. FACILITY MAINTENANCE

–The facilities manager:

1. **Ensures that exercise areas and equipment are clean, disinfected, and safe** for use during club hours.

2. **Maintains equipment in good working order** using a program of preventive maintenance and quick repair.

3. **Ensures that open walkways provide adequate clearance** for clients to pass with minimal risk of injury (including wheelchair clearance).

D. PARTICIPANT/CLIENT INTERACTION AND FEEDBACK

–The exercise program manager:

1. **Uses staff and client surveys** to determine needs and problems within the club.

2. Makes sure that there is a **timely response** to client needs, requests, and problems.

3. **Informs clients regularly.**

4. **Provides educational information and programs** for clients and staff on a variety of exercise and health issues.

5. **Maintains high visibility** by being present in the exercise area.

   –Stays in touch with clients.

   –Observes programs.

   –Observes staff.

   –Listens to ideas and offers feedback.

IV. BUDGETING AND FINANCIAL PLANNING

–**Appropriate and careful financial management** is important to the success of facilities, staff, and programs.

A. PURPOSES OF BUDGETS

1. A **financial plan** for a program or facility
2. To **control costs**
3. To **evaluate program performance**
4. A **tool for realistic planning**
5. To **determine program viability**
6. To **identify financial difficulties** early

B. DEVELOPING A BUDGET

1. **Establish budget periods and goals.**
   a. The **period** is **the time course of a program.**
   b. Use of a **time line to project goals** (i.e., revenue or class size) or assist with assessment.
   c. **Goals** may be the **number of participants** or **revenue level,** but should be **specific** and **measurable.**

2. **Collect pertinent information** by projecting all costs and revenues.

3. **Determine capital expenses** for equipment and facilities, which are usually higher to start programs.

4. **Project start-up costs** and include the following in the long-term budget:

   –Supplies

   –Space renovation

   –Uniforms

   –Equipment purchase or lease

   –Staff hiring and training

   –Insurance and related costs

5. Ensure **realistic budgeting** by comparison with other budgets and thorough review by other managers.

C. OPERATIONAL VERSUS CAPITAL BUDGETS

–**Operating budgets** (Table 10-1) reflect the **day-to day cost** of operating the program or facility, including **direct and indirect costs.**

–**Capital budgets** reflect the costs associated with the **equipment and facilities** needed to provide the program or services.

D. COST/BENEFIT ANALYSIS

1. **Net income** reflects all costs and revenues associated with the program—"the bottom line."

2. **Cost/benefit analysis** describes all benefits compared with costs or net income. These benefits may include:
   a. **Profit** status
   b. **Client satisfaction**
   c. **Satisfactory attendance**
   d. Providing a **health benefit** that can be marketed
   e. **Attracting new members**
   f. **Benefits to other programs and services** (directly or indirectly)
   g. **Enhancing club reputation**
   h. **Program expansion** or additional programs generated

Table 10-1. Sample Budget

ACSM Fitness Center

	Existing Clients	Monthly Fee($)	New	Average Fee($)	Cancellations	Total	Total Revenue
Jan	700	45	50	150	0	750	39,000
Feb	750	45	75	150	22	803	44,010
Mar	803	45	75	150	25	853	46,260
Apr	853	45	65	150	25	893	47,010
May	893	45	55	150	27	921	47,220
June	921	45	50	150	28	943	47,685
July	943	45	50	150	28	965	48,675
Aug	965	45	50	150	29	986	49,620
Sept	986	45	60	150	29	1,017	52,065
Oct	1,017	45	65	150	31	1,051	54,120
Nov	1,051	45	70	150	31	1,090	56,400
Dec	1,090	45	50	150	33	1,107	55,065
			TOTAL MEMBERSHIP REVENUE:				**587,130**

OTHER REVENUE:

Smoking Cessation	1,200
Massage	16,200
Guest Fees	35,000
1-1 Training	32,400
Weight Management	12,000
Pro-Shop	1,200
Rest	3,000
Wellness Programs	1,200
Misc.	10,000
TOTAL OTHER REVENUE	**112,200**
MEMBERSHIP REVENUE	587,130
TOTAL REVENUE	**699,330**

PAYROLL PROJECTIONS:

General Manager	35,000
Sales 1	35,000
Administrator	20,000
Fitness Director	26,000
FT Fitness 1	22,000
FT Fitness 2	20,000
PT Fitness	21,840
Receptionist	25,000
Aerobics	18,000
Nutrition	9,500
Cleaning	24,000
Bonus	8,000
TOTAL PAYROLL	**264,340**
TAXES	34,364
BENEFITS	18,240
TOTAL SALARIES	**316,944**

TOTAL OPERATING EXPENSES:

Salary, Tax, & Benefits	316,944
Marketing	48,000
Maintenance/Repair	
HVAC	1,500
Equipment	2,400
Exterminate	1,200
Other	500
TOTAL MAINTENANCE	5,600
Operating Supplies	
Cleaning	1,200
Locker Room	3,000
Other	1,500
Towels	2,000
TOTAL SUPPLIES	7,700
Utilities	
Electric	36,000
Gas	4,800
Water	2,000
TOTAL UTILITIES	42,800
Rent	70,705
Other Expenses	
Printing	3,600
Postage	3,000
Travel	2,000
Uniforms	6,000
Programs	500
Office Supplies	600
Telephone	7,200
Misc.	1,000
TOTAL OTHER EXPENSES	23,900
Corporate Expenses	
Amort/Dep	24,000
Debt	
Insurance	
Leasing	
Mgmt Fees	
TOTAL CORPORATE	108,400
TOTAL EXPENSES	**624,049**
NET PROFIT/(LOSS)	**75,281**

(With permission from McCarthy J. Fund Allocation has become critical. *Club Business International,* 1990.)

V. POLICIES AND PROCEDURES

–**Policies** are **general guidelines** for operating a program or department.

–Policies and procedures **establish control of the operations** of the facility.

–**Procedures describe how policies are enacted** or **how a program functions** within the policies.

A. **THE ROLE OF THE MANAGER IS TO ENSURE THAT POLICIES ARE ENFORCED AND PROCEDURES ARE FOLLOWED BY STAFF AND CLIENTS.**

B. **THE PRIMARY PURPOSES OF POLICIES AND PROCEDURES ARE:**

–to **clearly define operations.**

–to **ensure** that a facility or program is **operated safely and effectively.**

C. **ALL DEPARTMENTS AND PROGRAMS SHOULD HAVE POLICIES AND PROCEDURES. FOR PROGRAMS, THEY MAY BE CALLED "RULES AND REGULATIONS."**

D. **STAFF RESPONSIBILITIES INCLUDE:**

–**ensuring that clients understand** policies (and rules).

–**enforcement.**

E. **WRITTEN DISCIPLINARY PROCEDURES SHOULD BE IN PLACE FOR SITUATIONS IN WHICH A POLICY OR PROCEDURE IS NOT FOLLOWED.**

VI. LEGAL ISSUES IN EXERCISE PROGRAMMING

A. **OVERVIEW**

–Legal issues are the concern of fitness professionals involved in exercise testing, exercise prescription, and program administration.

–Legal concerns can develop with any of the following:

1. The **instructor-client relationship.**
2. The **exercises.**
3. The **exercise setting.**
4. The **purpose of the programs and exercises.**
5. The **procedures** used by the staff.

B. **TORT**

–is a type of **civil wrongdoing.**

1. **Negligence** is **failure to perform in a generally accepted standard.**

    –Fitness professionals have specific documented and understood responsibilities to ensure client safety and success in reaching predetermined goals. Negligence may result if the responsibilities are not fulfilled.

2. **Malpractice** is a **specific type of negligence.**

    –It involves **claims against a defined professional.**

    –It is **usually limited to those with public authority to practice** arising from their responsibilities to a client.

    –Charges usually claim a **breach of professional duties and responsibilities** toward a client.

C. **STATE LAWS AND REGULATIONS**

–The manager of the fitness facility must understand any written regulations or "practice acts" applicable to the fitness industry that control the behavior and actions of the fitness professional.

D. **DOCUMENTATION**

–A **written record** of agreements, waivers, releases, incidents, policies and procedures, and clearances is **critical for the understanding of client activities and to know who is protected** if problems occur.

1. **Agreements, releases, and consents**

    –clearly describe **client participation,** the **rights** of the client and the facility, and any **risks.**

    –**transfer some responsibility and risk** associated with participation **to the client** (see Chapter 7, Figure 7-2, for an example of a Participant Agreement).

2. All fitness facilities are strongly encouraged to have **program/service agreements** and **informed consents drafted by a lawyer** for their protection.

3. A client who does not meet the criteria for exercising or who wishes to break a policy in order to exercise can sign a **waiver** to be allowed to participate, thus **accepting risk.**

4. A **"Physician Clearance"** requires a medical opinion of the client's risk with exercise (**Figure 10-1**). This document **places much of**

SAMPLE

PHYSICIAN'S CLEARANCE FORM

Your patient, _____ is starting an exercise program at our center. Prior to beginning an exercise program each client completes a medical history questionnaire, resting heart rate and blood pressure measurements, a submaximal cardiovascular test, a body compostition test, and strength and flexibility tests. These evaluative tests are conducted by trained and certified fitness staff, and follow the American College of Sports Medicine exercise and testing guidelines. The information obtained is designed to determine the level of cardiac risk and the appropriate exercise program for your patient.

Your patient has a medical history that indicates potential risk to exercise. We are requiring your patient to acquire a physician's clearance prior to exercise. If you clear your patient, we ask that you indicate any restrictions or limits while exercising.

Reason(s) for clearance:

____ Hypertension   ____ Diabetes

____ Peripheral Vascular Disease   ____ COPD

____ Heart Surgery (PTCA, CABG)   ____ Medications

____ Myocardial Infarction   ____ Musculoskeletal Condition

____ Angina   ____ Other

_____

_____

_____

This patient is ____ CLEARED / ____ NOT CLEARED to exercise. I have listed my restrictions, limitations, recommendations and/or reasons below:

_____

_____

_____

We appreciate you cooperation. It is our intent to provide a safe and effective exercise program to your patient. If you would like, we will send you the results of the evaluation, progress notes, and/or blood pressure records.

Physician's signature: _____   Date: _____

Please check if you would like progress notes and records: ____

FIGURE 10-1. Sample of a physician's clearance form.

the risk on the medical professional rather than the fitness facility. A physician's clearance is recommended for:

   a. A client who has considerable risk with exercise as indicated by a medical history questionnaire or Par-Q.

   b. A client who exhibits signs or symptoms during exercise that indicate increased risk if exercise continues.

5. Incident reports are used to document a problem or incident; these

  –provide a **detailed description of the incident.**

–list all witnesses.

–include **witness statements** if possible.

–state the **results of the actions by the staff.**

–include a follow-up status of clients and/or staff involved in the incident.

6. **Malpractice insurance** provides coverage for staff in case a malpractice lawsuit is filed.

VII. RECORDS

–Records are helpful for many activities, including **program evaluation, client motivation, understanding the success of the business,** and **marketing.**

A. ATTENDANCE RECORDS

–may **clarify the levels of business** within the environment.

–may **include:**

1. The **percentage of members that use the facility**

2. Demographics **information for future program development**

3. Measurements of **success for specific programs** (e.g., revenue, numbers)

4. **Member retention data**

5. **Adherence information** that may help staff target clients' efforts

B. CLIENT PROGRESS RECORDS ARE EXERCISE-RELATED RECORDS TO EVALUATE INDIVIDUAL PROGRAMS AND PROVIDE FEEDBACK ON GOAL ATTAINMENT.

C. OUTCOME STUDIES MEASURE RESULTS FOR INDIVIDUALS WITHIN A PROGRAM.

1. Outcome studies **require measurable data.**

2. Change can be assessed with **objective measures** (e.g., weight change, body fat, functional capacity) and **subjective measures** (e.g., client satisfaction and quality of life).

3. Outcome studies can assist in **marketing efforts, member retention,** and **program/facility comparison.**

VIII. EDUCATION

A. PROFESSIONAL STAFF DEVELOPMENT

–Fitness facilities should provide a variety of opportunities for staff members.

1. Fitness and related **journals and texts** should be available.

2. Membership in reputable **fitness and exercise organizations** provides opportunities for all levels of staff. Organizations such as the **ACSM** and the American Alliance for Health, Physical Education, Recreation and Dance (**AAHPERD**) offer **basic and applied research** pertinent to the practice of the exercise professional.

3. Attendance at **conferences and workshops** should be encouraged.

4. **In-service programs** provide opportunity for staff education from local resources, such as physicians, nurses, physical and occupational therapists, athletes, psychologists, and business professionals.

5. **Certifications** enhance the knowledge base of the staff and add professional credibility.

B. CLIENT EDUCATION MAY INCLUDE:

–a **fitness newsletter.**

–**health and fitness fact sheets.**

–a **fitness library** with health and nutrition newsletters, books, and videos.

–a **bulletin board** with reprints of articles that address specific topics with facts and tips.

–**classes or lectures** on a variety of health, wellness, and fitness topics conducted by the staff or by local experts.

–a **computer** with access to fitness resources, program design, nutrition and health information, and equipment reviews.

IX. MARKETING FITNESS PROGRAMS

–Marketing can be **internal** (within the facility) or **external** (outside the facility).

–**Developing ideas** is the key to marketing; this requires **research** and an **understanding of the target audience**.

A. NEEDS ASSESSMENT

–A needs assessment is conducted to determine the **specific needs and interests of the target market**. It includes:

1. **Participant demographics**
2. **Knowledge of the competition**
3. **Understanding the market base:**
   –Geographic boundaries
   –Special populations
   –Location
   –Convenience
   –Proximity to other health services
4. **Targeting market surveys** to determine level of interest
5. **Current program evaluation** to determine whether programs are popular and effective
6. **Survey of staff and management**
7. **Costs** with comparison to other programs

B. MARKETING PLAN

–The marketing plan includes **detailed description of marketing strategies** and **justification for each action and program.**

C. STAFF TRAINING IN SALES AND MARKETING ENSURES THAT STAFF ARE ABLE TO IMPLEMENT THE PLAN. KEEPING PRESENT CUSTOMERS IS MORE IMPORTANT THAN GETTING NEW CUSTOMERS. COMMON SALES TECHNIQUES INCLUDE:

–**honesty.**

–knowledge of the client.

–**making people feel they belong.**

–selling the **whole organization.**

–**substance** (more important than "fluff").

D. THE BUSINESS PLAN IS A DETAILED DESCRIPTION OF THE MARKETING PLAN WITH JUSTIFICATION FOR EACH ACTION AND PROGRAM AND PROJECTIONS FOR PROGRAM SUCCESS, INCLUDING A COST/BENEFIT ANALYSIS.

E. PUBLIC RELATIONS (PR) IS THE PROMOTION OF THE FACILITY AND ITS PROGRAMS THROUGH NON-MARKETING TECHNIQUES.

1. PR programs include **public speaking, clinics, community service, donation of services,** and **charity work.**
2. The **professional staff** is most likely to be involved in PR programs and **must be skilled at group presentation.**

F. MARKETING AND PROMOTIONAL MATERIALS

1. Consider the **design, text, color, and type of paper** in preparing materials.
2. Prepare **high-quality materials** (e.g., print ads, radio ads, direct mail pieces, newsletters, flyers, posters).
3. **Research** helps to determine the effectiveness of individual pieces.

REVIEW TEST

DIRECTIONS: Carefully read all questions and select the BEST single answer.

1. Do fitness instructors need management skills?
   (A) Only if they wish to become floor supervisors or program managers
   (B) Yes, because of the natural progression of advancement into management
   (C) Yes, because, as instructors, they manage client programs and manage the floor with the clients
   (D) No, because they will be trained in management if they become managers

2. A fitness newsletter, fitness library, and bulletin boards
   (A) are part of staff news.
   (B) are part of client and staff education.
   (C) are part of the facility marketing.
   (D) require considerable money and must be budgeted carefully.

3. Why would a fitness facility be interested in public relations?
   (A) To increase exposure for the facility and sell services
   (B) To become involved in local politics
   (C) To improve staff morale
   (D) To make the staff work harder

4. Why would a fitness instructor have an interest in tort laws?
   (A) Negligence is breaking a tort law and can ruin an instructor's career.
   (B) State taxes are often related to profit, which is governed by tort laws.
   (C) Tort laws are related to worker's compensation regulations.
   (D) They relate to the Americans with Disabilities Act (ADA).

5. What is the best way that an administrator can educate the fitness staff?
   (A) Voicing his or her opinion
   (B) Joining fitness organizations and subscribing to fitness journals
   (C) Buying fitness videos
   (D) Reading the newspaper

6. What should the manager's involvement be in developing fitness programs?
   (A) The manager should maintain a hands-off approach.
   (B) The manager should be involved only in the budgeting and final approval.
   (C) The manager should be the only person involved in program development.
   (D) The manager should be active as a program developer, as well as a resource, supporter, and critic for programs developed by other staff.

7. Budgets are designed to
   (A) make management happy.
   (B) determine if a program is viable.
   (C) save money.
   (D) teach managers about cost analysis.

8. The rules and regulations of a facility are commonly referred to as
   (A) the law.
   (B) the client rights statement.
   (C) policies and procedures.
   (D) a check and balance for management and clients.

9. A physician's clearance
   (A) is not necessary if the client completes the medical history questionnaire.
   (B) is a communication tool with little exercise value.
   (C) provides information about the physician's attitude regarding your club.
   (D) provides a medical opinion about a client's risk with exercise.

10. Some of the duties in supervising a fitness staff include scheduling, implementing the policies and procedures, and
    (A) cleaning the equipment.
    (B) emergency procedures and evaluations.
    (C) marketing and promotions.
    (D) managing the fitness billing.

11. What is the primary reason that a manager or director should conduct a needs assessment?
    (A) To determine the specific needs and interests of the target market
    (B) To determine the quality of potential fitness instructors that could be hired in the area
    (C) To determine the needs of management before developing the budgets
    (D) To determine the need for new or different exercise equipment

12. Policies and procedures are important in a fitness center because they
    (A) explain how to properly use the fitness equipment.
    (B) clarify the rights and risks in being a fitness member.
    (C) are general guidelines for operating a fitness program or department.
    (D) explain the employee insurance plans and how to use them.

13. What are some of the common sales "rules" in promoting your fitness program?
    (A) Selling memberships at any cost is key.
    (B) You know more than they do, so be aggressive.
    (C) Honesty and an understanding of the needs of the potential member are always the best way.
    (D) Long-term agreements make more money than short-term agreements.

14. Program description, resource availability, and client interest are examples of
    (A) a business plan.
    (B) a survey.
    (C) management factors.
    (D) budget categories.

15. What do effective program administration and management create and/or reduce?
    (A) They create problems with staff egos.
    (B) They reduce memberships.
    (C) They create successful programs and reduce problems.
    (D) They create more work for the staff and reduce feedback.

16. Incident reports are important because
    (A) they inform the manager which employees are performing poorly.
    (B) they indicate which members are problematic and should be dismissed.
    (C) they document and give details of any incident or problem that occurs.
    (D) state laws often require them.

17. Why are records valuable to a fitness program?
    (A) They help in evaluation of a program.
    (B) They offer music not found in tapes or compact discs.
    (C) They help provide facts in any legal issues.
    (D) They help the front desk monitor paid and unpaid clients.

18. Examples of program records include
    (A) client progress and outcomes.
    (B) member needs.
    (C) performance of clients on selected exercises.
    (D) member suggestions and actions taken.

19. Which of the following is an example of participant interaction as part of the supportive role of a manager?
    (A) Offering a shoulder on which to cry
    (B) Conducting surveys and responding to client needs
    (C) Encouraging members to "let go" in exercise classes
    (D) Having members teach classes

20. The manager's role in staff education is
    (A) valuable because it looks good to the owners.
    (B) to create many opportunities for educating the staff.
    (C) to let the staff handle their own education, but encourage it.
    (D) not very valuable because member retention and sales are the key to any program.

21. Staff certification is
    (A) not important because members do not care.
    (B) important primarily because it adds spice to marketing materials.
    (C) not a good idea because certified staff increase your payroll.
    (D) important primarily because it adds a standard of knowledge and credibility to your facility.

22. Capital budgets
    (A) reflect the costs of implementing a program.
    (B) reflect the costs to operate a program.
    (C) are not necessary with fitness programs.
    (D) are part of the balance sheet in financial reports.

23. What do budgets determine?
    (A) Fitness equipment costs
    (B) If a company is making or losing money
    (C) Viability, identification of problems, and plan for the future of a program
    (D) Assets and liabilities of the financial plan

24. Why should a fitness operator be concerned with state practice laws?
    (A) State laws help identify illegal aliens who may apply for a job in your club.
    (B) State laws may control the number of minority employees working at your club.
    (C) They may affect how much may be charged for a membership.
    (D) Many states have practice acts that control the behavior and actions of fitness instructors.

25. Why is public relations important to a fitness program?
    (A) It helps promote the program and staff to the public.
    (B) It reduces the risk of legal action against your staff.
    (C) It lowers your malpractice insurance by promoting quality.
    (D) It makes sure your clients are happy and getting what they want.

ANSWERS AND EXPLANATIONS

1–C. The definition of a manager is someone who designs, implements, and monitors programs, which is what fitness instructors are responsible for as a natural part of their job. Managing a client's program fits the basic definition of a manager, so the skills of managing a person and his program fit the need for management training. A fitness instructor does not naturally become a manager.

2–B. Educating a fitness client on the principles of exercise, proper nutrition and good health is important; this information can be communicated in a variety of ways. Newsletters, libraries, and bulletin boards are some of the recommended ways to communicate with and educate members. Staff news should not necessarily be within the library or posted on a board. Marketing strategies often do not include the library or bulletin boards. These forms of education are usually inexpensive to develop and maintain.

3–A. Public relations (PR), a common form of promotion, is important for any business. It is very important to "get your name out" and increase exposure. PR activities can help people learn who you are and how good you are. PR has nothing to do with politics when it involves your facility. PR may improve the morale of your staff, but the intent is to generate exposure for your club. PR should not be considered a strategy for making the staff work harder.

4–A. A tort law refers to a civil wrong, such as negligence (failure to perform a generally accepted standard). Negligence in fitness often refers to the instructor giving bad instruction or advice that leads to an injury or accident. Clients often sue instructors for negligence, which can be very damaging. Tort laws do not involve state taxes, are not regulated by workers compensation insurance, and do not involve the ADA.

5–B. Fitness organizations and journals offer excellent opportunities for staff and management to learn about many aspects of fitness. Most fitness organizations and journals work with experts in fitness and provide accurate and up-to-date information. An administrator's opinion may not be an educated or unbiased one, which can make for poor education. Newspapers and videos often present misinterpreted or inaccurate information.

6–D. The manager's job is to manage programs by being a program developer, to act as a resource for staff and clients, to evaluate programs, and to provide constructive input to staff. A hands-off approach is not recommended because it often leads to poor program implementation and problems. Managing program development is an important role for managers, not just budgeting. It is important to involve the staff in the design and implementation of the programs; otherwise, the manager does all of the work.

7–B. One of the primary goals of a fitness business is to make a profit. Budgeting helps a manager and the owner understand if a program can make money and be successful (viable). Budgets are not designed to save money; the programs are designed to save money. Management is only happy if the budgets show a profit. Managers must learn cost analysis before developing budgets, so they know how to create a budget that will make management happy.

8–C. Policies and procedures are essentially the rules and regulations of a facility, plus the means of conducting and implementing the regulations correctly. Regulations can be considered the law, but are not often labeled that. The client rights statement is a different document. Management monitors the rules and makes sure that staff and members follow them; however, these regulations are not considered a balance measurement.

9–D. A fitness instructor will request or require a physician's clearance when there is concern regarding the risk of a medical crisis with exercise. The clearance is a medical opinion that it is safe for the client to exercise. The medical history will indicate if a concern with exercise is evident, but will not assure the fitness instructor that it is safe for the client to exercise. A physician's clearance is a very important tool for the safety of the exercising client and should not be an opinion statement about your facility.

10–B. Staff evaluations and developing emergency procedures are common duties in supervising staff. It is important that your staff know how to implement emergency procedures, and the supervisor must train the staff. The staff handles the equipment cleaning, not the supervisors. Marketing and billing are duties that are not involved with fitness staff supervision.

11–A. A needs assessment is designed to analyze your target market and determine what that market needs and wants. This assessment has nothing to do with assessing fitness staff, equipment, or management needs.

12–C. Policies and procedures provide general guidelines and how to enact those guidelines in implementing an exercise program. Polices and procedures help establish control of the operations of programs. Use of fitness equipment may be a part of a policy and procedure statement, but polices and procedures are much more than that. The rights and risks of a fitness member are written in the client rights statement. Insurance plans are presented in the employee handbook, not the policies and procedures.

13–C. Honesty and understanding are always the best policy. It is very important to know what the client needs and wants. This information can help you sell the programs that meet those needs and desires. Being honest enhances your reputation and client retention because clients get what you told them they would get. Selling memberships at any cost will often result in losing business over time because of dishonesty or giving away too much. Being aggressive and assuming the client does not know anything can alienate potential clients and they won't join your club. Short-term agreements tend to improve client retention.

14–C. Managing involves many characteristics or factors. Developing programs, being a resource to staff and members, and monitoring client interest are some of the factors of management. A business plan explains the business in detail, the target market, and marketing strategies, not resource availability. Surveys can assess client interest, but do not assess program descriptions. These examples are not part of a budget.

15–C. Effective management should create a successful facility that meets the needs of the clients, staff, and owners. Problems should be reduced, membership should increase, and feedback and communication should be enhanced, not reduced.

16–C. Incident reports provide a detailed record of what happened in any incident at the fitness facility. These records may be critical for a physician or emergency medical unit if there was an accident. The report also provides evidence, witnesses, and the results of actions by the staff. These reports are not intended to inform management of bad employees or members. State laws do not require incident reports, though they may recommend them.

17–A. Records help management in many ways, including the evaluation of a program. Recording the workouts, client attendance, feedback, and more can help determine if the program was successful. Records can help as evidence in a legal issue, but this value is not nearly as important as answer A. Records also help at the front desk, but are not part of a fitness program; instead, they are part of the facility management. Records, in this case, do not involve music.

18–A. Program records refer to the specific evaluation of an individual or group program. The progress of clients throughout the program and the outcomes following the program are very important factors to assess. Specific exercise records are part of the data in the program records, which are then used to chart progress and outcomes. Member needs and suggestions are not usually part of program recordings; these are usually recorded as part of a survey.

19–B. Fitness facilities constantly seek information on what their clients want, need, like, and don't like. Interacting with clients makes clients feel important and respected. Conducting surveys and responding to client input are two of the better ways to invite interaction. A shoulder to cry on is not a way to encourage interaction. Nor do you want to increase the risk of a problem by letting clients "let go" or teach your classes.

20–B. Creating opportunities for educating the staff is very important because it enhances their knowledge and provides a perk for them. A well-educated staff enhances the quality and safety of your programs, improves the facility's reputation, and increases respect and acceptance of your clients. It is not valuable to provide education only for the purpose of looking good to the owners, or to ignore the need for education.

21–D. Certification shows the clients that your staff members meet industry standards. The staff should have a certain level of skill and competency with certifications. Most members DO care, and payroll should be a secondary factor to the choice of certifying staff. Certified staff should bring more members, which can justify the increased cost. The marketing is also secondary to the value to the clients and the program.

22–A. Capital budgets refer to the budgeting of program or facility implementation. How much does it cost to start the program and implement the first stage of it? Capital budgets usually include equipment, staffing, initial marketing, etc., in the start-up. Operating a program is part of the operating budget, not the capital budget. Capital budgets are critical in determining whether to start a program or not. Capital budgets are not included in the balance sheet.

23–C. Budgets show what it will cost to run a program and whether the program will be profitable. Managers can review a budget and determine if there are financial problems with the program. Budgets are a future look at a program and should be developed with the idea of making money. Budgets also present only a part of the financial statement of the company. The company must include other financial information, such as assets and liabilities, in order to determine if it is making or losing money.

24–D. Each state may set its own laws in regulating fitness facilities and fitness staff. These laws differ from state to state. It is important to know these laws and be sure that your facility and staff follow them. Issues regarding illegal aliens, discrimination, and membership fees are not addressed in the laws governing the way in which fitness centers conduct programs.

25–A. Public relations (PR) is a way to promote your facility to various groups or communities. It shows the community who you are and what you offer. PR promotes quality, but this is no guarantee that you will not be negligent or sued, so malpractice insurance is not affected by PR. PR is designed to make those people who haven't joined yet familiar with you and want to join your facility, not to make your clients happy. Client participation programs (surveys, suggestion boxes, feedback opportunities) make clients happy and give them the opportunity to ask for what they want.

CHAPTER 11

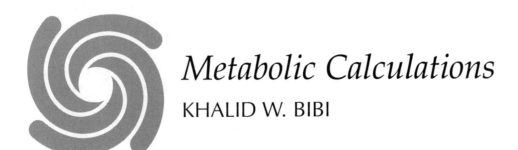

Metabolic Calculations

KHALID W. BIBI

I. OVERVIEW

A. RATIONALE FOR USE OF THE ACSM METABOLIC FORMULAE

–Fundamental to the application of proper exercise testing or prescription is the ability to measure or estimate energy expenditure.

1. **Direct measurement of $\dot{V}o_2$ is impractical.**

   –Actual oxygen consumption ($\dot{V}o_2$), using open-circuit spirometry, provides the health and fitness professional with the best measure of the energy cost of physical activity. Oxygen uptake values obtained during maximal exercise ($\dot{V}o_{2\,max}$) are commonly used as the index of cardiopulmonary fitness. Unfortunately, accurate $\dot{V}o_2$ measurement is arduous and costly, making it impractical for nonclinical purposes.

2. **$\dot{V}o_2$ can be estimated using the ACSM metabolic formulae.**

   –The American College of Sports Medicine (ACSM) introduced the ACSM metabolic formulae to provide health and fitness practitioners with a practical method to estimate the oxygen cost of the most common exercises. **Practical uses for the ACSM metabolic formulae are as follows:**

   a. Estimating the rate of oxygen uptake during exercise allows for an **estimate of the energy expenditure and hence caloric consumption** from fat associated with exercise.

   b. An estimate of the rate of oxygen uptake during maximal exercise ($\dot{V}o_{2\,max}$) indicates the maximal capacity for aerobic work, allowing for **fitness categorization, and inter- and intra-subject comparisons.** See the *ACSM's Guidelines for Exercise Testing*

   and Prescription, 6th edition, for more information about estimation of $\dot{V}o_{2\,max}$.

   c. Calculating the appropriate exercise intensity (**work rate**) needed to elicit the desired oxygen consumption will allow the health and fitness professional **to develop more effective exercise prescriptions.**

B. WHAT TO EXPECT REGARDING METABOLIC CALCULATION QUESTIONS ON THE ACSM WRITTEN EXAM

1. Expect from **6 to 10 metabolic calculation questions** on the examination. A few of these questions will be simple, requiring straightforward algebraic calculations. Some may be classified as moderately difficult, requiring simple mathematical substitution. One or two questions may be classified as difficult, requiring additional algebraic manipulation of these formulae.

2. A copy of the ACSM metabolic formulae (**Table 11-1**) is included in the written examination packet. You should be familiar with these formulae before you take the exam.

3. The **unit conversion factors** and the **energy equivalency factors** will **not** be provided with the examination. **Commit these numbers to memory.**

4. The written examination might contain metabolic calculation questions that will not require the use of the metabolic equations. However, a good understanding of energy expenditure and energy equivalency will be needed to arrive at the correct answer.

⟳ Table 11-1. Summary of Metabolic Calculations

Walking
$$\dot{V}o_2 = (0.1 \cdot S) + (1.8 \cdot S \cdot G) + 3.5$$

Treadmill and Outdoor Running
$$\dot{V}o_2 = (0.2 \cdot S) + (0.9 \cdot S \cdot G) + 3.5$$

Leg Ergometry
$$\dot{V}o_2 = (10.8 \cdot W \cdot M^{-1}) + 7$$

Arm Ergometry
$$\dot{V}o_2 = (18 \cdot W \cdot M^{-1}) + 3.5$$

Stepping
$$\dot{V}o_2 = (0.2 \cdot f) + (1.33 \cdot 1.8 \cdot H \cdot f) + 3.5$$

*Where $\dot{V}o_2$ is gross oxygen consumption in $ml \cdot kg^{-1} \cdot min^{-1}$; S is speed in $m \cdot min^{-1}$; M is body mass in kg; G is the percent grade expressed as a fraction; W is power in watts; f is stepping frequency in min^{-1}; H is step height in meters.

Note: These equations are presented in conventional units following each mode of exercise, simplifying the calculations.

(From *ACSM's Guidelines for Exercise Testing and Prescription*, 6th ed. Philadelphia, Lippincott Williams & Wilkins, 2000, p 303.)

C. EXPRESSIONS OF ENERGY

–Energy expenditure in humans can be expressed in many terms. Converting from one expression to another is simple. Be familiar with the following terms:

1. **Absolute oxygen consumption** L/min

    –This is the volume of oxygen consumed by the whole person, expressed in liters per minute ($L \cdot min^{-1}$) or milliliters per minute ($ml \cdot min^{-1}$).

    a. **Resting absolute oxygen consumption** for a 70-kg person is approximately $0.245 \ L \cdot min^{-1}$.

    b. In highly trained subjects, **maximal absolute oxygen consumption** as high as $4.9 \ L \cdot min^{-1}$ may be expected.

    c. Absolute oxygen consumption is useful because it allows for an easy **estimation of caloric expenditure.** Each liter of O_2 consumed expends 5 kilocalories (5 kcal), or 20.9 kilojoules (20.9 kJ).

2. **Relative oxygen consumption** ml/kg⁻¹/min

    –This is the measure of **oxygen consumption relative to body weight,** measured in $ml \cdot kg^{-1} \cdot min^{-1}$—in other words, the **volume of oxygen consumed by the cells of each kilogram of body weight every minute.**

    a. **For the purpose of the ACSM examination,** a given mass of lean body tissue requires the same amount of O_2 at rest, and at any given work rate, irrespective of gender, race, age, and level of fitness. The **resting relative oxygen consumption is always assumed to be 3.5 $ml \cdot kg^{-1} \cdot min^{-1}$.**

    b. In highly trained aerobic athletes, a maximal relative oxygen consumption ($\dot{V}o_{2\,max}$) may be as high as 75–80 $ml \cdot kg^{-1} \cdot min^{-1}$.

    c. **Relative** $\dot{V}o_2$ is commonly used to compare oxygen consumption of individuals who vary in size. Because $\dot{V}o_{2\,max}$ is also used as an index of cardiopulmonary fitness, **a higher value is indicative of greater aerobic fitness.**

    d. All ACSM formulae provide $\dot{V}o_2$ values in gross relative terms.

3. **Metabolic equivalents (METs)**

    –Physicians and clinicians commonly use the term **MET** as an expression of **energy expenditure or exercise intensity.** One MET is equivalent to the relative oxygen consumption at rest. Therefore, **1 MET = 3.5 $ml \cdot kg^{-1} \cdot min^{-1}$.**

    a. **METs are calculated by dividing the relative oxygen consumption by 3.5.** For example, an individual consuming $35 \ ml \cdot kg^{-1} \cdot min^{-1}$ during steady-state exercise is exercising at 10 METs.

    b. A MET is a useful expression because it allows for an easy **comparison of the amount of oxygen uptake during exercise with that at rest.**

4. **Calorie**

    –This expression of energy intake and expenditure is commonly used to quantify the **amount of energy derived from consumed foods** as well as the **amount of energy expended at rest and during physical activity** (see Chapter 9 Section II A, for more information about this topic).

5. **Fat stores**

    –The human body stores the majority of excess energy intake as fat.

    –It takes 3500 calories to make and store 1 pound of body fat.

    –Stated in reverse, **1 pound of fat can provide the body with 3500 calories**—the amount of energy needed to **walk or run about 35 miles!**

6. **Net vs. gross** $\dot{V}o_2$

    –**Humans** require about 3.5 $ml \cdot kg^{-1} \cdot min^{-1}$ (1 MET) of oxygen at rest. This amount of oxygen uptake is **vital for the survival of the body's cells, tissues, and systems.**

    –**Physical activity elevates oxygen consumption** above resting oxygen requirements.

    a. Net $\dot{V}o_2$ is the difference between the oxygen consumption value for exercise

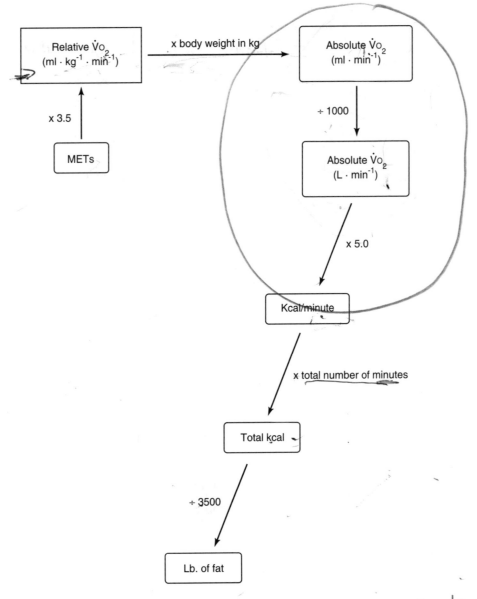

FIGURE 11-1 The energy equivalency chart: the 7 energy expressions.

NET $\dot{V}O_2$ = $\dot{V}O_2$ for exercise = Resting $\dot{V}O_2$

Gross $\dot{V}O_2$ = $\dot{V}O_2$ for exercise + Resting $\dot{V}O_2$

and the resting value. Net $\dot{V}O_2$ is used to assess the caloric cost of exercise.

  b. **Gross** $\dot{V}O_2$ is the sum of the oxygen cost of physical activity and the resting component.

  c. Hence,

net $\dot{V}O_2$ = *gross oxygen uptake – resting oxygen uptake*

  d. Net and gross oxygen uptake **can be expressed in relative or absolute terms.**

  e. The **ACSM metabolic formulae** in *ACSM's Guidelines for Exercise Testing and Prescription*, 6th edition, and those described in this chapter, were designed to provide you with **gross values.**

The ability to convert from one energy expression to another is fundamental. Do not proceed to the next section of this chapter until you master this task.

- Converting an expression merely requires the multiplication or division of that expression by a constant. For example, to convert from METs to relative oxygen consumption, multiply the MET value by 3.5. Conversely, to convert from relative oxygen consumption to METs, divide by 3.5 (**Figure 11-1**). *Commit these constants to memory.*
- **Figure 11-1**, **the Energy Equivalency Chart,** will help you to remember these conversions.
- **Figure 11-2** is a **practice sheet.** Duplicate this sheet and practice completing it from memory. Then answer the following questions.

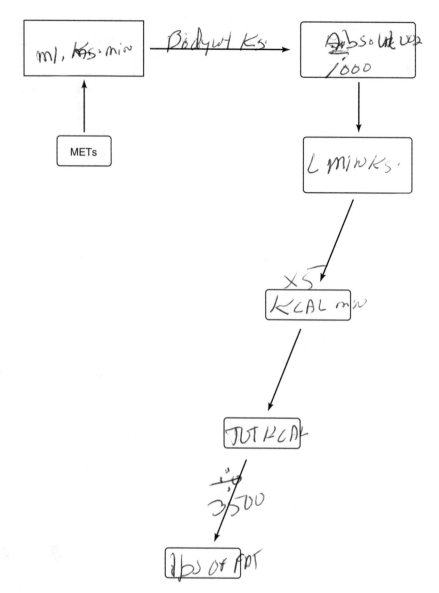

FIGURE 11-2 The energy equivalency chart practice sheet.

🌀 PRACTICE QUESTIONS: CONVERTING ENERGY EXPRESSIONS

1. What is the MET equivalent to 8.75 ml · kg⁻¹ · min⁻¹? *2.5/MET*

2. What is the absolute oxygen consumption equivalent to 10 METs for a 155-pound male? *2.45*

3. What is the equivalent total caloric expenditure of 2.5 pounds of fat? *8750*

4. A 70-kg male expends 7.5 kcal · min⁻¹ while exercising. What is the equivalent MET value? *6.12 MET*

5. How many pounds of fat will a 50-kg woman lose after 4 weeks of training if she exercises at a frequency of three days per week, a duration of 45 minutes per session, and an energy expenditure of 6.5 kcal · min⁻¹? Assume that there are no modifications in her eating habits during the 4 weeks of training.

6. Using the ACSM walking formula, you calculate a gross $\dot{V}O_2$ of 13.0 ml · kg⁻¹ · min⁻¹. What is the net oxygen uptake? *9.5*

SOLUTIONS

1. To convert from ml · kg⁻¹ · min⁻¹ to METs, divide 8.75 by 3.5. The correct answer is **2.5 METs.**

2. To convert from METs to $\dot{V}O_2$ in absolute terms, first multiply the MET value by 3.5 to convert METs to $\dot{V}O_2$ in relative terms (ml · kg⁻¹ · min⁻¹), then multiply the product (35 ml · kg⁻¹ · min⁻¹) by body weight in kg (155 pounds ÷ 2.2 = 70.5 kg). The correct answers are **2467.5 ml · min⁻¹** or **2.47 L · min⁻¹**.

3. To convert from pounds of fat to total kcal, multiply the fat weight (in pounds) by 3500. The correct answer is **8750 kcal.**

4. To convert from kcal · min⁻¹ to METs:

   a. First, convert the value to absolute $\dot{V}O_2$ in L · min⁻¹:

   $$7.5\ kcal \cdot min^{-1} \div 5.0 = 1.5\ L \cdot min^{-1}$$

   b. Then to absolute $\dot{V}O_2$ in ml · min⁻¹:

   $$1.5\ L \cdot min^{-1} \times 1000 = 1500\ ml \cdot min^{-1}$$

Table 11-2. Conversion Factors

To convert from:	to:	do this:
Centimeters (cm)	Meters (M)	÷ by 100
Inches (in)	Meters (M)	× by 0.0254
Inches (in)	Centimeters (cm)	× by 2.54
kg·m·min⁻¹	Watts (W)	÷ by 6.0
Liters (L)	Milliliters (ml)	× by 1000
Miles per hour (mph)	Meters per minute (m·min⁻¹)	× by 26.8
Miles per hour (mph)	Minutes per mile	÷ by 60
Pounds (lbs)	Kilograms (kg)	÷ by 2.2
Revolutions per minute (RPM) on a • Monark™ arm ergometer • Monark™ leg ergometer • Tunturi or BodyGuard cycle ergometer	Meters per minute (m·min⁻¹)	× by 2.4 × by 6 × by 3

c. Then to relative $\dot{V}O_2$:

1500 ml · min⁻¹ ÷ 70 kg = 21.43 ml · kg⁻¹ · min⁻¹

d. Then to METs:

21.43 ml · kg⁻¹ · min⁻¹ ÷ 3.5 = 6.12 METs

5. The first step to solving this conversion question is to calculate the total number of minutes spent exercising during the 4 weeks.

   a. Because she trained for 45 minutes per session, three times per week, she accumulated a total of 540 minutes of exercise during the 4 weeks:

   45 minutes/session × 3 sessions/week × 4 weeks = 540 minutes

   b. The second step is to calculate the total number of calories expended during exercise throughout the 4 weeks (540 minutes) of training:

   6.5 kcal · min⁻¹ × 540 minutes of exercise = 3510 kcal

   c. Finally, find the fat weight equivalent to the expended calories:

   3510 kcal ÷ 3500 = 1.003 pounds of fat

   or approximately 1 pound of fat.

6. Since gross $\dot{V}O_2$ = net $\dot{V}O_2$ + resting $\dot{V}O_2$, then net $\dot{V}O_2$ = gross $\dot{V}O_2$ – resting $\dot{V}O_2$:

Net $\dot{V}O_2$ = 13.0 ml · kg⁻¹ · min⁻¹ – 3.5 ml · kg⁻¹ · min⁻¹
Net $\dot{V}O_2$ = 9.5 ml · kg⁻¹ · min⁻¹

D. OTHER CONVERSION FACTORS

–You must also commit to memory some other important conversions. Practice writing out the conversions in **Table 11-2** from memory.

PRACTICE QUESTIONS: OTHER CONVERSION FACTORS

Convert the following values to the desired units:

1. 1.5 meters to cm
2. 59.1 inches to meters
3. 70 kg to pounds
4. 6.0 mph to meters per minute
5. 50 RPM on the Monark™ leg ergometer to meters per minute

SOLUTIONS

1. 1.5 meters × 100 = **150 cm**
2. 59.1 inches × 0.0254 = **1.5 meters**
3. 70 kg × 2.2 = **154 pounds**
4. 6.0 mph × 26.8 = **160.8 m · min⁻¹**
5. 50 RPM × 6 = **300 m · min⁻¹**

II. THE ACSM METABOLIC FORMULAE

–All ACSM formulae yield **gross** oxygen uptake in **relative** terms.

A. WALKING AND RUNNING FORMULAE
(Figure 11-3)

General Structure: ACSM Walking and Running Formulae

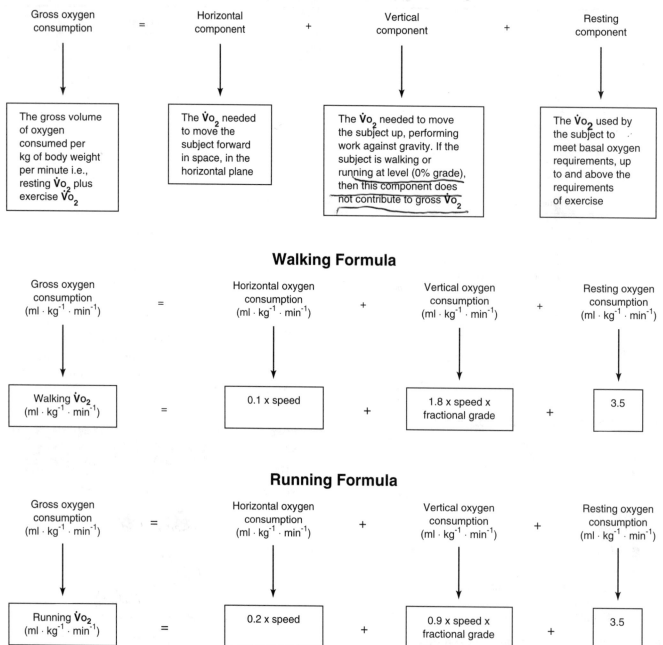

FIGURE 11-3 General structure of the walking and running formulae.

1. **Walking formula**

   –This formula applies to speeds of 50 to 100 m · min⁻¹ (1.9 to 3.7 mph).

   a. **Gross** $\dot{V}O_2$ is calculated in **relative terms** (ml · kg⁻¹ · min⁻¹).

   b. The **horizontal component** is the product of the speed of the treadmill, in meters per minute (m · min⁻¹), multiplied by 0.1 (the O_2 cost of walking). The product, the $\dot{V}O_2$ of walking forward, is in ml · kg⁻¹ · min⁻¹.

   c. The **vertical component** is the product of the grade of the treadmill multiplied by the speed of the treadmill (m · min⁻¹) multiplied by 1.8 (the O_2 cost of walking uphill). The product, the $\dot{V}O_2$ of walking uphill, is in ml · kg⁻¹ · min⁻¹. (Do not confuse the percent grade of the treadmill with the degree angle of inclination. **Percent grade of the treadmill** is the amount of vertical rise for 100 units of belt travel. For example, a client walking on a treadmill at a 12% grade travels

12 meters vertically for every 100 meters of belt travel.)

    d. The **resting component** is 3.5 ml · kg^{-1} · min^{-1}.

2. **Running formula**

   –This formula applies to treadmill and outdoor running speeds exceeding 134 m · min^{-1} (5.0 mph) and for true jogging speeds above 80.4 m · min^{-1} (3.0 mph).

   –This formula may also be used for off-the-treadmill level running, but not for running on a graded track.

    a. **Gross** $\dot{V}o_2$ is calculated in **relative terms** (ml · kg^{-1} · min^{-1}).

    b. The **horizontal component** is the product of the speed of the treadmill, in m · min^{-1} multiplied by 0.2 (the O_2 cost of running). The product, the $\dot{V}o_2$ of running forward, is in ml · kg^{-1} · min^{-1}.

    c. The **vertical component** is the product of the grade (elevation) of the treadmill multiplied by the speed of the treadmill (m · min^{-1}) multiplied by 0.9 (the O_2 cost of running uphill). The product, the $\dot{V}o_2$ of running uphill, is in ml · kg^{-1} · min^{-1}.

    d. The **resting component** is 3.5 ml · kg^{-1} · min^{-1}.

B. **LEG AND ARM ERGOMETRY FORMULAE**
    (**Figure 11-4**)

1. **Leg cycling**

   –This formula applies to work rates between 300 and 1200 kg · m· min^{-1}, or 50 to 200 watts (50–200 W).

    a. **Gross O$_2$** consumption is calculated in **relative terms** (ml · kg^{-1} · min^{-1}).

    b. **Oxygen cost of loaded leg cycling.** This is the product of the cost of cycling (1.8) multiplied by the work rate (kg · m · min^{-1}) divided by body weight (kg). The O_2 cost of loaded leg cycling may also be calculated using the following expression:

$$10.8 \times (\text{work rate (in watts)}) \div \text{body weight (in kg)}$$

Exam Note: Work Rate
The work rate may be provided to you in the question. You may also be expected to derive it from the cadence of the cycle ergometer and the resistance set on the flywheel.
- Work rate, also known as the **power output** or **workload,** is the product of the resistance set on the cycle ergometer and the speed of cycling (velocity):

Work rate = force (resistance set on the flywheel in kg) × velocity (in m · min^{-1})

The units for the resistance set on the flywheel, **kilogram-force (kgf) and kilopond (kp), can be used interchangeably: 1 kgf = 1 kp.**
- **Calculate velocity from revolutions per minute (RPM)** by multiplying the RPM value by **6 for a Monark cycle ergometer, or 3 for either a Tunturi or a BodyGuard.** For example, an individual cycling at 50 RPM on a Monark leg ergometer is pedaling at a velocity of 300 m · min^{-1}. If the same individual works against a resistance of 2 kp, then the work rate will be 2 × 50 × 6 = 600 kg · m · min^{-1}.
- **Work rate can also be expressed in watts:**

1 watt = 6.0 kg · m · min^{-1}

    c. **Oxygen cost of unloaded leg cycling.** Leg cycling incurs a small oxygen cost for the movement of the legs in space.

    d. The **resting O$_2$** component is 3.5 ml · kg^{-1} · min^{-1}.

2. **Arm cycling**

   –This formula applies to work rates between 150 and 750 kg · m · min^{-1} (25 to 125 W).

    a. **Gross O$_2$** consumption is calculated in relative terms (ml · kg^{-1} · min^{-1}).

    b. **Oxygen cost of loaded arm cycling.** This is the product of the cost of cycling (3) multiplied by the work rate (kg · m · min^{-1}) divided by body weight (kg). The O_2 cost of loaded arm cycling may also be calculated using the following expression:

18 × work rate (in watts) ÷ body weight (in kg)

Exam Note: Work Rate
The work rate may be provided to you in the question. You may also be expected to derive it from the cadence of the cycle ergometer and the resistance set on the flywheel.
- Work rate, also known as the power output or workload, is the product of the resistance set on the flywheel and the speed of cycling (velocity):

Work rate = force (resistance set on the flywheel in kg) × velocity (in m · min^{-1})

- Calculate velocity from RPM by multiplying the RPM value by **2.4 for a Monark arm ergometer.** The units for the resistance set on the flywheel, kilogram-force (kgf) and kilopond (kp), can be used interchangeably: *1 kgf = 1 kp*

For example, an individual arm cycling at 50 RPM on a Monark arm ergometer is pedaling at a velocity of 120 m · min^{-1}. If the same individual works against a resistance of 2 kp, then the work rate will be 2 × 50 × 2.4 = 240 kg · m · min^{-1}.
- Work rate can also be expressed in watts:

1 watt = 6.0 kg · m · min^{-1}

General Structure: ACSM Leg and Arm Ergonometry Formulae

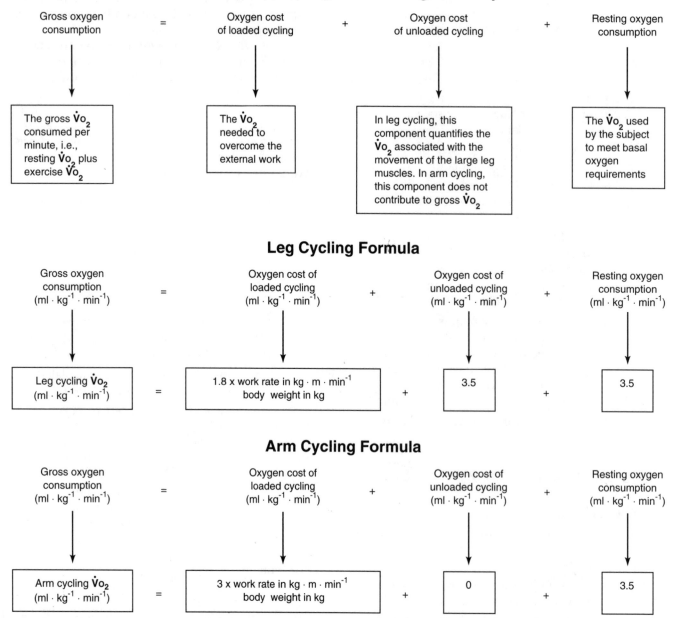

FIGURE 11-4 General structure of the leg and arm ergonometry formulae.

c. **Oxygen cost of unloaded arm cycling.** Arm cycling does not incur an oxygen cost of unloaded cycling.

d. The **resting component is 3.5 ml · kg^{-1} · min^{-1}.**

C. STEPPING FORMULA (Figure 11-5)

–This formula applies to stepping performed on a step box, a bleacher, or a similar stepping object where both concentric contractions (moving up against gravity) and eccentric contractions (moving down with gravity) are involved.

–The formula is appropriate for stepping rates between 12 and 30 steps · min^{-1}, and heights between 0.04 and 0.4 m (1.6 to 15.7 inches).

1. **Gross O$_2$** consumption is calculated in **relative terms** (ml · kg^{-1} · min^{-1}).

2. **Horizontal component.** This is the product of the rate of stepping per minute multiplied by 0.2. The product is O$_2$ consumption in ml · kg^{-1} · min^{-1}.

ACSM Stepping Formula

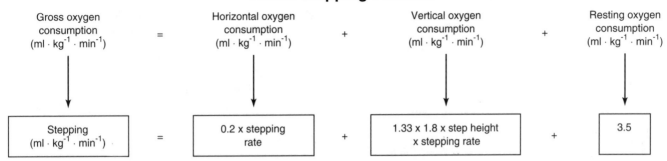

FIGURE 11-5 ACSM stepping formula.

3. **Vertical component.** This is the product of the height of each step (in meters) multiplied by the rate of stepping per minute multiplied by

1.33 multiplied by 1.8. The product is O_2 consumption in $ml \cdot kg^{-1} \cdot min^{-1}$.

4. **Resting component** is 3.5 $ml \cdot kg^{-1} \cdot min^{-1}$.

III. SOLVING THE ACSM METABOLIC FORMULAE

A. USING A SYSTEMATIC APPROACH

–The task of solving the ACSM formulae is made much easier using a systematic approach, which will help you avoid small but costly mistakes.

1. Read each question carefully and do not proceed until you know what you are expected to calculate. Remember that some questions may be solved without the use of a metabolic formula.

2. Extract the required information. Do not be misled with extraneous information. If, for example, a question wants you to calculate the $\dot{V}o_2$ for walking on a treadmill, volunteered data about the height, age, or the gender of the subject are irrelevant.

3. Select the correct metabolic equation. A common error committed by many candidates is choosing the wrong formula.

4. Write down each step. *Do not take shortcuts.* Going through all the steps once is faster than two shortcut attempts!

5. On the top left corner of a clean sheet of paper, write the known values and indicate what is the unknown.

6. Where needed, convert all values to the appropriate units (see Table 11-2).

   a. Convert the treadmill speed or cycling cadence to meters per minute ($m \cdot min^{-1}$).

   b. Convert body weight to kilograms (kg).

   c. Convert step height to meters (m).

   d. Convert work rate to $kg \cdot m \cdot min^{-1}$.

7. Write down the formula and plug in the known values and constants. Write clearly and place units after all variables.

8. Solve for the unknown. If the unknown is on the left side of the equation (i.e., the $\dot{V}o_2$ value), simply calculate the sum of the three components of the appropriate equation. If the unknown is on the right side of the equation, substitute and solve for the unknown. More on solving linear equations later.

9. Examine the answer. Is the answer logical? Does it fall within expected "normal" values and human abilities?

10. Examine the choices. Make sure that your answer is in the same units as the answer on the examination, especially if a question does not specify what energy expression is needed (i.e., relative or absolute $\dot{V}o_2$, METs, kcal).

B. SOLVING LINEAR EQUATIONS

–The ACSM metabolic formulae are simple linear regression equations.

–The process of arriving at an answer to a metabolic calculation question is greatly simplified if the unknown is the $\dot{V}o_2$ value.

–In instances where the $\dot{V}o_2$ value is known, you might be expected to calculate an unknown value on the right side of the equation, such as the resistance on the cycle ergometer, the speed of the treadmill, the height of the step bench, etc.

To solve an equation with an unknown on the right side of the equation, you must simplify the expression so that the unknown stands by itself on one side of the equation and all the known numbers on the other.

1. **Example 1**

   –Solve for χ in the following equation:

   $$\chi - 4 = 10$$

   Solution: Add 4 to both sides of the equation:

   $$\chi - 4 + 4 = 10 + 4$$
   $$\chi = 14$$

2. **Example 2**

   –Solve for α in the following equation:

   $$2\alpha + 7 = 3$$

   Solution: Subtract 7 from both sides of the equation:

   $$2\alpha = -4$$

   Divide both sides by 2:

   $$\alpha = -2$$

3. **Example 3**

   –Solve for β in the following equation:

   $$4\beta - \tfrac{3}{4} = \tfrac{7}{9}$$

   Solution: Add ¾ to both sides of the equation:

   $$4\beta = \tfrac{55}{36}$$

   Divide both sides by 4:

   $$\beta = \tfrac{55}{144}$$

4. **Helpful hint:** Substitute your answer for the unknown value in the original equation. If the left side equals the right side after the substitution, your answer is correct. For example, in the previous problem, plugging in $\tfrac{55}{144}$ in the place of β yields ⅞. Hence, $\tfrac{55}{144}$ is the correct answer.

⑨ SOLVING METABOLIC CALCULATIONS: EXAMPLES

1. What is the gross oxygen cost of walking on a treadmill at 3.5 mph and a 10% grade?

Solution: Choose the walking equation.

   a. On the top left corner of a clean sheet of paper, write down the knowns and convert all numbers to the appropriate units:

   Speed in m · min^{-1} = 3.5 mph × 26.8 = 93.8 m · min^{-1}

   b. Write down the ACSM walking formula:

   Walking (ml · kg^{-1} · min^{-1}) = (0.1 × *speed*) + (1.8 × *speed* × *fractional grade*) + 3.5 ml · kg^{-1} · min^{-1}

   c. Substitute the variable name with the known values:

   Walking (ml · kg^{-1} · min^{-1}) = 0.1 × **93.8** m · min^{-1} +1.8 × **93.8** m · min^{-1} × **0.1** + 3.5 ml ·kg^{-1} · min^{-1}

Math Reminder

Multiply and divide numbers **before** *adding or subtracting.* For example, in the following expression:

$$Y = 5 + 2 \times 5 + 7 \times 2$$

Multiply the 2 by the 5 (=10), the 7 by the 2 (=14), and then add the 10, the 14, and the 5 together. The correct answer is Y = 29, not 84.

---

   d. Multiply values:

   Walking (ml · kg^{-1} · min^{-1}) = 9.38 ml · kg^{-1} · min^{-1} +16.88 ml · kg^{-1} · min^{-1} + 3.5 ml · kg^{-1} · min^{-1}

   e. Then add numbers:

   Gross walking $\dot{V}o_2$ = **29.76 ml · kg^{-1} · min^{-1}**

2. A 176-lb client set the treadmill at 3.0 mph and 2% grade. While exercising, his heart rate was 140 beats · min^{-1} and his blood pressure was 160/80 mm Hg. What was his estimated oxygen consumption in relative terms?

Solution: The question is clearly asking for $\dot{V}o_2$ in relative terms (ml · kg^{-1} · min^{-1}).

   a. Extract the information you need (speed and elevation of the treadmill) and ignore extraneous information (HR and BP).

   b. Choose the walking equation.

   c. On the top left corner of a clean sheet of paper, write down the knowns and convert all numbers to the appropriate units:

   Weight = 176 lb ÷ 2.2 = 80.0 kg

   Speed = 3.0 mph × 26.8 = 80.4 m · min^{-1}

   Treadmill elevation = 2% grade = 2/100 = 0.02

   d. Plug the knowns into the formula and calculate the answer:

   Walking (ml · kg^{-1} · min^{-1}) = *speed* (m · min^{-1}) × 0.1 + *grade* (fraction) × *speed* (m · min^{-1}) × 1.8 + 3.5 (ml · kg^{-1} · min^{-1})

   Walking (ml · kg^{-1} · min^{-1}) = **80.4** (m · min^{-1}) × 0.1 + **0.02 × 80.4** (m · min^{-1}) × 1.8 + 3.5 (ml · kg^{-1} · min^{-1})

   Walking (ml · kg^{-1} · min^{-1}) = 8.04 ml · kg^{-1} · min^{-1} + 2.89 ml · kg^{-1} · min^{-1} + 3.5 ml · kg^{-1} · min^{-1}

   14.43 (ml · kg^{-1} · min^{-1}) = 8.04 ml · kg^{-1} · min^{-1} + 2.89 ml · kg^{-1} · min^{-1} + 3.5 ml · kg^{-1} · min^{-1}

   Relative $\dot{V}o_2$ = **14.43 ml · kg^{-1} · min^{-1}**

3. What resistance should you set a Monark cycle ergometer at to elicit a $\dot{V}o_2$ value of 2750 ml · min⁻¹ while cycling at 50 RPM? The subject is 65 inches tall and weighs 110 pounds?

Solution: Read the question carefully; know what the question is asking for. The question is providing you with the oxygen consumption (2750 ml · min⁻¹), but expects you to calculate the resistance (F) to be set on the cycle ergometer.

a. Extract the information you need. Only the weight of the subject and the speed of the cycle are needed.

b. Convert the known units:

$$110 \text{ pounds} = 50.0 \text{ kg}$$

c. Select the leg ergometer equation.

d. Calculate the gross relative $\dot{V}o_2$ from the given information:

$$\dot{V}o_2 \text{ ml} \cdot kg^{-1} \cdot min^{-1} = 2750 \text{ ml} \cdot min^{-1} \div 50.0 \text{ kg}$$
$$= 55.0 \text{ ml} \cdot kg^{-1} \cdot min^{-1}$$

$$\text{Leg cycling } (ml \cdot kg^{-1} \cdot min^{-1}) = 1.8 \times \text{work rate}$$
$$\div \text{ body weight} + 3.5 \ (ml \cdot kg^{-1} \cdot min^{-1})$$
$$+ 3.5 \ (ml \cdot kg^{-1} \cdot min^{-1})$$

e. Note that the unknown (resistance in kg) is part of the work rate. Write out the work rate as force (in kg) × speed (in m · min⁻¹):

$$55 \text{ ml} \cdot kg^{-1} \cdot min^{-1} = 1.8 \times F \times \text{speed} \div \text{body weight}$$
$$+ 3.5 \ (ml \cdot kg^{-1} \cdot min^{-1}) + 3.5 \ (ml \cdot kg^{-1} \cdot min^{-1})$$

f. From the given information, we also know that the speed of cycling is 300 m · min⁻¹ (50 RPM × 6). Plug all the knowns into the equation:

$$55 \text{ ml} \cdot kg^{-1} \cdot min^{-1} = 1.8 \times F \times 300 \text{ m} \cdot min^{-1} \div 50 \text{ kg}$$
$$+ 3.5 \ (ml \cdot kg^{-1} \cdot min^{-1}) + 3.5 \ (ml \cdot kg^{-1} \cdot min^{-1})$$

g. Move the unknown F to one side of the equation, all the knowns to the other side, and calculate for the unknown:

$$55 \text{ ml} \cdot kg^{-1} \cdot min^{-1} = 1.8 \times F \times 300 \text{ m} \cdot min^{-1} \div 50 \text{ kg}$$
$$+ 3.5 \ (ml \cdot kg^{-1} \cdot min^{-1}) + 3.5 \ (ml \cdot kg^{-1} \cdot min^{-1})$$

$$55 \text{ ml} \cdot kg^{-1} \cdot min^{-1} - 3.5 \text{ ml} \cdot kg^{-1} \cdot min^{-1} - 3.5 \text{ ml} \cdot kg^{-1}$$
$$\cdot min^{-1} = 1.8 \times F \cdot 300 \text{ m/min} \div 50 \text{ kg}$$

$$48 \text{ ml} \cdot kg^{-1} \cdot min^{-1} = 1.8 \times F \times 300 \text{ m/min} \div 50 \text{ kg}$$

$$\frac{48 \times 50}{1.8 \times 300} = F$$

$$4.44 \text{ kp} = F$$

REVIEW TEST

DIRECTIONS: Carefully read all questions and select the BEST single answer.

1. What is the relative oxygen consumption of walking on a treadmill at 3.5 mph and 0% grade?
   (A) 9.38 ml · kg^{-1} · min^{-1}
   (B) 12.88 ml · kg^{-1} · min^{-1}
   (C) 18.76 ml · kg^{-1} · min^{-1}
   (D) 22.26 ml · kg^{-1} · min^{-1}

2. A client is walking on a treadmill at 3.4 mph up a 5% grade. What is her $\dot{V}o_2$ in relative terms?
   (A) 9.11 ml · kg^{-1} · min^{-1}
   (B) 11.9 ml · kg^{-1} · min^{-1}
   (C) 24 ml · kg^{-1} · min^{-1}
   (D) 20.81 ml · kg^{-1} · min^{-1}

3. A 70-kg client is running on a treadmill at 5 mph set at a 5% grade. What is his caloric expenditure rate?
   (A) 12.7 kcal · min^{-1}
   (B) 1.271 kcal · min^{-1}
   (C) 3.633 kcal · min^{-1}
   (D) 36.33 kcal · min^{-1}

4. What is the relative oxygen consumption of walking on a treadmill at 3.5 mph up a 10% grade?
   (A) 181.72 ml · kg^{-1} · min^{-1}
   (B) 18.17 ml · kg^{-1} · min^{-1}
   (C) 29.76 ml · kg^{-1} · min^{-1}
   (D) 27.96 ml · kg^{-1} · min^{-1}

5. What is the MET equivalent to level walking on a treadmill at 3.0 mph?
   (A) 5.59 METs
   (B) 3.30 METs
   (C) 2.30 METs
   (D) 3.02 METs

6. What is the relative oxygen consumption of running on a treadmill at 6.5 mph and 0% grade?
   (A) 34.84 ml · kg^{-1} · min^{-1}
   (B) 34.48 ml · kg^{-1} · min^{-1}
   (C) 38.34 ml · kg^{-1} · min^{-1}
   (D) 43.83 ml · kg^{-1} · min^{-1}

7. What is the relative oxygen consumption of running on a treadmill at 5.5 mph and 12% grade?
   (A) 29.48 ml · kg^{-1} · min^{-1}
   (B) 45.4 ml · kg^{-1} · min^{-1}
   (C) 47.2 ml · kg^{-1} · min^{-1}
   (D) 48.9 ml · kg^{-1} · min^{-1}

8. A 150-pound male sets the treadmill speed at 5.0 mph and a 5.2% grade. Calculate his MET value.
   (A) 36.57 METs
   (B) 10.45 METs
   (C) 12.25 METs
   (D) Not enough information to answer the question

9. What is a subject's work rate in watts if he pedals on a Monark cycle ergometer at 50 RPM at a resistance of 2.0 kiloponds?
   (A) 50 watts
   (B) 100 watts
   (C) 200 watts
   (D) 300 watts

10. A 110-pound female pedals a Monark™ cycle ergometer at 50 RPM against a resistance of 2.5 kiloponds. Calculate her absolute oxygen consumption.
    (A) 300 ml · min^{-1}
    (B) 750 ml · min^{-1}
    (C) 1.25 L · min^{-1}
    (D) 1.7 L · min^{-1}

11. How many calories will a 110-pound woman expend if she pedals on a Monark™ cycle ergometer at 50 RPM against a resistance of 2.5 kiloponds for 60 minutes?
    (A) 12.87 calories
    (B) 31.28 calories
    (C) 510 calories
    (D) 3500 calories

12. A 55-kilogram woman trains on a cycle ergometer by pedaling at 60 RPM against a resistance of 1.5 kiloponds. What is her absolute oxygen consumption?
    (A) 1.36 L · min^{-1}
    (B) 2.47 L · min^{-1}
    (C) 3.62 L · min^{-1}
    (D) 3600 ml · min^{-1}

13. The same 55-kilogram woman also trains on a Monark arm ergometer at 60 RPM against a resistance of 1.5 kiloponds. What is her absolute oxygen consumption?
    (A) 1.52 L · min^{-1}
    (B) 773.0 ml · min^{-1}
    (C) 0.840 L · min^{-1}
    (D) 0.774 L · min^{-1}

14. If a 70-kilogram man runs on a treadmill at 8 mph and 0% grade for 45 minutes, what is his caloric expenditure?
    (A) 1067.07 calories
    (B) 392.18 calories
    (C) 730.48 calories
    (D) Not enough information to answer the question

15. What is the relative oxygen cost of bench stepping at a rate of 24 steps per minute up a 10-inch stepping box? The individual weighs 140 pounds.
    (A) 12.91 ml · kg^{-1} · min^{-1}
    (B) 14.61 ml · kg^{-1} · min^{-1}
    (C) 16.41 ml · kg^{-1} · min^{-1}
    (D) 18.11 ml · kg^{-1} · min^{-1}

16. What stepping rate should a client use if she wishes to exercise at 5 METs? The step box is 6 inches high and she weighs 50 kilograms.
    (A) 12 steps per minute
    (B) 32 steps per minute
    (C) 35 steps per minute
    (D) 96 steps per minute

17. A 143-pound woman regularly exercises on a treadmill at a speed of 5.5 mph and a 2% elevation. What is her caloric expenditure?
    (A) 6.78 kcal · min^{-1}
    (B) 11.58 kcal · min^{-1}
    (C) 20.85 kcal · min^{-1}
    (D) 25.47 kcal · min^{-1}

18. A 143-pound woman regularly exercises on a treadmill at a speed of 5.5 mph and a 2% elevation. How much weight will she lose weekly if she exercises for a duration of 45 minutes per session, a frequency of 3 sessions per week?
    (A) 1.5 kilograms
    (B) 2.07 kilograms
    (C) 0.25 pounds
    (D) 0.45 pounds

19. What resistance would you set a cycle ergometer at if your 80-kilogram client needs to train at 6 METs? Assume a 50 RPM cycling cadence.
    (A) 1.5 kilograms
    (B) 2.07 kilograms
    (C) 0.25 pounds
    (D) 0.45 pounds

20. What running speed would you set a level treadmill at to elicit an oxygen consumption of 40 ml · kg^{-1} · min^{-1}?
    (A) 5.0 mph
    (B) 6.8 mph
    (C) 18.25 m · min^{-1}
    (D) 18.25 mph

21. If a healthy young man exercises at an intensity of 45 ml · kg^{-1} · min^{-1} three times per week for 45 minutes each session, how long would it take him to lose 10 pounds of fat?
    (A) 4 weeks
    (B) 7.14 weeks
    (C) 16.5 weeks
    (D) 19 weeks

22. A 35-year-old female reduced her caloric intake by 1200 kcal per week. How much weight will she lose in 26 weeks?
    (A) 8.9 pounds
    (B) 12.0 pounds
    (C) 26.0 pounds
    (D) 34.3 pounds

23. From question 22, how much weight will she lose in 26 weeks if she integrated a 1-mile walk three times per week into her weight loss program?
    (A) 3 pounds
    (B) 6 pounds
    (C) 11 pounds
    (D) 15 pounds

ANSWERS AND EXPLANATIONS

1–B. The steps are as follows:
   a. Choose the ACSM walking formula.
   b. Write down your knowns and convert the values to the appropriate units:
     Knowns: 3.5 mph × 26.8 m · min^{-1}
        = 93.8 m · min^{-1}
        0% grade = 0.0
   c. Write down the ACSM walking formula:

Walking = (0.1 × speed) + (1.8 × speed × fractional grade) + (3.5 ml · kg^{-1} · min^{-1})

   d. Substitute the known values for the variable name:

ml · kg^{-1} · min^{-1} = (0.1 × 93.8) + (1.8 × 93.8 × 0) + (3.5)
ml · kg^{-1} · min^{-1} = (9.38) + (0) + (3.5)

   e. Solve for the unknown:
     ml · kg^{-1} · min^{-1} = (9.38) + (3.5)
   Gross walking V̇o$_2$ = 12.88 ml · kg^{-1} · min^{-1}

2–D. The steps are as follows:
   a. Choose the ACSM walking formula.
   b. Write down your knowns and convert the values to the appropriate units:
     Knowns: 3.4 mph × 26.8 m · min^{-1}
        = 91.12 m · min^{-1}
        5% grade = 0.05
   c. Write down the ACSM walking formula:

Walking = (0.1 × speed) + (1.8 × speed × fractional grade) + (3.5)(ml · kg^{-1} · min^{-1})

d. Substitute the known values for the variable name:

$ml \cdot kg^{-1} \cdot min^{-1} = (0.1 \times 91.12) + (1.8 \times 91.12 \times .05) + (3.5)\ ml \cdot kg^{-1} \cdot min^{-1} = (9.112) + (8.2008) + (3.5)$

e. Solve for the unknown:

$ml \cdot kg^{-1} \cdot min^{-1} = (9.112) + (8.2008) + (3.5)$

Gross walking $\dot{V}o_2 = 20.81\ ml \cdot kg^{-1} \cdot min^{-1}$

3–A. The steps are as follows:

a. Choose the ACSM running formula.
b. Write down your knowns and convert the values to the appropriate units:
   Knowns: 5 mph × 26.8 = 134 m · min^{-1}
   5% grade = 0.05
c. Write down the ACSM running formula:

Running $= (0.2 \times speed) + (0.9 \times speed \times fractional\ grade) + (3.5)(ml \cdot kg^{-1} \cdot min^{-1})$

d. Substitute the known values for the variable name:

$ml \cdot kg^{-1} \cdot min^{-1} = (0.2 \times 134) + (0.9 \times 134 \times .05) + (3.5)$

$ml \cdot kg^{-1} \cdot min^{-1} = (26.8) + (6.03) + (3.5)$

e. Solve for the unknown:

$ml \cdot kg^{-1} \cdot min^{-1} = (26.8) + (6.03) + (3.5)$

Gross running $\dot{V}o_2 = 36.33\ ml \cdot kg^{-1} \cdot min^{-1}$

f. The question is asking you to find the client's caloric expenditure rate, which means that you need to first determine his O_2 consumption in absolute terms:

Absolute $\dot{V}o_2\ (ml \cdot min^{-1}) = relative\ \dot{V}o_2\ (ml \cdot kg^{-1} \cdot min^{-1}) \times body\ weight\ in\ kg$

$ml \cdot min^{-1} = 36.33\ ml \cdot kg^{-1} \cdot min^{-1} \times 70\ kg$

Absolute $\dot{V}o_2\ (ml \cdot min^{-1}) = 2543.1\ ml \cdot min^{-1}$

Now, divide by 1000 to get L · min^{-1}:

$2543.1 \div 1000 = 2.54\ L \cdot min^{-1}$

g. Multiply absolute $\dot{V}o_2$ by 5.0 to determine his caloric expenditure rate:

$2.54\ L \cdot min^{-1} \times 5.0 = 12.7\ kcal \cdot min^{-1}$

4–C. The steps are as follows:

a. Choose the ACSM walking formula.
b. Write down your knowns and convert the values to the appropriate units:
   Knowns: 3.5 mph × (26.8) = 93.8 m · min^{-1}
   10% grade = 0.10
c. Write down the ACSM walking formula:

Walking $= (0.1 \times speed) + (1.8 \times speed \times fractional\ grade) + (3.5)(ml \cdot kg^{-1} \cdot min^{-1})$

d. Substitute the known values for the variable name:

$ml \cdot kg^{-1} \cdot min^{-1} = (0.1 \times 93.8) + (1.8 \times 93.8 \times 0.1) + (3.5)$

$ml \cdot kg^{-1} \cdot min^{-1} = (9.38) + (16.884) + (3.5)$

e. Solve for the unknown:

$ml \cdot kg^{-1} \cdot min^{-1} = (9.38) + (16.884) + (3.5)$

Gross walking $\dot{V}o_2 = 29.76\ ml \cdot kg^{-1} \cdot min^{-1}$

5–B. The steps are as follows:

a. Choose the ACSM walking formula.
b. Write down your knowns and convert the values to the appropriate units:
   Knowns: 3.0 mph × (26.8) = 80.4 m · min^{-1}
   0% grade (level walking) = 0.0
c. Write down the ACSM walking formula:

Walking $(ml \cdot kg^{-1} \cdot min^{-1}) = (0.1 \times speed) + (1.8 \times speed \times fractional\ grade) + (3.5)$

d. Substitute the known values for the variable name:

$ml \cdot kg^{-1} \cdot min^{-1} = (0.1 \times 80.4) + (1.8 \times 80.4 \times 0) + (3.5)$

e. Solve for the unknown:

$ml \cdot kg^{-1} \cdot min^{-1} = (8.04) + (0) + (3.5)$

Gross walking $\dot{V}o_2 = 11.54\ ml \cdot kg^{-1} min^{-1}$

f. Because this question wants you to find the MET equivalent, we must divide our gross walking $\dot{V}o_2$ by the constant 3.5:

$METs = relative\ \dot{V}o_2\ (ml \cdot kg^{-1} \cdot min^{-1}) \div 3.5$

$METs = 11.54\ ml \cdot kg^{-1} \cdot min^{-1}) \div 3.5$

$= 3.30\ METs$

6–C. The steps are as follows:

a. Choose the ACSM running formula.
b. Write down your knowns and convert the values to the appropriate units:
   Knowns: 6.5 mph × 26.8 = 174.2 m · min^{-1}
   0% grade = 0.0
c. Write down the ACSM running formula:

Running $= (0.2 \times speed) + (0.9 \times speed \times fractional\ grade) + (3.5)(ml \cdot kg^{-1} \cdot min^{-1})$

d. Substitute the known values for the variable name:

$ml \cdot kg^{-1} \cdot min^{-1} = (0.2 \times 174.2) + (0.9 \times 174.2 \times 0) + (3.5)$

e. Solve for the unknown:

$ml \cdot kg^{-1} \cdot min^{-1} = (34.84) + (0) + (3.5)$

Gross running $\dot{V}o_2 = 38.34\ ml \cdot kg^{-1} \cdot min^{-1}$

7–D. The steps are as follows:

a. Choose the ACSM running formula.
b. Write down your knowns and convert the values to the appropriate units:
   Knowns: 5.5 mph × 26.8 = 147.4 m · min^{-1}
   12% grade = 0.12
c. Write down the ACSM running formula:

Running $= (0.2 \times speed) + (0.9 \times speed \times fractional\ grade) + (3.5)(ml \cdot kg^{-1} \cdot min^{-1})$

d. Substitute the known values for the variable name:

$$ml \cdot kg^{-1} \cdot min^{-1} = (0.2 \cdot 147.4)$$
$$+ (0.9 \cdot 147.4 \cdot 0.12) + (3.5)$$

e. Solve for the unknown:

$$ml \cdot kg^{-1} \cdot min^{-1} = (29.48) + (15.92) + (3.5)$$

Gross running $\dot{V}o_2 = 48.9 \, ml \cdot kg^{-1} \cdot min^{-1}$

8–B. The steps are as follows:
   a. Choose the ACSM running formula.
   b. Write down your knowns and convert the values to the appropriate units:
   Knowns: 5.0 mph × 26.8 = 134 m · min⁻¹
          5.2% grade = 0.052
   c. Write down the ACSM running formula:

Running = (0.2 × speed) + (0.9 × speed × fractional grade) + (3.5)(ml · kg⁻¹ · min⁻¹)

   d. Substitute the known values for the variable name:

$$ml \cdot kg^{-1} \cdot min^{-1} = (0.2 \times 134)$$
$$+ (0.9 \times 134 \times 0.052) + (3.5)$$

   e. Solve for the unknown:

$$ml \cdot kg^{-1} \cdot min^{-1} = (26.8) + (3.5)$$

Gross running $\dot{V}o_2 = 36.57 \, ml \cdot kg^{-1} \cdot min^{-1}$

   f. This question asks us for his MET value so we must divide his gross funning $\dot{V}o_2$ (ml · kg⁻¹ · min⁻¹) by the constant 3.5 (we can ignore his weight—this is extraneous information):

METs = relative $\dot{V}o_2$ (ml · kg⁻¹ · min⁻¹) ÷ 3.5

METs = 36.57 ml · kg⁻¹ · min⁻¹ ÷ 3.5

$$= 10.45 \, METs$$

9–B. This question does not require the use of a metabolic formula because it is asking for the subject's work rate. The steps are as follows:
   a. Write down your knowns and convert the values to the appropriate units:
   Knowns: 50 RPM × 6 meters = 300 m · min⁻¹ (each revolution on a Monark cycle ergometer = 6 m)
   2.0 kiloponds = 2.0 kilograms
   b. Write down the formula for work rate:

Work rate = force × distance ÷ time

   c. Substitute the known values for the variable name:

Work rate = 2.0 kg × 300 m · min⁻¹

Work rate = 600 kg · m · min⁻¹

   d. The question asks for watts, so we must divide the work rate (kg⁻¹ · m · min⁻¹) by 6:

W = kg · m · min⁻¹ ÷ 6 watts = 600 kg · m · min⁻¹ ÷ 6

$$= 100 \, W$$

10–D. The steps are as follows:
   a. Choose the ACSM leg cycling formula.
   b. Write down your knowns and convert the values to the appropriate units:
   Knowns: 110 pounds ÷ 2.2 = 50kg
         50 RPM × 6 meters = 300 m · min⁻¹
         2.5 kp = 2.5 kg
   c. Write down the ACSM leg cycling formula:

Leg cycling (ml · kg⁻¹ · min⁻¹) = (1.8 × work rate ÷ body weight) + (3.5) + (3.5)

   d. Calculate work rate:

Work rate = kg · m ÷ min

$$= 2.5 \, kg \times 300 \, m \cdot min^{-1}$$

$$= 750 \, kg \cdot m \cdot min^{-1}$$

   e. Substitute the known values for the variable name:

$$ml \cdot kg^{-1} \cdot min^{-1} = (1.8 \times 750 \div 50) + (3.5) + (3.5)$$

   f. Solve for the unknown:

$$ml \cdot kg^{-1} \cdot min^{-1} = (27) + (3.5) + (3.5)$$

Gross leg cycling $\dot{V}o_2 = 34 \, ml \cdot kg^{-1} \cdot min^{-1}$

   g. This question is asking for her absolute oxygen consumption, so we must multiply her gross $\dot{V}o_2$ (in relative terms) by her body weight:

Absolute $\dot{V}o_2$ = relative $\dot{V}o_2$ × body weight

$$= 34 \, ml \cdot kg^{-1} \cdot min^{-1} \times 50 \, kg$$

$$= 1700 \, ml \cdot min^{-1}$$

   h. To get L · min⁻¹, divide by 1000:

1700 ml · min⁻¹ ÷ 1000 = 1.7 L min⁻¹

11–C. The steps are as follows:
   a. Choose the ACSM leg cycling formula.
   b. Write down your knowns and convert the values to the appropriate units:
   Knowns: 110 pounds ÷ 2.2 = 50 kg
         50 RPM × 6 meters = 300 m · min⁻¹
         2.5 kp = 2.5 kg
         60 minutes of cycling
   c. Write down the ACSM formula:

Leg cycling (ml · kg⁻¹ · min⁻¹) = (1.8 × work rate ÷ body weight) + (3.5) + (3.5) (ml · kg⁻¹ · min⁻¹)

   d. Calculate work rate:

work rate = kg · m/min = 2.5 kg · 300 m · min⁻¹

$$= 750 \, kg^{-1} \cdot m \cdot min^{-1}$$

   e. Substitute the known values for the variable name:

$$ml \cdot kg^{-1} \cdot min^{-1} = (1.8 \times 750 \div 50) + (3.5) + (3.5)$$

   f. Solve for the unknown:

Gross leg cycling $\dot{V}o_2 = 34 \, ml \cdot kg^{-1} \cdot min^{-1}$

g. To find out how many calories she expends, we must first convert her oxygen consumption to absolute terms:

$$Absolute\ \dot{V}O_2 = relative\ \dot{V}O_2 \times body\ weight$$
$$= 34\ ml \cdot kg^{-1} \cdot min^{-1} \times 50\ kg$$
$$= 1700\ ml \cdot min^{-1}$$

h. Convert $ml \cdot min^{-1}$ to $L \cdot min^{-1}$ by dividing by 1000:

$$1700\ ml \cdot min^{-1} \div 1000 = 1.7\ L \cdot min^{-1}$$

i. Next we must see how many calories she expends in one minute by multiplying her absolute $\dot{V}O_2$ (in $L \cdot min^{-1}$) by the constant 5.0:

$$1.7\ L \cdot min^{-1} \times 5.0 = 8.5\ kcal \cdot min^{-1}$$

j. Finally, multiply the number of calories she expends in one minute by the number of minutes she cycles:

$$8.5\ kcal \cdot min^{-1} \times 60\ min = 510\ total\ calories$$

12–A. The steps are as follows:

a. Choose the ACSM leg cycling formula.
b. Write down your knowns and convert the values to the appropriate units:
   Knowns: 55 kg = body weight
   60 RPM × 6 meters = 360 m · min⁻¹
   1.5 kp = 1.5 kg
c. Write down the ACSM formula:

$$Leg\ cycling\ (ml \cdot kg^{-1} \cdot min^{-1}) = (1.8 \times work\ rate \div body\ weight) + (3.5) + (3.5)$$

d. Calculate work rate:

$$Work\ rate = kg \cdot m \div min = 1.5\ kg \times 360\ m \cdot min^{-1}$$
$$= 540\ kg \cdot m \cdot min^{-1}$$

e. Substitute the known values for the variable name:

$$ml \cdot kg^{-1} \cdot min^{-1} = (1.8 \times 540 \div 55) + (3.5) + (3.5)$$

f. Solve for the unknown:

$$ml \cdot kg^{-1} \cdot min^{-1} = (17.67) + (3.5) + (3.5)$$
$$Gross\ leg\ cycling\ \dot{V}O_2 = 24.67\ ml \cdot kg^{-1} \cdot min^{-1}$$

g. To get her absolute oxygen consumption, multiply by her body weight:

$$Absolute\ \dot{V}O_2 = relative\ \dot{V}O_2 \cdot body\ weight$$
$$= 24.67\ ml \cdot kg^{-1} \cdot min^{-1} \times 55\ kg$$
$$= 1356.85\ ml \cdot min^{-1}$$

h. To get absolute $\dot{V}O_2$ in $L \cdot min^{-1}$, divide $ml \cdot min^{-1}$ by 1000:

$$1356.85\ ml \cdot min^{-1} \div 1000 = 1.36\ L \cdot min^{-1}$$

13–C. The steps are as follows:

a. Choose the ACSM arm cycling formula.

b. Write down your knowns and convert the values to the appropriate units:
   Knowns: 55 kg = body weight
   60 RPM × 2.4 meters (each revolution on a Monark arm ergometer = 2.4 m)
   = 144 m · min⁻¹
   1.5 kp = 1.5 kg
c. Write down the ACSM formula:

$$Arm\ cycling\ (ml \cdot kg^{-1} \cdot min^{-1}) = (3 \times work\ rate \div body\ weight) + (0) + (3.5)\ (ml \cdot kg^{-1} min^{-1})$$

d. Calculate work rate:

$$Work\ rate = kg \cdot m \div min$$
$$= 1.5\ kg \times 144\ m \cdot min^{-1}$$
$$= 216\ kg \cdot m \cdot min^{-1}$$

e. Substitute the known values for the variable name:

$$ml \cdot kg^{-1} \cdot min^{-1} = (3 \times 216 \div 55) + (0) + (3.5)$$

f. Solve for the unknown:

$$ml \cdot kg^{-1} \cdot min^{-1} = (11.78) + (0) + (3.5)$$
$$Gross\ arm\ cycling\ \dot{V}O_2 = 15.28\ ml \cdot kg^{-1} \cdot min^{-1}$$

g. To get her absolute oxygen consumption, multiply her relative oxygen consumption by her body weight:

$$Absolute\ \dot{V}O_2 = relative\ \dot{V}O_2 \times body\ weight$$
$$= 15.28\ ml \cdot kg^{-1} \cdot min^{-1} \times 55\ kg$$
$$= 840.4\ ml \cdot min^{-1}$$

h. To get her absolute oxygen consumption in $L \cdot min^{-1}$, divide $ml \cdot min^{-1}$ by 1000:

$$840.4\ ml \cdot min^{-1} \div 1000 = 0.8404\ L \cdot min^{-1}$$

14–C. The steps are as follows:

a. Choose the ACSM running formula.
b. Write down your knowns and convert the values to the appropriate units:
   Knowns: 8 mph × 26.8 = 214.4 m · min⁻¹
   70 kg = body weight
   45 minutes of running
   0% grade
c. Write down the ACSM running formula:

$$Running = (0.2 \times speed) + (0.9 \times speed \times fractional\ grade) + (3.5)\ (ml \cdot kg^{-1} \cdot min^{-1})$$

d. Substitute the known values for the variable name:

$$ml \cdot kg^{-1} \cdot min^{-1} = (0.2 \times 214.4) + (0.9 \times 214.4 \times 0) + (3.5)$$

e. Solve for the unknown:

$$ml \cdot kg^{-1} \cdot min^{-1} = (42.88) + (0) + (3.5)$$
$$Gross\ running\ \dot{V}O_2 = 46.38\ ml \cdot kg^{-1} \cdot min^{-1}$$

f. To find out his total caloric expenditure, we must first put his gross running $\dot{V}O_2$ in absolute terms by multiplying by his body weight:

Absolute $\dot{V}_{O_2}$ = relative $\dot{V}_{O_2}$ × body weight

$= 46.38 \ ml \cdot kg^{-1} \cdot min^{-1} \times 70 \ kg$

$= 3246.6 \ ml \cdot min^{-1}$

g. Next we must convert $ml \cdot min^{-1}$ to $L \cdot min^{-1}$ by dividing by 1000:

$3246.6 \ ml \cdot min^{-1} \div 1000 = 3.2466 \ L \cdot min^{-1}$

h. We must then multiply $L \cdot min^{-1}$ by the constant 5.0 to get $kcal \cdot min^{-1}$:

$3.2466 \ L \cdot min^{-1} \times 5.0 = 16.233 \ kcal \cdot min^{-1}$

i. Finally, we multiply $kcal \cdot min^{-1}$ by the total number of minutes to get total caloric expenditure:

$16.233 \ kcal \cdot min^{-1} \times 45 \ min = 730.48 \ calories$

15–C. The steps are as follows:
   a. Choose the ACSM stepping formula.
   b. Write down your knowns and convert the values to the appropriate units:
      Knowns: Rate = 24 steps per minute
      Step height = 10 in × 0.0254 = 0.254 meters
      (The body weight is irrelevant in this problem.)
   c. Write down the ACSM stepping formula:

Stepping = (0.2 × stepping rate) + (1.33 × 1.8 × step height × stepping rate) + (3.5)

   d. Substitute the known values for the variable name:

$ml \cdot kg^{-1} \cdot min^{-1} = (0.2 \times 24)$
$+ (1.33 \times 0.254 \times 24) + (3.5)$

   e. Solve for the unknown:

$ml \cdot kg^{-1} \cdot min^{-1} = (4.8) + (8.11) + (3.5)$

Gross stepping $\dot{V}_{O_2}$ = 16.41 $ml \cdot kg^{-1} \cdot min^{-1}$

16–C. The steps are as follows:
   a. Choose the ACSM stepping formula.
   b. Write down your knowns and convert the values to the appropriate units:
      Knowns: 5 METs × 3.5 = 17.5 $ml \cdot kg^{-1} \cdot min^{-1}$
      (This gives us the relative $\dot{V}_{O_2}$ equivalent, which we will need for the stepping formula.)
      6 inches × 0.0254 = 0.1524 meters
      (Her body weight is irrelevant.)
   c. Write down the ACSM stepping formula:

Stepping = (0.2 × stepping rate) + (1.33 × 1.8 × step height × stepping rate) + (3.5)

   d. Substitute the known values for the variable name:

$17.5 = (0.2 \times stepping \ rate) + (1.33 \times 0.1524$
$\times stepping \ rate) + (3.5)$

   e. Move all of the knowns on one side of the equation and keep the unknown on the other:

$17.5 - 3.5 = (0.2 \times stepping \ rate) + (0.203 \times stepping \ rate)$

$14 = 0.403 \ (stepping \ rate)$

   f. Divide by 0.403 to get the stepping rate:

$34.7 = stepping \ rate$

About 35 steps per minute = stepping rate

17–B. The steps are as follows:
   a. Choose the ACSM running formula.
   b. Write down your knowns and convert the values to the appropriate units:
      Knowns: 143 pounds ÷ 2.2 = 65 kg
      5.5 mph = 147.4 $m \cdot min^{-1}$
      2% grade = 0.02
   c. Write down the ACSM running formula:

Running ($ml \cdot kg^{-1} \cdot min^{-1}$) = (0.2 × speed) + (0.9 × speed × fractional grade) + (3.5)

   d. Substitute the known values for the variable name:

$ml \cdot kg^{-1} \cdot min^{-1} = (0.2 \times 147.4)$
$+ (0.9 \times 147.4 \times 0.02) + (3.5)$

   e. Solve for the unknown:

$ml \cdot kg^{-1} \cdot min^{-1} = (29.48) + (2.65) + (3.5)$

Gross running $\dot{V}_{O_2}$ = 35.63 $ml \cdot kg^{-1} \cdot min^{-1}$

   f. To find out how many calories per minute she is expending, we must first convert her gross running $\dot{V}_{O_2}$ (in relative terms) to absolute $\dot{V}_{O_2}$ by multiplying by her body weight:

Absolute $\dot{V}_{O_2}$ = relative $\dot{V}_{O_2}$ × body weight

$= 35.63 \ ml \cdot kg^{-1} \cdot min^{-1} \times 65 \ kg$

$= 2315.95 \ ml \cdot min^{-1}$

   g. Convert $ml \cdot min^{-1}$ to $L \cdot min^{-1}$ by dividing by 1000:

$2315.95 \ ml \cdot min^{-1} \div 1000 = 2.31595 \ L \cdot min^{-1}$

   h. Finally, we can find out how many calories she is expending per minute by multiplying 2.31595 by the constant 5.0:

$2.31595 \ L \cdot min^{-1} \times 5.0 = 11.58 \ kcal \cdot min^{-1}$

18–D. This problem expands on problem #17. We established that she is expending 11.58 kcal per minute. The steps are as follows:
   a. Multiply 11.58 kcal per minute by the total number of minutes she exercises (45 minutes × 3 sessions per week = 135 total minutes):

11.58 kcal per minute × 135 total minutes = 1563.3 total calories expended

   b. To find out how many pounds of fat she will lose per week, divide the total calories expended by 3500 (because there are 3500 kcal in one pound of fat):

1563.3 kcal ÷ 3500 = 0.4466 pounds of fat per week of exercise

19–B. The steps are as follows:
   a. Choose the ACSM leg cycling formula.
   b. Write down your knowns and convert the values to the appropriate units:
   Knowns: 6 METs × 3.5 = 21 ml · kg^{-1} · min^{-1}
   80 kg = body weight
   c. Write down the ACSM leg cycling formula:
   Leg cycling (ml · kg^{-1} · min^{-1}) = [(1.8 × work rate) ÷ body weight] + (3.5) + (3.5)
   d. Substitute the known values for the variable name:
   21 = [(1.8 × work rate) ÷ 80] + 7
   Assuming that he cycles at 50 RPM (or 300 m · min^{-1}):
   21 = [(1.8 × 300 × F) ÷ 80] + 7
   e. Move all of the knowns to one side of the equation and solve for the unknown.
   21 – 7 = 540F
   14 × 80 = 540F
   1120 ÷ 540 = F
   2.07(kg) = F
   About 2.0 kg of force (F) is needed

20–B. The steps are as follows:
   a. Choose the ACSM running formula.
   b. Write down your knowns and convert the values to the appropriate units:
   Knowns: 40 ml · kg^{-1} · min^{-1} = relative $\dot{V}O_2$
   Level treadmill = 0% grade
   c. Write down the ACSM running formula:
   Running (ml · kg^{-1} · min^{-1}) = (0.2 × speed) + (0.9 × speed × fractional grade) + (3.5)
   d. Substitute the known values for the variable name:
   40 = (0.2 × speed) + (0) + (3.5)
   e. Solve for the unknown:
   36.5 = 0.2 (speed)
   182.5 m · min^{-1} = speed
   f. Convert m · min^{-1} to mph by dividing m · min^{-1} by 26.8:
   182.5 m · min^{-1} ÷ 26.8 = 6.8 mph

21–C. The steps are as follows:
   a. Convert relative $\dot{V}O_2$ to absolute $\dot{V}O_2$ by multiplying relative $\dot{V}O_2$ (ml · kg^{-1} · min^{-1}) by his body weight. We are not given his body weight so we cannot finish this problem.

   b. Assuming that he is an average 70-kg man:
   Absolute $\dot{V}O_2$ = relative $\dot{V}O_2$ × body weight
   = 45 ml · kg^{-1} · min^{-1} × 70 kg
   = 3150 ml · min^{-1}
   c. To get L · min^{-1}, divide ml · min^{-1} by 1000:
   3150 ml · min^{-1} ÷ 1000 = 3.15 L · min^{-1}
   d. Multiply 3.150 L · min^{-1} by the constant 5.0 to get kcal · min^{-1}:
   3.15 L · min^{-1} × 5.0 = 15.75 kcal · min^{-1}
   e. Multiply 15.75 kcal per minute by the total number of minutes he exercises (45 minutes × 3 times per week = 135 total minutes) to get the total caloric expenditure:
   15.75 kcal per minute × 135 minutes = 2126.25 total kcal per week
   f. Divide by 3500 to get pounds of fat:
   2126.25 kcal ÷ 3500 = 0.6075 pounds of fat per week
   g. Divide 10 pounds by 0.6075 pounds of fat per week to get how many weeks it will take him to lose 10 pounds of fat:
   10 ÷ 0.6075 = 16.46 weeks ≈ 16.5 weeks

22–A. No metabolic formula is needed. The steps are as follows:
   a. Multiply the number of calories per week she is eliminating by the number of weeks:
   1200 kcal per week × 26 weeks = 31200 total kcal
   b. Now divide by 3500 to get the total pounds she will lose:
   31200 ÷ 3500 total kcal = 8.9 or about 9 pounds over 26 weeks

23–C. No metabolic formula is needed for this question either. The steps are as follows:
   a. One mile of walking or running expends about 100 kcal. Since she walks 1 mile 3 times per week, she expends about 300 kcal per week. Multiply 300 kcal by 26 weeks to determine the total amount of calories she expends by walking:
   300 kcal per week × 26 weeks = 7800 kcal
   b. Divide 7800 kcal by 3500 to see how many pounds of fat this represents:
   7800 kcal ÷ 3500 = 2.22 pounds or about 2 pounds
   So she would lose about 11 pounds over 26 weeks if she incorporated walking into her weight loss program.

Recommended Readings

Chapter 1—Functional Anatomy and Biomechanics

ACSM's Resource Manual for Guidelines for Exercise Testing and Prescription, 3rd ed. Baltimore, Williams & Wilkins, 1998, Chapters 7–13.

Marieb EN: *Human Anatomy and Physiology,* 4th ed. Menlo Park, CA, Benjamin Cummings/Addison Wesley Longman, Inc., 1998.

Nordin M, Frankel VH: *Basic Biomechanics of the Musculoskeletal System,* 2nd ed. Philadelphia, Lea & Febiger, 1989.

Chapter 2—Nutrition and Weight Management

ACSM's Resource Manual for Guidelines for Exercise Testing and Prescription, 3rd ed. Baltimore, Williams & Wilkins, 1998, Chapters 7–13.

Brooks G, Fahey T, White T: *Exercise Physiology: Human Bioenergetics and Its Applications,* 2nd ed. Mountain View, CA, Mayfield Publishing Co., 1996.

Fox E, Bowers R, Foss M: *The Physiological Basis for Exercise and Sport,* 5th ed. Madison, WI, Brown and Benchmark, 1993.

McArdle W, Katch F, Katch V: *Exercise Physiology. Energy, Nutrition and Human Performance,* 4th ed. Baltimore, Williams & Wilkins, 1996.

Chapter 3—Human Development and Aging

Blimkie CJR, Oded B-O, Eds: *New Horizons in Pediatric Exercise Science.* Champaign, IL, Human Kinetics, 1995.

Skinner JS, ed: *Exercise Testing and Exercise Prescription for Special Cases: Theoretical Basis and Clinical Application.* Philadelphia, Lea & Febiger, 1993.

Chapter 4—Pathophysiology/Risk Factors

Campaigne BN, Lampman RI: *Exercise in the Clinical Management of Diabetes Mellitus.* Champaign, IL, Human Kinetics Publishers, Inc., 1994.

Fuster V, Gotto AM, Libby P, et al: Task Force 1. Pathogenesis of coronary disease: The biologic role of risk factors. *Journal of the American College of Cardiology* 27:964–976, 1996.

Hagberg JM: *Physical Activity, Physical Fitness, and Blood Pressure.* NIH Consensus Development Conference: Physical Activity and Cardiovascular Health. Bethesda, MD: Office of the Director, National Institutes of Health, 1995.

Pasternak RC, Grundy SM, Levy D, et al: Task Force 3: Spectrum of risk factors for coronary heart disease. *Journal of the American College of Cardiology* 27:978–990, 1996.

Second Report of the National Cholesterol Education Program (NCEP) Expert Panel on Detection, Evaluation, and Treatment of High Blood Cholesterol in Adults (Adult Treatment Panel II.) 1993. NIH Publication No. 93.

Chapter 5—Human Behavior / Psychology

Prochaska JO, Norcross JC, DiClemente CC: *Changing for Good: A Revolutionary Six-Stage Program for Overcoming Bad Habits and Moving Your Life Positively Forward.* New York, Avon Books, 1994.

Sallis J, Owen N: *Physical Activity and Behavioral Medicine.* Thousand Oaks, CA, Sage Publications, 1999.

US Department of Health and Human Services, Public Health Service. Centers for Disease Control and Prevention. National Center for Chronic Disease Prevention and Health Promotion. Division of Nutrition and Physical Activity. *Physical Activity: A Guide for Community Action.* Champaign, IL, Human Kinetics, 1999.

US Department of Health and Human Services. *Physical activity and health: A report of the Surgeon General.* Atlanta, US Department of Health and Human Services, Centers for Disease Control and Prevention, National Center for Chronic Disease Prevention and Health Promotion, 1996.

Chapter 6—Health Appraisal and Fitness Testing

Heyward VH: *Advanced Fitness Assessment and Exercise Prescription,* 3rd ed. Champaign IL, Human Kinetics, 1998.

Howley ET, Franks BD: *Health Fitness Instructor's Handbook,* 3rd ed. Champaign, IL, Human Kinetics, 1997.

Nieman DC: *Fitness and Sports Medicine: A Health-Related Approach,* 3rd ed. Palo Alto, CA, Bull Publishing, 1995.

Chapter 7—Safety, Injury Prevention, and Emergency Care

Franklin BA (ed): *ACSM's Guidelines for the Exercise Testing and Prescription,* 6th ed. Philadelphia, Lippincott Williams & Wilkins, 1999.

Roitman JL (ed): *ACSM's Resource Manual for Guidelines for Exercise Testing and Prescription,* 3rd ed. Baltimore, MD, Williams & Wilkins, 1998.

Tharrett SJ, Peterson JA (eds): *ACSM's Health/Fitness Facility Standards and Guidelines,* 2nd ed. Champaign, IL, Human Kinetics, 1997.

Chapter 8—Exercise Programming

American College of Sports Medicine: *ACSM's Exercise Management for Persons with Chronic Diseases and Disabilities.* Champaign, IL, Human Kinetics, 1997.

Carpinelli RN, Otto RM: Strength training: Single vs multiple sets. *Sports Medicine* 26(2):73–84, 1998.

Goldberg L, Elliot DL: *Exercise for Prevention and Treatment of Illness.* Philadelphia, FA Davis, 1994.

Pollock ML, Wilmore JH: *Exercise in Health and Disease: Evaluation and Prescription for Prevention and Rehabilitation,* 2nd ed. Philadelphia, WB Saunders, 1990.

Chapter 9—Nutrition and Weight Management

Clarkson PM: Nutrition for improved sports performance. Current issues on ergogenic aids. *Sports Med* 21:393–401,1996.

Grilo C, Brownell KD: Interventions for weight management. In *ACSM's Resource Manual for Guidelines for Exercise Testing and Prescription,* 3rd ed. Edited by Roitman JF. Baltimore, Lippincott Williams & Wilkins, 1998.

National Cholesterol Education Program: Summary of the second report of the National Cholesterol Education Program (NCEP) expert panel on detection, evaluation, and treatment of high blood cholesterol in adults (Adult Treatment Panel II). *JAMA* 269:3015–3023, 1993.

Position Stand of the American College of Sports Medicine. Exercise and fluid replacement. *Med Sci Sports Exerc* 28(1):i–vii, 1996.

Position Stand of The American College of Sports Medicine. The female athlete triad. *Med Sci Sports Exerc* 29(5):i–ix, 1997.

Position Stand of The American College of Sports Medicine: Osteoporosis and exercise. *Med Sci Sports Exerc* 27(4):i–vii, 1995.

Position Stand of The American College of Sports Medicine: Heat and Cold Illnesses During Distance Running. *Med Sci Sports Exerc* 28(12):i–x, 1996.

Position Stand of The American College of Sports Medicine: Proper and Improper Weight-Loss Programs. *Med Sci Sports Exerc* 15(1):ix–xiii, 1983.

Position of The American Dietetic Association and The Canadian Dietetic Association: Nutrition for physical fitness and athletic performance for adults. *JADA* 93:691–697, 1993.

Riley R: Nutrition and weight management. In *ACSM's Resource Manual for Guidelines for Exercise Testing and Prescription,* 3rd ed. Edited by Roitman JF. Baltimore, Lippincott Williams & Wilkins, 1998.

Shape Up America, American Obesity Association: *Guidance for Treatment of Adult Obesity.* Bethesda, Shape Up America, 1996.

U.S. Department of Agriculture, U.S. Department of Health and Human Services: *Dietary Guidelines for Americans.* 1995.

Chapter 10–Program Administration / Management

American College of Sports Medicine: *ACSM's Resource Manual for Guidelines for Exercise Testing and Prescription,* 3rd ed. Baltimore, Williams & Wilkins, 1998.

Cleverly WO: *Essentials of Health Care Finance.* Gaithersburg, MD, Aspen Publishers, 1997.

Grantham WC, Patton RW, York TD, Winick ML: *Health Fitness Management.* Champaign, IL, Human Kinetics, 1998.

Langley TD, Hawkins JD: *Administration for Exercise Related Professions.* Englewood, CO, Morton Publishing, 1999.

Patton RW, Grantham WC, Gerson RF, Gettman LR: *Developing and Managing Health/Fitness Facilities.* Champaign, IL, Human Kinetics, 1989.

Tharrett SJ, Peterson JA (eds): *ACSM's Health/Fitness Facility Standards and Guidelines,* 2nd ed. Champaign, IL, Human Kinetics, 1997.

COMPREHENSIVE EXAMINATION

Directions: Each of the numbered items or incomplete statements in this section is followed by answers or by completions of the statement. Select the **one** lettered answer or completion that is **best** in each case.

1. Which of the following exercise modes allows buoyancy to reduce the potential for musculoskeletal injury and even allow an injured person an opportunity to exercise without further injury?
   (A) Cycling
   (B) Walking
   (C) Skiing
   (D) Water exercise

2. Which of the following energy systems has the ability to assist the muscle with maximal power?
   (A) ATP–PC
   (B) Anaerobic glycolysis
   (C) Oxidative phosphorylation
   (D) Free-fatty acid metabolism

3. Which of the following types of medications is designed to control blood lipids, especially cholesterol?
   (A) Nitrates
   (B) Alpha-blockers
   (C) Antihyperlipidemics
   (D) Beta-blockers

4. Which of the following represents more than 90% of the fat stored in the body and is a glycerol molecule connected to three fatty acids?
   (A) Phospholipids
   (B) Cholesterol
   (C) Triglycerides
   (D) Free fatty acids

5. Limited flexibility of which of the following muscle groups increases the risk of low back pain?
   (A) Quadriceps
   (B) Hamstrings
   (C) Hip flexors
   (D) Biceps femoris

6. Calcium, phosphorus, magnesium, potassium, sulfur, sodium, and chloride are examples of
   (A) macrominerals.
   (B) microminerals.
   (C) proteins.
   (D) vitamins.

7. Which of the following terms represents an imaginary horizontal plane passing through the midsection of the body and dividing it into upper and lower portions?
   (A) Sagittal plane
   (B) Frontal plane
   (C) Transverse plane
   (D) Superior plane

8. Which of the following is a function of bone?
   (A) Provides structural support for the entire body
   (B) Serves as levers that can change the magnitude and direction of forces generated by skeletal muscles
   (C) Protects organs and tissues
   (D) All of the above

9. An elevation of either the systolic or diastolic blood pressure is classified as hypertension. The elevation must be measured on two different days, preferably several days apart. To be classified as hypertension, the blood pressure should be more than
   (A) 100/60.
   (B) 110/70.
   (C) 120/80.
   (D) 140/90.

10. The term "risk stratification" refers to the
    (A) ability of the client to take airplane rides.
    (B) ability of the client to perform high-intensity exercise.
    (C) identification of diseases that place the client into certain categories.
    (D) identification of latent or overt coronary artery disease.

11. Uncoordinated gait, headache, dizziness, vomiting and elevated body temperature are signs and symptoms of
    (A) acute exposure to the cold.
    (B) hypothermia.
    (C) heat exhaustion and heat stroke.
    (D) acute altitude sickness.

12. Fitness newsletters, health and fitness fact sheets, a fitness library, and bulletin boards are all ways to
    (A) educate the client.
    (B) inform the client when payments are due.
    (C) advertise new products for purchase.
    (D) certify clients as Health/Fitness Instructors.

13. The movement that decreases the joint angle, bringing the bones closer together is called
    (A) flexion.
    (B) extension.
    (C) abduction.
    (D) adduction.

14. Which of the following energy systems is capable of using all three fuels (carbohydrates, fats, and proteins)?
    (A) anaerobic glycolysis
    (B) lactic acid system
    (C) phosphagen system
    (D) oxygen system

15. How many calories will a 116.6-pound woman expend if she pedals on a Monark cycle ergometer at 50 RPMs against a resistance of 2.5 kiloponds for 30 minutes?
    (A) 226.7 calories
    (B) 258.3 calories
    (C) 512 calories
    (D) 216 calories

16. Relative proportions of fat and fat-free (lean) tissue can be assessed and are reported as
    (A) percent body fat.
    (B) body composition.
    (C) hydrodensitometry.
    (D) near-infrared interactance.

17. Which of the following is/are characteristic(s) of an effective exercise leader or Health/Fitness Instructor?
    (A) The Health/Fitness Instructor should be a resource for up-to-date, accurate information regarding health and fitness.
    (B) The Health/Fitness Instructor should be able to dispel myths and quackery regarding exercise.
    (C) The Health/Fitness Instructor is able to create an atmosphere and an opportunity for learning.
    (D) All of the above

18. Surrounding each myofibril is a series of interconnected sacs and tube in which is stored calcium. These are referred to as
    (A) terminal cisternae.
    (B) sarcomeres.
    (C) myofilaments.
    (D) sarcoplasmic reticulum.

19. Anaerobic glycolysis is also known as the
    (A) phosphagen system.
    (B) aerobic metabolism.
    (C) lactic acid system.
    (D) none of the above

20. Which of the following is true regarding cardiac output changes during submaximal exercise as a result of regular, chronic exercise?
    (A) Cardiac output increases.
    (B) Cardiac output decreases.
    (C) Cardiac output stays the same.
    (D) Cardiac output increases only during dynamic exercise.

21. Which of the following is a condition characterized by a decrease in bone mass and density producing bone porosity and fragility?
    (A) Osteoarthritis
    (B) Osteomyelitis
    (C) Epiphyseal osteomyelitis
    (D) Osteoporosis

22. Studies designed to measure the success of a program based upon some quantifiable data that can be analyzed are called
    (A) incomes.
    (B) outcomes.
    (C) client progress notes.
    (D) attendance records.

23. The Rating of Perceived Exertion scale is considered to be an adjunct to using heart rate as a guide to exercise intensity. When using the original Borg scale, intensity should be maintained between
    (A) 7 and 10.
    (B) 12 and 16.
    (C) 16 and 20.
    (D) 18 and 21.

24. Muscle fibers that can produce a large amount of tension in a very short period of time but fatigue quickly are referred to as
    (A) slow-twitch glycolytic.
    (B) fast-twitch glycolytic.
    (C) fast-twitch oxidative.
    (D) slow-twitch oxidative.

25. Rotation of the anterior surface of a bone toward the midline of the body is called
    (A) medial rotation.
    (B) lateral rotation.
    (C) supination.
    (D) pronation.

26. As each primary bronchus enters the lung, secondary bronchi branch off with smaller and smaller branches continuing to branch until the smallest narrow passage is formed, called the
    (A) lobes.
    (B) trachea.
    (C) bronchiole.
    (D) nasopharynx.

27. Cardiac output can be calculated by multiplying
    (A) heart rate and stroke volume.
    (B) stroke volume and the difference between the oxygen carrying capacity of the arterial blood and venous blood.
    (C) oxygen consumption and heart rate.
    (D) heart rate and blood volume.

28. The initial cause of coronary artery disease is thought to be an irritation of, or injury to the tunica intima (innermost of the three layers in the wall) of the blood vessel. A source or sources of this initial injury may be
    (A) dyslipidemia.
    (B) hypertension.
    (C) turbulence of blood flow within the vessel.
    (D) all of the above

29. Which of the following is NOT considered to be an independent risk factor in the development of cardiovascular disease?
    (A) Age (older than 55 years of age)
    (B) Cigarette smoking
    (C) Being overweight
    (D) Hypertension

30. Signs and/or symptoms of cardiopulmonary disease or metabolic disease, or more than two risk factors for the development of coronary artery disease place the client in the
    (A) apparently healthy risk category.
    (B) increased risk category.
    (C) known disease category.
    (D) all of the above

31. A second person assisting a weight lifter in initially lifting the weight into position, correcting incorrect movements, and assisting in lifting or stretching is called a
    (A) buddy.
    (B) spotter.
    (C) friend.
    (D) housekeeper.

32. Which of the following vitamins functions to maintain bone and teeth health and have a dietary source of dairy products?
    (A) Vitamin A
    (B) Vitamin D
    (C) Vitamin K
    (D) Thiamine

33. Each cusp of the atrioventricular valves in the heart is braced by tendinous fibers called chordae tendinae, which, in turn, are connected to special muscles on the inner surface of the ventricle, which are called
    (A) myocardial muscles.
    (B) papillary muscles.
    (C) endocardial muscles.
    (D) epicardial muscles.

34. An individual's maximal oxygen consumption or $\dot{V}O_{2\,max}$ is a measure of the power of the aerobic energy system. This value is generally regarded as the best indicator of aerobic fitness. What is the average $\dot{V}O_{2\,max}$ of college-age males and females, respectively?
    (A) 35 and 45 ml/kg/min
    (B) 45 and 35 ml/kg/min
    (C) 55 and 65 ml/kg/min
    (D) 45 ml/kg/min

35. Cardiac muscle tissue is similar to skeletal muscle except for its ability to
    (A) summate.
    (B) tetanize.
    (C) contract.
    (D) relax.

36. Which of the following is NOT true regarding the psychological benefits of regular exercise in the elderly?
    (A) Older people who exercise regularly have a more positive attitude toward their work, and are generally in better health than sedentary persons.
    (B) Strong correlations have been reported between the activity level of older adults and self-reported happiness.
    (C) Older persons taking part in exercise programs commonly report that they find everyday tasks more difficult than before they began the exercise program.
    (D) Older adults improve their score on self-concept questionnaires following participation in an exercise program.

37. A condition resulting from temporary or permanent reduction in blood flow in one or more coronary arteries may cause
    (A) pectoralis excavatum.
    (B) angina pectoris.
    (C) pectoralis reductum.
    (D) dysrhythmia.

38. To determine program effectiveness, psychological theories provide a conceptual framework for assessment and
    (A) development of programs or interventions.
    (B) application of cognitive-behavioral or motivational principles.
    (C) evaluation.
    (D) all of the above.

39. Information gathered by way of an appropriate health screening allows the health/fitness instructor to develop specific exercise programs appropriate to the individual needs and goals of the client. This is called the
    (A) exercise prescription.
    (B) heart rate.
    (C) blood pressure.
    (D) graded exercise test.

40. In order to maximize safety during a physical fitness assessment, which of the following items should be addressed?
    (A) The hospital emergency room services
    (B) Emergency evacuation plan
    (C) Client's financial status
    (D) All of the above

41. Some externally applied forces, such as exercise pulleys, do not act in a vertical direction as do weights attached to the body because
    (A) a distractive force is sometimes used to promote normal joint movement.
    (B) the angle of application changes in different parts of the range of motion, causing a change in the magnitude of the rotary component of the force and thus the torque.
    (C) weights applied to the body behave as weights of body segments, thus changing the torque and altering the difficulty of an exercise when weight is applied.
    (D) by shifting the mass of the weight more proximally up the arm, less effort on the part of the stabilizing muscles is required so that torque produced at the glenohumeral joint is reduced.

42. If a motor unit is continuously stimulated without adequate time for relaxation to occur, what will be accomplished?
    (A) Tetanus
    (B) Summation
    (C) Twitch
    (D) None of the above

43. Heart rate can be measured by counting the number of pulses in a specified time period at one of several locations, including the radial, femoral, and carotid arteries. Which of the following is a special precaution when taking the carotid pulse?
    (A) When heart rate is measured by palpation, the first two fingers should be used and not the thumb because it has its own pulse.
    (B) Heart rates taken during exercise sometimes reach beyond 200 beats per minute, making it too difficult to feel at the carotid artery.
    (C) If heart rate is taken at the carotid artery, care should be taken not to press too hard or a reflex slowing of the heart may occur and cause dizziness.
    (D) Heart rate should never be taken at the carotid artery.

44. As a result of regular exercise training, which of the following is NOT affected during maximal exercise?
    (A) Cardiac output
    (B) Stroke volume
    (C) Heart rate
    (D) None of the above

45. When exercise testing children
    (A) most ergometers used in adult exercise testing can be used for children, with the treadmill generally preferred to cycle ergometers.
    (B) only strength should be measured.
    (C) flexibility should be stressed.
    (D) use only heart rate as an indicator of cardiovascular fitness.

46. Which of the following risk factors for the development of coronary artery disease has the greatest likelihood of being influenced by regular exercise?
    (A) Smoking
    (B) Cholesterol
    (C) Type I diabetes
    (D) Hypertension

47. At a minimum, professionals performing fitness assessments on others should possess which combination of the following?
    (A) CPR and ACSM Health/Fitness Instructor
    (B) Advanced Cardiac Life Support and ACSM Program Director
    (C) Advanced Cardiac Life Support and ACSM Health/Fitness Director
    (D) Only physicians can perform fitness assessments.

48. For an exercise prescription, which of the following combinations work inversely with each other?
    (A) Intensity and duration
    (B) Mode and intensity
    (C) Mode and duration
    (D) Duration and frequency

49. Which of the following types of muscle stretching alternates contraction and relaxation of both agonist and antagonist muscle groups, may cause residual muscle soreness, is time consuming and typically requires a partner?
    (A) Static stretching
    (B) Ballistic stretching
    (C) Proprioceptive neuromuscular facilitation (PNF) stretching
    (D) All of the above

50. Glucose, fructose, and sucrose are commonly referred to as
    (A) proteins.
    (B) complex carbohydrates.
    (C) simple carbohydrates.
    (D) fats.

51. Failure of a Health/Fitness Instructor to perform in a generally acceptable standard is called
    (A) malpractice.
    (B) malfeasance.
    (C) negligence.
    (D) none of the above

52. All energy for muscular contraction must come from the breakdown of a chemical compound called
    (A) ATP.
    (B) STP.
    (C) NADH + H^+.
    (D) $FADH_2$.

53. Actin is a muscle protein (sometimes called the thin filament) that can be visualized as looking like a twisted strand of beads. Actin also contains two other proteins,
    (A) epimysium and perimysium.
    (B) perimysium and endomysium.
    (C) troponin and tropomyosin.
    (D) myosin and troponin.

54. From rest to maximal exercise, the systolic blood pressure should _____ with an increasing workload.
    (A) increase
    (B) decrease
    (C) stay the same
    (D) decrease with isometric or increase with isotonic contractions

55. The majority of sedentary people are not motivated to initiate exercise programs, and if exercise is initiated, it is likely to stop within
    (A) 1–2 days.
    (B) 3–6 weeks.
    (C) 1 month.
    (D) 3–6 months.

56. Reasons for fitness testing for the older adult include
    (A) evaluation of progress.
    (B) exercise prescription.
    (C) motivation.
    (D) all of the above.

57. Body weight 15 percent below expected, a morbid fear of fatness, preoccupation with food, and an abnormal body image are symptoms of
    (A) bulimia nervosa.
    (B) dieting.
    (C) anorexia nervosa.
    (D) obesity.

58. If a motor unit receives a second stimulation before it is allowed to relax, the two impulses are added and the tension developed is greater. This is called
    (A) twitch.
    (B) tetanus.
    (C) summation.
    (D) motor unit.

59. What is the energy cost of running at 6.5 miles per hour up a grade of 5%?
    (A) 13.2 METs
    (B) 15.2 METs
    (C) 10.2 METs
    (D) 8.2 METs

60. Feeling good about being able to perform an activity or skill, such as finally being able to run 1 mile or to increase the speed of walking 1 mile, is an example of
    (A) extrinsic rewards.
    (B) intrinsic rewards.
    (C) external stimulus.
    (D) internal stimulus.

61. Albuterol, terbutaline, glucocorticosteroids, cromolyn sodium, and theophylline are effective drugs to prevent or reverse
    (A) coronary artery disease.
    (B) emphysema.
    (C) asthma.
    (D) cancer.

62. Safety in the fitness center is very important to the welfare of the client. Specifically, exercise equipment should be
    (A) flexible enough to allow for different body sizes.
    (B) large enough to accommodate small and large clients.
    (C) inexpensive to allow for changing out equipment periodically.
    (D) placed on the floor with wheels so that it can be moved easily.

63. The American College of Sports Medicine recommendation for intensity, duration, and frequency of physical activity for apparently healthy individuals includes
    (A) intensity of 60% to 90% maximal heart rate, duration of 20 to 60 minutes, frequency of 3 to 5 days a week.
    (B) intensity of 85% to 90% maximal heart rate, duration of 30 minutes, frequency of 3 days a week.
    (C) intensity of 50% to 70% maximal heart rate, duration of 15 to 45 minutes, frequency of 5 days a week.
    (D) intensity of 60% to 90% maximal heart rate reserve, duration of 20 to 60 minutes, frequency of 7 days a week.

64. A method of strength and power training that involves an eccentric loading of muscles and tendons followed immediately by an explosive concentric contraction is called
    (A) plyometrics.
    (B) periodization.
    (C) super-sets.
    (D) isotonic reversals.

65. Which of the following are characteristics of a good manager?
    (A) Designs programs and monitors the implementation of the program
    (B) Guides staff or clients through the program
    (C) Strong communicator
    (D) All of the above

66. Agreements, releases, and consents are documents that clearly describe
    (A) what the client is participating in, the risks involved, and the rights of the client and the facility.
    (B) what the client can and cannot do in your facility.
    (C) the relationship between the facility operator and the Health/Fitness Instructor.
    (D) the rights and responsibilities of the club owner to reject an application of a prospective client.

67. There is enough ATP stored in a given skeletal muscle to fuel how much activity?
    (A) 2–3 seconds
    (B) 5–10 seconds
    (C) 10–20 seconds
    (D) 1 hour

68. The sliding filament theory of muscle contraction depends upon the interaction of actin and myosin. At rest, there is no interaction. When called upon to contract, these two create an interdigitation and the muscle contracts. This process is dependent upon the presence of
    (A) magnesium.
    (B) manganese.
    (C) creatine.
    (D) calcium.

69. After age 30, skeletal muscle strength begins to decline primarily due to
    (A) a gain in fat tissue.
    (B) a gain in lean tissue.
    (C) a loss of muscle mass caused by a loss of muscle fibers.
    (D) myogenic precursor cell inhibition.

70. The rate of an acute cardiovascular event occurring during exercise for men is
    (A) 1 in 20,000 hours.
    (B) 1 in 57,000 hours.
    (C) 1 in 187,500 hours.
    (D) 1 in a million hours.

71. Which of the following is a complex carbohydrate that is not digestible by the body and passes straight through the digestive system?
    (A) Fats
    (B) Proteins
    (C) Sugars
    (D) Fiber

72. The Health Belief Model assumes that people will engage in a behavior (e.g., exercise) when
    (A) there is a perceived threat of disease.
    (B) there is a belief of susceptibility to disease.
    (C) the threat of disease is severe.
    (D) all of the above

73. The "informed consent" document
    (A) is a legal document.
    (B) provides immunity from prosecution.
    (C) provides an explanation of the test to the client.
    (D) is all of the above.

74. A measure of muscular endurance is
    (A) one-repetition maximum.
    (B) three-repetition maximum.
    (C) number of sit-ups in 1 minute.
    (D) treadmill testing.

75. If an exerciser starts to exercise too much and either does not take a rest day at all and/or develops a minor injury and does not stop and rest so that the injury might heal, what can occur?
    (A) An overuse injury
    (B) A fatal or near fatal automobile accident
    (C) Sleep deprivation
    (D) Decreased physical conditioning

76. The American College of Sports Medicine recommends that exercise intensity be prescribed within what percentage of maximal heart rate?
    (A) 40% and 50%
    (B) 50% and 70%
    (C) 60% and 90%
    (D) 70% and 100%

77. The American College of Sports Medicine recommends how many repetitions of each exercise for muscular strength and endurance?
    (A) 5–6
    (B) 8–12
    (C) 12–20
    (D) More than 20

78. For higher intensity activities,
    (A) the benefit outweighs any potential risk.
    (B) the risk of orthopedic and cardiovascular complications are increased.
    (C) the risk of orthopedic and cardiovascular complications are minimal.
    (D) there is no increased risk of orthopedic and cardiovascular complications.

79. "Auscultation" of the heart rate refers to
    (A) feeling the pulse at the radial artery.
    (B) listening to the sounds of the heart through the chest.
    (C) counting the pulse rate at the carotid artery.
    (D) counting the pulse rate at the carotid, radial, or femoral arteries.

80. Which of the following are changes seen as a result of regular, chronic exercise?
    (A) Decreased heart rate at rest
    (B) Increased stroke volume at rest
    (C) No change in cardiac output at rest
    (D) All of the above

81. The heart has its own capability of producing an action potential (unlike skeletal muscle). If an electrical impulse is not received from higher level brain centers, cardiac muscle will stimulate itself. This is called
    (A) tetany.
    (B) simulated contraction.
    (C) diastole.
    (D) autorhythmicity.

82. Maximal exercise testing has been labeled by some medical experts as a dangerous situation for most people. Actually, the death rate during maximal exercise testing is approximately
    (A) 0.01%.
    (B) 1%.
    (C) 10%.
    (D) 5%.

83. Which of the following is an example of a cognitive process in the Transtheoretical Model?
    (A) Counterconditioning
    (B) Reinforcement management
    (C) Dramatic relief
    (D) Self-liberation

84. The purpose of the fitness assessment is to
    (A) develop the exercise prescription.
    (B) evaluate progress.
    (C) motivate.
    (D) all of the above

85. RICES means
    (A) dietary supplements.
    (B) *Rest* and *ICE* are the best treatment for injury.
    (C) *Rest, Ice, Compression, Elevation, Stabilization.*
    (D) none of the above.

86. Resistance exercises performed either in an ascending (increasing the resistance within a set of repetitions from one set to the next) or descending (decreasing the resistance within a set of repetitions from one set to the next) order are called
    (A) circuit weight training.
    (B) super-sets.
    (C) split routines.
    (D) pyramids.

87. The American College of Sports Medicine recommendation for the maximal rate of weight loss is
    (A) 10–15 pounds per week (4.5–7 kg).
    (B) 8–10 pounds per week (4–4.5 kg).
    (C) 5–8 pounds per week (2.3–4 kg).
    (D) 1–2 pounds per week (0.5–1 kg).

88. New and expensive equipment is called what in a line-item budget?
    (A) Capital expense
    (B) Supplies
    (C) Disposables
    (D) All of the above

89. Which of the following assumes that an overall complex behavior arises from many small simple behaviors?
    (A) Learning Theories
    (B) Health Belief Model
    (C) Transtheoretical Model
    (D) Stages of Motivational Readiness

90. Individuals who choose to begin a self-directed exercise program (i.e., on their own) should be advised to complete, at a minimum, a quick screening of their health status using something like the
    (A) MMPI.
    (B) Borg scale.
    (C) PAR-Q.
    (D) all of the above

91. When a test battery of fitness assessments is administered to a client in a single session, the following order of tests is recommended.
    (A) Resting measurements, flexibility, cardiorespiratory fitness, body composition, muscular fitness
    (B) Flexibility, resting measurements, body composition, muscular fitness, cardiorespiratory fitness
    (C) Resting measurements, body composition, cardiorespiratory fitness, muscular fitness, flexibility
    (D) It makes no difference which order these tests are done in as long as they are all done.

92. Implementing emergency procedures must include the fitness center
    (A) management.
    (B) staff.
    (C) clients.
    (D) management and staff.

93. Which of the following is a possible medical emergency a client can experience during an exercise session?
    (A) Hypoglycemia
    (B) Hypotension
    (C) Hypertension
    (D) All of the above

94. During a graded exercise test, blood pressure must be taken at least
    (A) twice.
    (B) twice during each stage.
    (C) once during each stage.
    (D) every minute.

95. Which of the following muscle actions occurs when the length of the muscle does not change, but muscle tension is increased through enhanced neuromuscular recruitment patterns?
    (A) Concentric isotonic
    (B) Eccentric isotonic
    (C) Isokinetic
    (D) Isometric

96. Which of the following is the only nutrient that contains nitrogen?
    (A) Fats
    (B) Proteins
    (C) Simple carbohydrates
    (D) Complex carbohydrates

97. Which of the following activities provides for the greatest improvement in aerobic fitness for someone who is beginning an exercise program?
    (A) Weight training
    (B) Downhill snow skiing
    (C) Dieting
    (D) Walking

98. In commercial settings, clients should be more extensively screened for potential health risks. The information solicited should include information about which of the following
    (A) Personal medical history
    (B) Present medical status
    (C) Medication
    (D) All of the above

99. Generally, persons of poor fitness may benefit from
    (A) longer duration, higher intensity, lower frequency exercise.
    (B) longer duration, lower intensity, lower frequency exercise.
    (C) shorter duration, lower intensity, higher frequency exercise.
    (D) shorter duration, higher intensity, higher frequency exercise.

100. A document that details the marketing plan and justification for each action in the program as well as an analysis of each aspect of the research plus projections for success is called a
    (A) public relations plan.
    (B) marketing plan.
    (C) market research.
    (D) business plan.

ANSWERS AND EXPLANATIONS

1–D. Water exercise has gained in popularity because the buoyancy properties of water help to reduce the potential for musculoskeletal injury and may even allow an injured person an opportunity to exercise without further injury. A variety of activities may be offered in a water exercise class. Walking, jogging, and dance activity all may be adapted for water. Water exercise classes should typically combine the benefits of the buoyancy properties of water with the resistive properties. In this regard, both an aerobic stimulus may be provided as well as activity to enhance muscular strength and endurance.

2–A. Because the number of reactions is small (basically only two), the ATP–PC system can provide ATP at a very fast rate. The ATP–PC system is ranked number one in power. There is enough phosphocreatine stored in skeletal muscle for approximately 25 seconds of high-intensity work. Therefore, the ATP–PC system will last for about 30 seconds (5 seconds for stored ATP, 25 seconds for PC). [Chapter 2]

3–C. Nitrates and nitroglycerine are antianginals (used to reduce chest pain associated with angina pectoris). Alpha-blockers are antihypertensives (reduce blood pressure by inhibiting the action of adrenergic neurotransmitters at the alpha-receptor, thereby promoting peripheral vasodilation). Beta-blockers also are designed to reduce blood pressure by inhibiting the action of adrenergic neurotransmitters at the beta-receptors, thereby decreasing cardiac output. Antihyperlipidemics control blood lipids, especially cholesterol. [Chapter 4]

4–C. Dietary fats include triglycerides, cholesterol, and phospholipids. Triglycerides represent more than 90% of the fat stored in the body. A triglyceride is a glycerol molecule connected to three fatty acid molecules. The fatty acids are identified by the amount of "saturation" or the number of single or double bonds that link the carbon atoms. Saturated fatty acids only have single bonds. Monounsaturated fatty acids have one double bond and polyunsaturated fatty acids have two or more double bonds. [Chapter 9]

5–B. An adequate range of motion or joint mobility is requisite for optimal musculoskeletal health. Specifically, limited flexibility of the low back and hamstring regions may be related to an increased risk for the development of chronic low back pain and disability. Activities that will enhance or maintain musculoskeletal flexibility should be included as a part of a comprehensive preventive or rehabilitative exercise program.

6–A. Minerals are inorganic substances that perform a variety of functions in the body. Many play an important role in assisting enzymes (or co-enzymes) that are necessary for the proper functioning of body systems. They are also found in cell membranes, hormones, muscles, and connective tissues, and as electrolytes in body fluids. Minerals are considered to be either macrominerals (needed in relatively large doses), such as calcium, phosphorus, magnesium, potassium, sulfur, sodium, and chloride, or microminerals (needed in very small amounts), such as iron, zinc, selenium, manganese, molybdenum, iodine, copper, chromium and fluoride. [Chapter 9]

7–C. There are three cardinal planes of the body, and each plane is perpendicular to each of the other two. Movement occurs along these planes. The sagittal plane divides the body into right and left parts, and the midsagittal plane is represented by an imaginary vertical plane passing through the midline of the body, dividing it into right and left halves. The frontal plane is represented by an imaginary vertical plane passing through the body, dividing it into front and back halves. The transverse plane represents an imaginary horizontal plane passing through the midsection of the body and dividing it into upper and lower portions. [Chapter 1]

8–D.   The bones of the skeletal system perform five functions: They provide structural support for the entire body, serve as levers that can change the magnitude and direction of forces generated by skeletal muscles, protect organs and tissues, provide storage (calcium salts of bone serve as mineral reservoirs for maintaining concentrations of calcium and phosphate ions in body fluids, and fat cells in yellow bone marrow store lipids as energy reserve), and produce red blood cells and other elements within the bone marrow. [Chapter 1]

9–D.   To be classified as hypertensive, the systolic blood pressure must exceed 140/90 mm Hg measured on two separate occasions, preferably days apart. An elevation of either the systolic or diastolic pressure is classified as hypertension. [Chapter 4]

10–C. The purpose of risk stratification is to identify high-risk individuals (persons with contraindications leading to potential exclusion from testing or exercise; individuals with disease symptoms or risk factors that require medical evaluation prior to testing or exercise; individuals with clinically significant disease that requires medical supervision during testing or exercise; or individuals with special testing or exercise needs) and to select the appropriate activities for those persons. Risk categories include apparently healthy, increased risk, and known disease. [Chapter 6]

11–C. Heat exhaustion and heat stroke are serious conditions that result from a combination of the metabolic heat generated from exercise accompanied by dehydration and electrolyte loss from sweating. Signs and symptoms include uncoordinated gait, headache, dizziness, vomiting, and elevated body temperature. If these conditions are present, exercise must be stopped. Attempts to rehydrate, perhaps intravenously, should be attempted and the body must be cooled by any means possible. The person should be placed in the supine position, with the feet elevated.

12–A. Educating the client on the benefits of exercise should be part of the mission of any fitness facility. Educational materials and programs are very popular with clients. Some educational opportunities include a fitness newsletter, health and fitness fact sheets, a fitness library (for clients with health and nutrition newsletters, books, and videos), bulletin boards, and education classes or lectures on a variety of topics.

13–A. Angular movements decrease or increase the joint angle produced by the articulating bones. There are four types of angular movements, flexion (a movement that decreases the joint angle, bringing the bones closer together), extension (the movement opposite to flexion decreasing the joint angle between two bones), abduction (the movement of a body part away from the midline in a lateral direction), and adduction (the opposite of abduction, the movement toward the midline of the body). [Chapter 1]

14–D. The oxygen system is capable of using all three fuels (carbohydrate, fat, and protein). Significant amounts of protein, however, are not used as a source of ATP energy during most types of exercise. Although all three can be used, the two that are most important are carbohydrate and fat. When fat is used as a fuel, significantly more energy is released. This requires, however, that more oxygen be supplied to produce this energy. If proteins are used, the amount of energy is comparable to that of carbohydrate. The carbohydrate, fat, and small amount of protein used by this energy system during exercise are completely metabolized, leaving only carbon dioxide (which is exhaled) and water. The nitrogen found in the protein is excreted as urea. [Chapter 2]

15–B. Choose the ACSM Leg cycling formula
Write down your knowns and convert the values to the appropriate units
knowns: 110 pounds ÷ 2.2 = 53 kg
50 RPMs × 6 meters = 300 m · min^{-1}
2.5 kp = 2.5 kg
60 minutes of cycling
Write down the ACSM formula:
Leg cycling = (1.8 × Work Rate ÷ Body Weight) + (3.5) + (3.5) (ml · kg^{-1} · min^{-1})
Calculate work rate:

$$\text{work rate} = \frac{\text{kg} \cdot \text{m}}{\text{min}}$$
$$= 2.5 \text{ kg} \cdot 300 \text{ m} \cdot \text{min}^{-1}$$
$$= 750 \text{ kg}^{-1} \cdot \text{min}^{-1}$$

Substitute the known values for the variable name:

$$ml \cdot kg^{-1} \cdot min^{-1} = (1.8 \times 750 \div 53) + (3.5) + (3.5)$$

Solve for the Unknown:

$$ml \cdot kg^{-1} \cdot min^{-1} = (25.47 + 3.5) + (3.5)$$

Gross Leg cycling $VO_2 = 32.47$ ml $\cdot$ kg^{-1} $\cdot$ min^{-1}

To find out how many Calories she expends we must first convert her oxygen consumption to Absolute terms:

$$\begin{aligned}
\text{Absolute } VO_2 &= \text{Relative } VO_2 \cdot \text{Body Weight} \\
&= 32.47 \text{ ml} \cdot kg^{-1} \cdot min^{-1} \times 53 \text{ kg} \\
&= 1721 \text{ ml} \cdot min^{-1}
\end{aligned}$$

Convert ml $\cdot$ min^{-1} to L $\cdot$ min^{-1} by dividing by 1000:

$$\frac{1721 \text{ ml} \cdot min^{-1}}{1000} = 1.721 \text{ L} \cdot min^{-1}$$

Next we must see how many Calories she expends in one minute by multiplying her Absolute VO2 (in L $\cdot$ min^{-1}) by the constant 5.0:

$$1.721 \text{ L} \cdot min^{-1} \times 5.0 = \underline{8.61} \text{ Kcal} \cdot min^{-1}$$

Finally, multiply the number of Calories she expends in one minute by the number of minutes she cycles:

$$8.61 \text{ Kcal} \cdot min^{-1} \times 30 \text{ min} = \underline{258.3 \text{ Calories}}$$

[Chapter 11]

16–B. Body composition refers to the relative proportions of fat and fat-free (lean) tissue in the body. It is commonly reported as "percent body fat," thereby identifying the proportion of the total body mass composed of fat. Fat-free mass is then determined as the balance of the total body mass. Hydrodensitometry and near-infrared interactance are ways to measure body composition. *[Chapter 6]*

17–D. Exercise leadership is a skill that requires an understanding of the scientific concepts of exercise; the ability to interpret and teach these concepts effectively; and the ability to motivate individuals toward continued exercise participation. The ability to identify the level of supervision required for individuals based on their health/fitness status is also a key to safe and effective exercise leadership. It is incumbent on the Health/Fitness Instructor to stay abreast of current information regarding exercise. He or she should be a resource for up-to-date and accurate information regarding health and fitness and to dispel myths and quackery. The Health/Fitness Instructor should also be able to create an atmosphere and an opportunity for learning by presenting a clear set of goals. Communication skills are also fundamental to effective teaching.

18–D. Surrounding each myofibril is the sarcoplasmic reticulum, specialized endoplasmic reticulum consisting of a series of interconnected sacs and tubes. Calcium is stored in portions of the sarcoplasmic reticulum called terminal cisternae. Myofibrils contain the myofilaments, which are contractile proteins consisting primarily of actin and myosin. *[Chapter 1]*

19–C. Anaerobic glycolysis is also known as the lactic acid system. The human stores carbohydrate in the body as muscle (or liver) glycogen. Glycogen is simply a long string of glucose molecules hooked end-to-end. Anaerobic glycolysis can use only carbohydrate as a fuel, not fat or protein. This system will use muscle glycogen, which is broken down to glucose and then enters anaerobic glycolysis. Only a small amount of ATP is produced, and the end-product is lactic acid (or lactate). If lactate is allowed to accumulate significantly in the muscle, it will eventually cause fatigue. Because no oxygen is required, this system is anaerobic. *[Chapter 2]*

20–C. Cardiac output does not change significantly primarily because the person is performing the same amount of work so he or she responds with the same cardiac output. It should be noted, however, that the same cardiac output is now being generated with a lower heart rate and higher stroke volume compared with when the person was untrained. *[Chapter 2]*

21–D. Every population that has been studied exhibits a decline in bone mass with aging. Therefore, bone loss is considered by most clinicians to be an inevitable consequence of aging. Osteoporosis refers to a condition characterized by a decrease in bone mass and density, producing bone porosity and fragility, and refers to the clinical condition of low bone mass and the accompanying increase in susceptibility to fracture from minor trauma. The age at which bone loss begins, and the rate at which it occurs varies greatly between males and females. Risk factors for age-related bone loss and the development of clinical osteoporosis include being a white or Asian female, being thin-boned or petite, having a low peak bone mass at maturity, having a family history of osteoporosis, premature or surgically induced menopause, alcohol abuse and/or cigarette smoking, sedentary lifestyle, and inadequate dietary calcium intake. *[Chapter 3]*

22–B. Outcomes are designed to measure the success of a program based upon the outcome for a patient or client. Outcome studies require quantifiable data that can be analyzed, data that study the success of a program in terms of quantifiable measures (e.g., change in body composition). Measuring client satisfaction, level of change, length of time for change to occur, or percentage of clients that reached their goals are other examples of outcomes. Outcomes can be very helpful in marketing programs as well as for comparing one facility to another.

23–B. Although some learning is required on the part of the participant, the Rating of Perceived Exertion (RPE) should be considered as an adjunct to heart rate measures. The RPE can be used as a reliable barometer of exercise intensity. The RPE is particularly useful when participants are incapable of monitoring their pulse accurately or when medications such as beta-blockers alter the heart rate response to exercise. The American College of Sports Medicine recommends an exercise intensity that will elicit an RPE within a range of 12 to 16 on the original 6–20 Borg scale.

24–B. Fast-twitch (Type II) muscle fibers can be subdivided into fast-twitch aerobic (Type IIa) and fast-twitch glycolytic (Type IIb). Although classified as a fast-twitch fiber, the Type IIa fiber does have the capability of performing some amounts of aerobic work. The motor nerve supplying fast-twitch fibers is larger than slow-twitch muscle fibers. Fast-twitch fibers are recruited when performing high-intensity, short-duration activities. Examples include weight lifting, sprints, jumping, and other similar activities. These fibers can produce large amounts of tension in a very short period; however, they fatigue quickly. [Chapter 2]

25–A. Rotation is the turning of a bone around its own longitudinal axis or around another bone. Rotation of the anterior surface of the bone toward the midline of the body is medial rotation, whereas rotation of the same bone away from the midline is lateral rotation. Supination is a specialized rotation of the forearm that results in the palm of the hand being turned forward (anteriorly). Pronation, the opposite of supination, is the rotation of the forearm that results in the palm of the hand being directed backward (posteriorly). [Chapter 1]

26–C. The trachea branches within the mediastinum to form the right and left primary bronchi. As each primary bronchus enters the lung, secondary bronchi branch off, with smaller and smaller branches continuing to branch until the smallest narrow passage is formed, called the bronchiole. Terminal bronchioles are the smallest diameter bronchioles and supply air to the lobules of the lung. Varying the diameter of the bronchioles gives control over the resistance to airflow and distribution of air to the lungs. [Chapter 1]

27–A. Cardiac output is calculated by multiplying heart rate and stroke volume. During dynamic exercise, cardiac output increases with increasing exercise intensity. Stroke volume increases only until about 40%–50% of maximal oxygen consumption. Above this point, increases in cardiac output are accounted for only by an increase in heart rate. During static exercise, cardiac output may fall as a result of a drop in venous return. When the contraction is released, there is a rapid increase in cardiac output as venous return increases. [Chapter 2]

28–D. Initial causes of coronary artery disease are thought to be an irritation of, or injury to the tunica intima (innermost of the three layers in the wall) of the blood vessel. Sources of this initial injury are thought to be caused by dyslipidemia (elevated total blood cholesterol); hypertension (chronic high blood pressure—either an elevation of systolic blood pressure or diastolic blood pressure, measured on two different days); immune responses; smoking; tumultuous, nonlaminar blood flow in the lumen of the coronary artery (turbulence); vasoconstrictor substances (chemicals that cause the smooth muscle cells in the walls of the vessel to contract, resulting in a reduction in the diameter of the lumen); and viral infections. [Chapter 4]

29–C. Risk factors that contribute to the development of coronary artery disease include age (men over 45 years and women over 55 years), a family history of myocardial infarction or sudden death (male first-degree relatives under 55 years of age and first-degree female relatives under 65 years of age), cigarette smoking, hypertension (arterial blood pressure greater than 140/90 mm Hg, measured on two separate occasions), hypercholesterolemia (total cholesterol greater than 200 mg/dl or 5.2 mmol/L, or HDL less than 35 mg/dl or 0.9 mmol/L), diabetes mellitus in individuals over 30 years of age or in individuals who have had Type I diabetes more than 15 years or Type II diabetes in individuals over age 35 years. Other risk factors contribute to the development of coronary artery disease but are not primary risk factors. [Chapter 4]

30–B. The apparently healthy risk category is asymptomatic and has one or less than one major risk factor for coronary artery disease. A person is placed in the increased risk category if he or she has any or all of the following: signs and/or symptoms of cardiopulmonary disease, signs and/or symptoms of metabolic disease, or two or more major risk factors for coronary artery disease. A person with known disease is someone with any or all of the following criteria: cardiac disease, pulmonary disease or metabolic disease. [Chapter 6]

31–B. The use of weights, whether on a machine or using dumbbells and barbells, increases the risk of injury because of the amount of weight used, improper technique, fatigue, fooling around, and other lifters. A second person assisting the lifter in initially lifting the weight into position, correcting incorrect movements, and most importantly, assisting in lifting the weight to safety if the lifter is unable to handle the weight is called spotting. *[Chapter 7]*

32–B. Vitamin A promotes healthy skin, resists infection, and improves night vision. Vitamin D helps build strong bones and teeth. Sources of vitamin D include fortified milk, fish oils and egg yolk. Vitamin K improves normal blood clotting. Thiamine is important in energy-releasing reactions. *[Chapter 9]*

33–B. Each atrium communicates with the ventricle on the same side via an atrioventricular (A-V) valve, which allows one-way flow of blood from the atrium to the ventricle. The right A-V valve is also known as the tricuspid valve because of the three cusps, or flaps, of fibrous tissue that constitute the valve. The left A-V valve is called the bicuspid valve (or mitral valve) because it contains a pair of cusps rather than a trio. Each cusp is braced by tendinous fibers called chordae tendinae, which, in turn, are connected to special papillary muscles on the inner surface of the ventricle. *[Chapter 1]*

34–B. The oxygen system is very complicated and involves many reactions. The oxygen system takes 2–3 minutes to adjust to a new exercise intensity. This system is ranked number three in power. An individual's maximal oxygen consumption or $\dot{V}O_{2\,max}$ is a measure of the power of the aerobic energy system. This value is generally regarded as the best indicator of aerobic fitness. The average $\dot{V}O_{2\,max}$ of college-age males is approximately 45 ml/kg/min. The average $\dot{V}O_{2\,max}$ of college-age females is 35 ml/kg/min. *[Chapter 2]*

35–B. The action potential in cardiac muscle is much longer in duration when compared with skeletal muscle. This prevents the cardiac muscle from being tetanized. If cardiac muscle was tetanized, no relaxation (diastole) of heart muscle would occur, preventing ventricular filling from occurring for the next contraction. *[Chapter 2]*

36–C. Older people who exercise regularly report greater life satisfaction (older people who exercise regularly have a more positive attitude toward their work, and are generally in better health than sedentary persons), greater happiness (strong correlations have been reported between the activity level of older adults and self-reported happiness), higher self-efficacy (older persons taking part in exercise programs commonly report that they are able to do everyday tasks more easily than before they began exercising), improved self-concept and self-esteem (older adults improve their score on self-concept questionnaires following participation in an exercise program), and reduced psychological stress (exercise has been shown to be effective in reducing psychological stress without unwanted side effects). *[Chapter 3]*

37–B. Angina pectoris is a heart-related chest pain caused by ischemia, which is insufficient blood flow resulting from a temporary or permanent reduction of blood flow in one or more coronary arteries. Angina-like symptoms often are felt in the chest area, neck, shoulder, or arm. *[Chapter 4]*

38–D. Psychological theories are the foundation for effective use of strategies and techniques of effective counseling and motivational skill-building for exercise adoption and maintenance. Theories provide a conceptual framework for assessment, development of programs or interventions, application of cognitive-behavioral or motivational principles, and evaluation of program effectiveness. Within the field of behavior change, a theory is a set of assumptions that account for the relationships between certain variables and the behavior of interest. *[Chapter 5]*

39–A. A-well designed health screening provides the exercise leader or health/fitness instructor with information that can lead to identification of those individuals for whom exercise is contraindicated. From that information, a proper exercise prescription can be developed. A graded exercise test can be useful to measure heart rate and blood pressure responses. *[Chapter 6]*

40–B. Regularly scheduled practices of responses to emergency situations, including a minimum of one announced and one unannounced drill should take place. Emergency plans should include written, posted emergency plans and posted emergency numbers. The equipment and floor space should be arranged to allow safe egress from the facility in an emergency situation and to prevent accidental upsetting of equipment. A written maintenance procedures document that includes all daily, weekly, and monthly activities associated with each piece of equipment should be developed. *[Chapter 6]*

41–B. Some externally applied forces do not act in a vertical direction as do weights attached to the body. The forces exert effects that vary according to their particular angle of application. In the case of exercise pulleys, the angle of application changes in different parts of the range of motion. Each change in angle or force causes a change in the magnitude of the rotary component of the force and thus the torque. In addition to the rotary component, weights applied to the extremities frequently exert traction on joint structures. This is known as a distractive force. *[Chapter 1]*

42–A. If a motor unit is continuously stimulated without adequate time for relaxation to occur, tetanus will occur. When a motor unit is in tetany, there will be sustained tension until the stimulus is removed or fatigue occurs. *[Chapter 2]*

43–C. Heart rate is simply the total number of times the heart contracts in 1 minute. Normal resting heart rate is approximately 70–80 beats per minute. Heart rates during maximal exercise can exceed 200 beats per minute, depending on the age of the participant. Heart rate can be measured by counting the number of pulses in a specified time period at one of several locations. These locations commonly include the radial, femoral and carotid arteries. The number of pulses is counted for 1 minute. If heart rate is taken at the carotid artery, caution should be taken not to press too hard, or a reflex slowing of the heart may occur and cause dizziness. *[Chapter 2]*

44–C. Maximal heart rate does not change significantly with exercise training. Maximal heart rate does decline, however, with age. Maximal stroke volume increases after training as a result of an increase in contractility and/or an increase in the size of the heart. Because maximal heart rate is unchanged and maximal stroke volume increases, maximal cardiac output must increase. *[Chapter 2]*

45–A. Because of the relatively underdeveloped musculature of the legs and difficulty following the pace of a metronome, the treadmill is generally preferred over cycle ergometers and step tests. However, ergometers used in adult exercise testing can be used for children. Protocols to measure maximal aerobic power should last between 6 and 10 minutes, consisting of a progressively increasing load. Testing protocols developed for adults can easily be modified for children by lowering the initial power output and subsequent incremental increases. Protocols designed to predict maximal aerobic capacity from submaximal exercise should be interpreted cautiously because several congenital conditions and diseases can cause peak heart rate to be reduced. *[Chapter 3]*

46–D. Exercise has no effect on age, family history of heart disease and no direct effect on cigarette smoking. While regular endurance exercise does increase HDL, it has no influence on total cholesterol. There is no direct effect of exercise on Type I diabetes but exercise can improve glucose tolerance for Type II diabetics. Regular exercise will decrease systolic blood pressure and will decrease diastolic blood pressure. *[Chapter 4]*

47–A. At the very minimum, professionals performing fitness assessments on others should possess CPR and ACSM Health/Fitness Instructor. Other certifications are available for other responsibilities. *[Chapter 6]*

48–A. Intensity and duration of exercise must be considered together and are inversely related to one another. Similar improvements in aerobic fitness may be realized if a person exercises at a low intensity for a longer duration or at a higher intensity for less time.

49–C. Three different stretching techniques are typically practiced and have associated risks and benefits. Static stretching is the most commonly recommended approach to stretching. It involves slowly stretching a muscle to the point of individual discomfort and holding that position for a period of 10 to 30 seconds. There is minimal risk of injury and it has been shown to be effective. Ballistic stretching uses repetitive bouncing type movements to produce muscle stretch. These movements may produce residual muscle soreness or acute injury. Proprioceptive neuromuscular facilitation (PNF) stretching alternates contraction and relaxation of both agonist and antagonist muscle groups. This technique is effective; however, it may cause residual muscle soreness and is time consuming. Additionally, a partner is typically required and the potential for injury exists when the partner-assisted stretching is applied too vigorously.

50–C. Carbohydrates are compounds made up of carbon, hydrogen, and oxygen. They are commonly known as simple carbohydrates (sugars) or complex carbohydrates (starch). Glucose, fructose, and sucrose are examples of sugars or simple carbohydrates. Some sources are refined sugar (white or brown) and fruits. Food sources for complex carbohydrates are grains, breads, cereals, pastas, potatoes, beans, and legumes. Proteins have nitrogen in them as well as carbon, hydrogen, and oxygen, and may be found in such food sources as meats and nuts. Fats are found in foods such as butter and oils. *[Chapter 9]*

51–C. Legal issues abound for fitness professionals involved in exercise testing, exercise prescription, and program administration. Legal concerns can develop with the instructor-client relationship, the exercises involved, the exercise setting, the purpose of the programs and exercises used, and the procedures used by the staff. A tort law is simply a type of civil wrong. Negligence is the failure to perform in a generally accepted standard. Fitness professionals have certain documented and understood responsibilities to ensure the client's safety and to succeed in reaching predetermined goals. If these responsibilities are not followed, it is possible that one could be considered negligent.

52–A. All energy for muscular contraction must come from the breakdown of a chemical compound called adenosine triphosphate or ATP. The energy is stored in the bonds between the last two phosphates. When work is performed, a biceps curl, for example, the last phosphate is split (forming ADP), releasing heat energy. Some (but not all) of this heat energy is converted to mechanical energy to perform the curl. Because we are not 100% efficient at converting this heat energy to mechanical energy, the rest of the heat is released to the environment. *[Chapter 2]*

53–C. A muscle is composed of muscle fibers (or cells). Each muscle fiber is composed of many myofibrils. Each myofibril is composed of sarcomeres. The sarcomere is the smallest part of muscle that will still contract. The contractile (or muscle) proteins are contained in the sarcomere. Actin is a muscle protein (sometimes called the thin filament) that can be visualized as looking like a twisted strand of beads. Actin also contains two other proteins called troponin and tropomyosin. Tropomyosin is a long string-like molecule that wraps around the actin filament. Troponin is a specialized protein found at the ends of the tropomyosin filament. *[Chapter 2]*

54–A. Systolic blood pressure is an indicator of cardiac output (the amount of blood pumped out of the heart in 1 minute) in a healthy vascular system. Cardiac output normally increases as workload increases because the peripheral and central stimuli that control cardiac output normally increase with an increase in workload. Thus, systolic blood pressure should increase with an increase in workload. Failure of the systolic blood pressure to increase as workload increases indicates that cardiac output is not increasing, thus indicating an abnormal response to increasing workload. Additionally, an abnormally elevated systolic blood pressure response to aerobic exercise is indicative of an unhealthy vascular system. *[Chapter 4]*

55–D. The majority of sedentary people are not motivated to initiate exercise programs, and if exercise is initiated, it is likely to stop within 3–6 months. In general participants in earlier stages benefit most from cognitive strategies such as listening to lectures and reading books without the expectation of actually engaging in exercise, whereas individuals in later stages depend more on behavioral techniques such as reminders to exercise and developing social support to help them establish a regular exercise habit and be able to maintain it. *[Chapter 5]*

56–D. Fitness testing is conducted in older adults for the same reasons as in younger adults, including exercise prescription, evaluation of progress, motivation, and education. *[Chapter 6]*

57–C. Disordered eating covers a continuum from the preoccupation with food and body image to the syndromes of anorexia nervosa and bulimia. Anorexia nervosa is defined by the symptoms including body weight that is 15% below expected, a morbid fear of being or becoming fat, a preoccupation with food, and an abnormal body image (the thin person feels "fat"). Bulimia nervosa is defined by symptoms that include binge eating twice a week for at least 3 months, a loss of control over eating, purging behavior, and an over-concern with body weight. Although specific psychiatric criteria must be met for a diagnosis to be made by a specialist, any degree of disordered eating may affect the eating pattern of the exerciser and place her or him at risk for nutritional deficiencies. *[Chapter 9]*

58–C. A motor unit consists of the efferent (motor) nerve and all of the muscle fibers supplied (or innervated) by that nerve. The total number of motor units varies between different muscles. In addition, the total number of fibers in each motor unit varies between and within muscles. Different degrees of contraction can be achieved by varying the total number of motor units stimulated (or recruited) in a particular muscle. The major determinants of how much force is produced when a muscle contracts are the number of motor units that are recruited and the number of muscle fibers in each motor unit. When a motor unit is stimulated by a single nerve impulse, it responds by contracting one time and then relaxing. This is called a twitch. If a motor unit is continuously stimulated without adequate time for relaxation to occur, tetanus will occur. If a motor unit receives a second stimulation before it is allowed to relax, the two impulses are added (or summated) and the tension developed is greater. *[Chapter 2]*

59–A. Write out the running equation (accurate for speeds in excess of 5 miles per hour):

$\dot{V}_{O_2}$ (ml/kg/min) = horizontal + vertical + resting

$\dot{V}_{O_2}$ (ml/kg/min) = (speed x 0.2) + (speed x grade x 0.9) + 3.5

Convert speed (6.5 miles per hour) to meters per minute (6.5 x 26.8 = 174.2 meters per minute)

Solve for the unknown:

$\dot{V}_{O_2}$ (ml $\cdot$ kg^{-1} $\cdot$ min^{-1}) = (174.2 x 0.2) + (174.2 x 0.05 x 0.9) + 3.5

$\dot{V}_{O_2}$ (ml $\cdot$ kg^{-1} $\cdot$ min^{-1}) = 46.18 ml $\cdot$ kg^{-1} $\cdot$ min^{-1}

Convert 48.18 ml $\cdot$ kg^{-1} $\cdot$ min^{-1} to METs (1 MET = 3.5 ml $\cdot$ kg^{-1} $\cdot$ min^{-1})

48.18 ÷ 3.5 = 13.2 METs

[Chapter 11]

60–B. Reinforcement is the positive or negative consequence for performing or not performing a behavior. Positive consequences are rewards that motivate behavior. This can include both intrinsic and extrinsic rewards. Intrinsic rewards are the benefits gained because of the rewarding nature of the activity. Extrinsic or external rewards are the positive outcomes received from others, which may include encouragement and praise or material reinforcements such as T-shirts and money. [Chapter 5]

61–C. Exercise-induced asthma is a reversible airway obstruction that is a direct result of the ventilatory response to exercise. Hyperventilation causes an individual to breathe more through the mouth than the nose and actually inhale deconditioned (cool, dirty, dry) air. The nose serves to warm, clean, and humidify the air. Deconditioned air triggers an immune or allergic response primarily in the small and medium-sized airways in some individuals and may manifest in bronchoconstriction or bronchospasm. Medications are available that may prevent or reverse asthma attacks. These are usually administered in a tablet or aerosol form. Albuterol, terbutaline, glucocorticosteroids, cromolyn sodium and theophylline are effective drugs to prevent or reverse asthma.

62–A. Creating a safe environment in which to exercise is a primary responsibility for any fitness facility. In developing and operating facilities and equipment for use by exercisers, the managers and staff are obligated to meet a standard of care for exerciser safety. The equipment to be used not only includes testing, cardiovascular, strength, and flexibility pieces, but also rehabilitation, pool, locker room and emergency equipment. You must evaluate a number of criteria when selecting equipment. These criteria include correct anatomic positioning, ability to adjust to different body sizes, quality of design and materials, durability, repair records, and then price. [Chapter 7]

63–A. The ability to take in and utilize oxygen is dependent on the health and integrity of the heart, lungs, and circulatory systems. Efficiency of the aerobic metabolic pathways is also necessary to optimize cardiorespiratory fitness. The degree of improvement that may be expected in cardiorespiratory fitness is directly related to the frequency, intensity, duration, and mode or type of exercise. Maximal oxygen uptake may improve between 5 and 30 percent with training. The exercise prescription may be altered for different populations to achieve the same results. However, for the apparently healthy person, the American College of Sports Medicine recommends an intensity of 60% to 90% maximal heart rate, duration of 20 to 60 minutes, frequency of 3 to 5 days a week.

64–A. Plyometrics is a method of strength and power training that involves an eccentric loading of muscles and tendons followed immediately by an explosive concentric contraction. This stretch-shortening cycle may allow for an enhanced force-generation during the concentric (shortening) phase. Most well-controlled studies have shown no significant difference in power improvement when comparing plyometrics with high-intensity strength training. The explosive nature of this type of activity may increase the risk for musculoskeletal injury. Plyometrics should not be considered a practical resistance exercise alternative for health/fitness applications, but may be appropriate for select athletic/performance needs.

65–D. The characteristics of a good manager include designing programs and monitoring the implementation of the program. He or she also guides the staff or clients through the program. He or she is a good communicator who also purchases equipment and supplies. A good manager monitors the safety of the program or facility and surveys clients and staff to assess the success and value of the program.

66–A. Agreements, releases, and consents are documents that clearly describe what the client is participating in, the risks involved, and the rights of the client and the facility. If signed by the client, he or she is accepting some of the responsibility and risk by participating in this program. All fitness facilities are strongly encouraged to have program/service agreements and informed consents drafted by a lawyer for their protection.

67–B. The stores of ATP energy in skeletal muscle are very limited (5–10 seconds of high-intensity work). After this time another high-energy source called phosphocreatine (PC) begins to break down. PC has only one high-energy phosphate bond. The energy from the breakdown of PC is used to re-form ATP, which then breaks down to provide energy for exercise. Only energy released from the breakdown of ATP, however, can provide energy for biologic work such as exercise. [Chapter 2]

68–D. The sliding filament theory defines how skeletal muscles are believed to contract. These steps can best be described as what occurs during rest, stimulation, contraction, and then relaxation of the muscle. At rest, there is no nerve activity (except normal resting tone). Calcium is stored in a network of tubes in the muscle called the sarcoplasmic reticulum. If no calcium is present, the active sites (where the myosin cross-bridges can attach) are kept covered. If the active sites are uncovered, the enzyme that causes ATP to break down and release energy is kept inactive. During conditions when a nerve impulse is present, this impulse causes calcium to be released. The calcium binds to the troponin on the actin filament. When this occurs, the active sites are uncovered. Now the myosin cross-bridges bind the active sites and form actomyosin (a connection between the actin and myosin proteins), and contraction occurs. [Chapter 2]

69–C. After the age of 30 years, skeletal muscle strength begins to decline. However, the loss of strength is not linear, with most of the decline occurring after the age of 50 years. By age 80, strength loss is usually in the range of 30%–40%. The loss of strength with aging is due primarily to a loss of muscle mass, which, in turn, is caused by both the loss of muscle fibers and the atrophy of the remaining fibers. [Chapter 3]

70–C. There are specific risks associated with exercise for men and for women (although the statistics for women are not yet known). The rate of acute cardiovascular events is 1 in 187,500 hours of exercise. The rate of death during exercise for men is 1 in 396,000 hours. In addition, deaths during exercise are more common among men with more than one risk factor for coronary artery disease. The risk of cardiovascular events or death is lower among habitually active men. [Chapter 4]

71–D. Fiber is a type of complex carbohydrate that is undigestible by the body. This means it will pass straight through the digestive system and is commonly referred to as "adding bulk to the diet." Fiber can be either water-soluble (pectin or gums) or water-insoluble (cellulose, hemicellulose, and lignin). Dietary fiber has been linked to the prevention of certain diseases. [Chapter 9]

72–D. The Health Belief Model assumes that people will engage in a behavior (e.g., exercise) when there is a perceived threat of disease, there is a belief of susceptibility to disease, and the threat of disease is severe. This model also incorporates cues to action as critical to adopting and maintaining behavior. The concept of self-efficacy (confidence) is also added to this model. [Chapter 5]

73–C. The informed consent is not a legal document. It does not provide legal immunity to a facility or individual in the event of injury to a client. It simply provides evidence that the client was made aware of the purposes, procedures, and risks associated with the test or exercise program. The consent form does not relieve the facility/individual of the responsibility to do everything possible to ensure the safety of the client. Negligence, improper test administration, inadequate personnel qualifications, and insufficient safety procedures are all items that are expressly not covered by informed consent. Because of the limitations associated with informed consent documents, legal counsel should be sought during the development of the document. [Chapter 6]

74–C. Three common assessments for muscular endurance include the bench press—upper body endurance (a weight is lifted in cadence with a metronome or other timing device; the total number of lifts performed correctly and in time with the cadence is counted); push-up—upper body endurance (the client assumes a standardized beginning position with the body held rigid and supported by the hands and toes for men and the hands and knees for women; the body is lowered to the floor, then pushed back up to the starting position; the score is the total number of properly performed push-ups completed without a pause by the client with no time limit); and the sit-up—abdominal muscular endurance (the client begins in the bent-knee sit-up starting position with the hands resting on the floor and no foot restraint; the client then curls the upper body upward so that the hands slide along the floor a distance of 123 centimeters, with sit-ups performed at a cadence of 25 per minute until the client is no longer able to complete the action at the prescribed cadence). [Chapter 6]

75–A. Overuse injuries become more common when people participate in more cardiovascular exercise. An exerciser starts to exercise too much and either does not take a rest day at all and/or develops a minor injury and does not stop and rest so that the injury might heal. [Chapter 7]

76–C. There are several methods available to objectively define exercise intensity. The American College of Sports Medicine recommends that exercise intensity be prescribed within a range of 60% to 90% of maximum heart rate or between 50% and 85% of $\dot{V}o_{2\,max}$, maximum METs, or heart rate reserve. Lower intensities will elicit a favorable response in individuals with very low fitness levels. Due to the variability in estimating maximal heart rate from age, it is recommended that whenever possible, an actual maximal heart rate from a graded exercise test be used. Factors to consider when determining appropriate exercise intensity include age, fitness level, medications, overall health status, and individual goals.

77–B. The American College of Sports Medicine recommends that one set of 8–12 repetitions of each exercise should be performed to volitional fatigue. A 5- to 10-minute warm-up of aerobic activity or a light set (50%–75% of the training weight) of the specific resistance exercise should precede the resistance exercise program. The ACSM recommends these exercises be performed at least 2 days per week. Training two times per week will yield approximately 80% of the strength improvement seen with training three times per week, provided the intensity is the same.

78–B. The risk of orthopedic and perhaps cardiovascular complications may be increased with high-intensity activity. Factors to consider when determining intensity include the individual's level of fitness, presence of medications that may influence exercise performance, risk of cardiovascular or orthopedic injury, and individual preference for exercise and individual program objectives.

79–B. During auscultation, a stethoscope is placed over the left aspect of the midsternum, or just under the pectoralis major. Care should be taken to avoid placing the stethoscope bell over fat or muscle tissue because this may interfere with the clarity of the sound. When measuring heart rate by auscultation, the initial sound is counted as zero. The longer the time for which heart sounds are counted the less the error introduced by inadvertently missing a single beat, yet the greater the risk of miscounting. [Chapter 6]

80–D. The effects of regular (chronic) exercise can be classified or grouped into those that occur at rest,

during moderate (or submaximal) exercise, and during maximal effort work. For example, you can measure an untrained individual's resting heart rate, train the person for several weeks or months, and then measure resting heart rate again to see what change has occurred. Resting heart rate declines with regular exercise probably because of a combination of decreased sympathetic tone, increased parasympathetic tone, and a decreased intrinsic firing rate of the sinoatrial node. Stroke volume increases at rest as a result of an increase in myocardial contractility. There is little or no change in cardiac output at rest because the decline in heart rate is compensated for by the increase in stroke volume. [Chapter 2]

81–D. Heart muscle has the capability of producing its own action potential (autorhythmicity). In other words, if an impulse is not received from higher level brain centers, cardiac muscle will stimulate itself. [Chapter 2]

82–A. The rate of death, during or immediately after exercise testing, is 0.5 in 10,000 (or, approximately 0.01%). The rate of myocardial infarction during or immediately after exercise testing is 3.6 in 10,000 (approximately 0.04%). Complications during testing that require hospitalization are approximately 0.1%. [Chapter 4]

83–C. Key components of the Transtheoretical Model are the Processes of Behavior Change. These processes include five cognitive processes (consciousness raising, dramatic relief, environmental reevaluation, self-reevaluation, and social liberation) and five behavioral processes (counterconditioning, helping relationships, reinforcement management, self-liberation, and stimulus control). [Chapter 5]

84–D. The purpose of the fitness assessment is to develop a proper exercise prescription (the data collected through appropriate fitness assessments assists the health/fitness instructor to develop safe, effective programs of exercise based on the individual client's current fitness status), to evaluate the rate of progress (baseline and follow-up testing indicate progression toward fitness goals), and to motivate (fitness assessments provide information needed to develop reasonable, attainable goals). Progress toward or attainment of a goal is a strong motivator for continued participation in an exercise program. [Chapter 6]

85–C. Basic principles of care for musculoskeletal injuries include the objectives for care of exercise-related injuries, which are to decrease pain, reduce swelling, and prevent further injury. These objectives can be met in most cases by RICES (rest, ice, compression, elevation, stabilization). Rest will prevent further injury and ensure that the healing process will begin. Ice is used to reduce swelling, bleeding, inflammation, and pain. Compression also helps reduce swelling and bleeding. Compression is achieved by the use of elastic wraps or tape. Elevation helps to decrease the blood flow and excessive pressure to the injured area. Stabilization reduces muscle spasm by assisting in relaxation of associated muscles. *[Chapter 7]*

86–D. There are various systems of resistance training that differ in their combinations of sets, repetitions, and resistance applied, all in an effort to overload the muscle. Circuit weight training uses a series of exercises performed in succession with minimal rest between exercises. Various health benefits as well as modest improvements in aerobic capacity have been demonstrated as a result of circuit weight training. Super-sets refer to consecutive sets for antagonistic muscle groups with no rest between sets or multiple exercises for a specific muscle group with little or no rest. Split routines entail exercising different body parts on different days or during different sessions. Pyramids are performed either in an ascending (increasing the resistance within a set of repetitions or from one set to the next) or a descending (decreasing the resistance within a set of repetitions or from one set to the next) fashion.

87–D. The goal of the exercise component of a weight reduction program should be to maximize caloric expenditure. Frequency, intensity, and duration must be manipulated in conjunction with a dietary regimen in an attempt to create a caloric deficit of 500–1000 calories per day. The recommended maximal rate for weight loss is 1–2 pounds per week.

88–D. A budget is a financial plan for a program or facility. Eventually, most fitness professionals will have to understand and develop budgets. Budgets are designed to help determine if a program is viable, help control costs, help identify financial difficulties early, and allow one to plan for the future in a realistic manner. When developing a budget, equipment and facilities are the primary capital expense and are higher at the start of the program.

89–A. Learning theories assume that an overall complex behavior arises from many small simple behaviors. By reinforcing partial behaviors and modifying cues in the environment, it is possible to shape the desired behavior. *[Chapter 5]*

90–C. The PAR-Q is a screening tool for self-directed exercise programming. The MMPI is a psychological scale. The Borg scale is used to measure or to rate perceived exertion during exercise or during an exercise test. *[Chapter 6]*

91–C. In order to get the best information in the state the individual may be in prior to exercise or during exercise, the following order is recommended: resting measurements (heart rate, blood pressure, blood analysis, etc.); body composition (some methods of assessing body composition are sensitive to the hydration status of the individual; because some tests of cardiorespiratory or muscular fitness may have an acute effect on hydration, it is inappropriate to conduct such assessments prior to the body composition assessment); cardiorespiratory fitness (assessments of cardiorespiratory fitness often utilize measurements of heart rate as a predictive measurement; because assessing muscular fitness or flexibility often results in an increase in heart rate, it would be inappropriate to conduct such tests prior to the test of cardiorespiratory fitness, as the heart rate responses during the cardiorespiratory assessment would be affected by the elevated heart rate produced by the muscular fitness or flexibility assessment). *[Chapter 6]*

92–D. When an emergency or injury occurs, the safe and effective management of the situation will assure the best care for the member. Implementing emergency procedures is an important part of the training of the staff. In-services, safety plans, and emergency procedures should be a part of the staff training. In addition, all exercise staff should be CPR certified and trained in first aid. Therefore, the fitness center management, staff and clients are all included in the implementation of an emergency plan. *[Chapter 7]*

93–D. Possible medical emergencies during exercise include heat exhaustion or heat stroke, fainting, hypoglycemia, hyperglycemia, simple or compound fractures, bronchospasm, hypotension or shock, seizures, bleeding, and other cardiac symptoms. *[Chapter 7]*

94–C. During most graded exercise tests, the following measurements are taken: heart rate (during a 2-minute stage, every minute; during a 3-minute stage, at minutes 2 and 3, and additionally at every subsequent minute until steady state is achieved), blood pressure (once during each stage, toward the end of the stage), and rating of perceived exertion (once during each stage, toward the end of the stage). For most graded exercise tests for which the stages are 3 minutes in length, it is practical to take the measurements according to the following schedule: minute 2—heart rate; minute 2:15—rating of perceived exertion; minute 2:30—blood pressure; minute 3—heart rate. [Chapter 6]

95–D. Resistance exercise may be performed by incorporating exercises requiring different muscle actions. Isometric muscle action occurs when the length of the muscle does not change, but muscle tension is increased through enhanced neuromuscular recruitment patterns. These actions occur when we attempt to push or pull against an immovable object. Although isometric activities have been shown to elicit improvements in muscular strength, these improvements seem to be limited to the joint angle(s) at which the action is applied. It would therefore require many isometric contractions at many joint angles for isometrics to be considered effective. Additionally, exaggerated increases in blood pressure may accompany isometric muscle actions. This type of exercise has some application in the management of select musculoskeletal injury.

96–B. Protein is made up of carbon, hydrogen, and oxygen, but also uniquely includes nitrogen. The building blocks of protein are the more than twenty amino acids. The amino acids make specific long-sequenced chains of proteins. There are eight essential amino acids that the human body cannot manufacture from other sources. These are necessary for protein production and they must be provided in the dietary intake. [Chapter 9]

97–D. Large muscle group activity performed in rhythmic fashion over prolonged periods facilitates the greatest improvements in aerobic fitness. Walking, running, cycling, swimming, stair climbing, aerobic dance, rowing, and cross-country skiing are examples of these types of activities. Weight training should not be considered an appropriate activity for enhancing aerobic fitness, but should be employed in a comprehensive exercise program to improve muscular strength and anaerobic muscular endurance. The mode(s) of activity should be selected based on the principle of specificity, that is, with attention to the desired outcomes and to maintain the participation and enjoyment of the individual.

98–D. Different types of health screenings are used for various purposes. In commercial settings, clients should be screened more extensively for potential health risks. At a minimum, a personal medical history should be taken. In addition, present medical status should be examined and questions asked regarding the use of medications (both prescription and over-the-counter), family history of heart disease and other medical conditions, and other lifestyle health habits (nutritional habits, exercise history, stress, and smoking). [Chapter 6]

99–C. The number of times per day or per week that a person exercises is interrelated with both the intensity and the duration of activity. Generally, persons of poor fitness may benefit from multiple short-duration, low-intensity exercise sessions per day. Individual goals, preferences, limitations, and time constraints will also determine frequency and the relationship between duration, frequency, and intensity.

100–D. Marketing and promoting a program is one of the significant functions of a manager. Promotions can be internal (within the facility to generate member interest) or external (bring new members into the club). Developing ideas is a key component to a marketing plan. Idea development requires preparation, research, and an understanding of your audience. Ideas for marketing strategies often come from studying the market (research). A business plan is the next step. The plan describes in detail the marketing plan and justification for each action and program. Analysis of each aspect of the research is made and projections of the success of the plan, including a cost/benefit analysis. The decision to accept the marketing plan by management is made by the information found in the business plan.

Index